Malaria Parasites: Diverse Topics

Malaria Parasites: Diverse Topics

Edited by **Jamie Spooner**

FOSTER ACADEMICS

New Jersey

Published by Foster Academics,
61 Van Reypen Street,
Jersey City, NJ 07306, USA
www.fosteracademics.com

Malaria Parasites: Diverse Topics
Edited by Jamie Spooner

International Standard Book Number: 978-1-63242-265-1 (Hardback)

Printed in China.

Contents

Preface

Malaria is a global disease today but most common in underdeveloped countries of the world. Nearly 90% of deaths due to this fatal disease occur in Sub-Saharan Africa. This book presents information regarding global endeavors undertaken by scientists from across the world. Collaborated efforts such as symbiont based malaria control, latest applications in avian malaria studies, advancement of humanized mice to study P. falciparum (the most virulent species of malaria parasite) and contemporary issues in laboratory diagnosis will aid efficient treatment of malaria. Research has been progressing rapidly in the quest for providing an effective vaccine for the prevention of malaria. This book presents research aimed at bringing forward abiding solutions to malaria issues and the methods and procedures that should be followed for combating these issues for better implementation of health policies in contemporary times as well as future.

This book is a comprehensive compilation of works of different researchers from varied parts of the world. It includes valuable experiences of the researchers with the sole objective of providing the readers (learners) with a proper knowledge of the concerned field. This book will be beneficial in evoking inspiration and enhancing the knowledge of the interested readers.

In the end, I would like to extend my heartiest thanks to the authors who worked with great determination on their chapters. I also appreciate the publisher's support in the course of the book. I would also like to deeply acknowledge my family who stood by me as a source of inspiration during the project.

Editor

Part 1

Introduction and Biology of Malaria

1

Biology of Malaria Parasites

John C. Igweh
Delta State University, Abraka Nigeria, Nigeria

1. Introduction

Plasmodium is a genus of parasitic protists. Infection by these organisms in known as malaria. The genus *plasmodium* was described in 1885 by Ettore Marchiafava and Angelo Celli. Currently over 200 species of this genus are recognized and new species continue to be described.[1]

Of the over 200 known species of *plasmodium.* At least 11 species infect humans. Other species infect other animals, including monkeys, rodents, and reptiles. The parasite always has two hosts in its life cycle: a mosquito vector and a vertebrate host.[2]

2. History

The organism itself was first seen by Lavern on November 6, 1880 at a military hospital in Constantine, Algeria, when he discovered a microgametocyte exflagellating. In 1885, similar organisms were discovered within the blood of birds in Russia. There was brief speculation that birds might be involved in the transmission of malaria; in 1894 Patrick Manson hypothesized that mosquito could transmit malaria. This hypothesis was independently confirmed by the Italian physician Giovanni Battista Grassi working in Italy and the British physician Ronald Ross working in India, both in 1898. [3] Ross demonstrated the existence of *Plasmodium* in the wall of the midgut and salivary glands of a Culex mosquito using bird species as the vertebrate host. For this discovery he won the Noble Prize in 1902. Grassi showed that human malaria could only be transmitted by *Anopheles* mosquito. It is worth noting, however, that for some species the vector may not be mosquito.[4]

3. Biology

The genome of four *plasmodium* species – *plasmodium falciparum, Plasmodium knowlest, Plasmodium vivax* and *Plasmodium yoelii* – have been sequenced. All these species have genomes of about 25 megabase organized into 14 chromosomes consistent with earlier estimates. The chromosomes vary in length from 500 kilobases to 3.5 megabases and it is presumed that this is the pattern throughout the genus.[5]

4. Diagnostic characteristics of the genus *Plasmodium*

- Merogony occur both in erythrocytes and other tissues

- Merozites, schizonts or gametocytes can be seen within erythrocytes and may displace the host nucleus
- Merzoites have a "signet-ring" appearance due to a large vacuole that forces the parasite's nucleus to one pole
- Schizonts are round to oval inclusions that contain the deeply staining merozoites
- Forms gamonts in erythrocytes
- Gametocytes are "halter-shaped" similar *Haemoproteus* but the pigment granules are more confined
- Hemozoin is present
- Vectors are either mosquito's or sand flies
- Vertebrate hosts include mammals, bird and reptiles

5. Life cycle

The life cycle of *Plasmodium* while complex is similar to several other species in the Haemosporidia.

All the *Plasmodium* species causing malaria in humans are transmitted by mosquito species of the genus *Anopheles.* Species of the mosquito genera *Aedes, Culex, Mansonia* and *Theobaldia* can also transmitted malaria but not to humans. Bird malaria is commonly carried by species belonging to the genus *Culex.* The life cycle of *Plasmodium* was discovered by Ross who worked with species from the genus *Culex.*[6]

Both sexes of mosquito live on nectar. Because nectar's protein content alone is insufficient for oogenesis (egg production) one or more blood meals is needed by the female. Only female mosquito bite.

Sporozoites from the saliva of a biting female mosquito are transmitted to either the blood or the lymphatic system of the recipient. It has been known for some time now that parasites block the salivary ducts of the mosquito and as a consequence the insect normally requires multiple attempts to obtain blood. The reason for this has not been clear. It is not known that the multiple attempts by the mosquito may contribute to immunological tolerance of the parasite.[4] The majority of sporozoites appear to be injected into the subcutaneous tissue from which they migrate into the capillaries. A proportion is ingested by macrophages and still others are taken up by the lymphatic system where they are presumably destroyed. 10% of the parasites inoculated by the mosquitoes may remain in the skin where they may develop into infective merozoites.[5,7,8]

6. Hepatic stages

The majority of sporozoites migrate to the liver and invade hepatocytes. For reasons that is currently unclear sporozoites typically penetrate several hepatocytes before choosing one to reside within.[9] The sporozoite then matures in the hepatocyte to a schizont containing many merozoites in it. In some *Plasmodium* species, such as *Plasmodium* vivax and *Plasmoduim ovale,* the parasite in the hepatocyte may not achieve maturation to a schizont immediately but remain as a latent or dormant form and called a hypnozoite. Although *Plasmodium falciparum* is not considered to have a hypnozoite form. This may not be entirely correct . This stage may be as short as 48 hours in the rodent parasite and as long as 15 days in *P. malaria* in humans.[10,11]

There is considerable variation in the appearance of the blood between individuals experimentally inoculated at the same time. Even within a single experimental individual there may be considerable variation in the maturity of the hepatic forms seen on liver biopsy.[12]

A proportion of the hepatic stages may remain within the liver for considerable time – a form known as hypnozoites. Reactivation of the hynozoites have been reported for up to 30 years after the initial infection in humans. The factors precipitating this reactivation are not known. In the species *Plasmodium ovale* and *Plasmodium vivax*. It is not yet known if hypnozoite reactivation occurs with any of the remaining species that infect humans but this is presumed to be the case.[13,14]

The development from the hepatic stages to the erythrocyte stages have, until very recently, been obscure. In 2006 it was showed that the parasite buds off the hepatocytes in merosomes containing hundreds of thousand of merozoties. These merosomes lodge in the pulmonary capillaries and slowly disintegrate there over 48 – 72 hours releasing merozoites. Erythrocyte invasion is enhanced when blood flow is slow and the cells tightly packed: both of these conditions are found in the alveolar capillaries.[15,16]

7. Erythrocyte stage

After entering the erythrocyte, the merozoite lose one of their members, the apical rings, conoid and the rhopteries. Phagotropy commences and both smooth and granular endoplasmic reticulum because prominent. The nucleus may become lobulated.[16]

Within the erythrocytes the merozoite grow first to a ring-shaped form and then to a larger trophozoite form. In the schizont stage, the parasite divides several times to produce new merozoites. Which leave the red blood cells and travel within the bloodstream to invade new red blood cells. The parasite feeds by ingesting hemoglobin and other materials from red blood cells and serum. The feeding process damages the erythrocytes. Details of process have not been studied in species other than *Plasmodium falciparum.* so generalization may be premature at this time.

Erythrocytes infected by *Plasmodium falciparum* tend to form clumps – rosettes – and these have been linked to pathology caused by vascular occlusion. This rosette formation may be inhibited by heparin. This agent has been used in the past as part of the treatment of malaria but was abandoned because of an increased risk of haemorrhage. Low molecular weight heparin also disrupts rosette formation and may have a lower risk of bleeding in malaria.[17]

8. Merozoites

The budding of the merozoites from interconnected cytoplasmic masses (pseudocytomeres) is a complex process. At the tip of each bud a thickened region of pellicle gives rise to the apical rings and conoid. As development proceeds an aggregation of smooth membranes and the nucleus enter the base of the bud. The cytoplasm contains numerous large ribosomes. synchronous multiple cytoplasmic cleavage of the mature schizont results in the formation of numerous uninucleate merozoites.

Escape of the merozoites from the erythrocyte has also been studies. The erythrocyte swells under osmotic pressure. A pore opens in the erythrocyte membrane and 1-2 meorozites escape. This is followed by an eversion of the entire erythrocyte membrane. An action that propels the merozoites into the blood stream.

Invasion of erythrocyte precursors has only recently been studied. The earliest stage susceptible to infection were the erythroblasts - the stage immediately preceding the reticulocyte stage which in turn is the immediate precursor to the mature erythrocyte. Invasion of the erythrocyte is inhibited by angiotensin 2. This is normally metabolized by erythrocytes to angiotensin (Ang) IV and Ang – (1-7). Parasite infection decreased the Ang – (1-7) levels and completely abolished Ang IV formation. Ang - (1-7), like its parent molecule, is capable of decreasing the level of infection. The mechanism of inhibition seems likely to be an inhibition of protein Kinase A activity within the erythrocyte.

9. Placental malaria

More than a hundred late-stage trophozoites or early schizont infected erythrocytes of *P. falciparum* in a case of placental malaria of a Tanzanian woman were found to form a nidus in an intervillous space of placenta. While such a concentration of parasite in placental malaria is rare, placental malaria cannot give rise to persistent infection as pregnancy in humans normally lasts only 9 months. We have also found this kind of placental infection in our own studies.[18]

10. Gametocytes

Most merozoites continue this explicative cycle but some merozoites differentiate into male or female sexual forms (gametocytes) (also in the blood), which are taken up by the female mosquito. This process of differentiation into gametocytes occur in the bone marrow. Five distinct morphological stages have recognized (stage I-V). Female gametocytes are produced about four times as commonly as male. In chonic infections in humans the gametocytes are often the only forms found in the blood. Incidentally the characteristic form of the female gametocytes in *Plasmodium falciparum* gave rise to this specie's name.

Gametocytes appear in the blood after a number of days post infection. In *P. falciprum* infections they appear after 7 to 15 days while on others they appear after 1 to 3 days. The ratio of asexual to sexual forms is between 10:1 and 156:1. The half life of the gametocytes has been estimated to be between 2 and 3 days but some are known to persist for up to four weeks.[18,19]

The five recognized morphological stages were first described by Field and Shute in 1956.

One constant feature of the gametocytes in all stages that distinguishes them from the asexual forms is the presence of a pellicular complex. This originates in small membranous vesicle observed beneath the gametocytes plasmalemma in late stage I. The structure itself consists of a subpellicular membrane vacuole. Deep to this is an array of longitudinally oriented microtubules. This structure is likely to be relatively inflexible and may help to explain the lack of amoeboid forms observed in asexual parasites.

Early stage one gametocytes are very difficult to distinguish from small round trophozoites. Later stages can be distinguished by the distribution of pigment granulues. Under the electron microscope the formation of the subpellicular membrane and a smooth plasma membrane are recognizable. The nuclei are recognizably dimorphic into male and female. These forms may be found between 0 and 2 in *P falciprum* infections.

In stage two gametocytes becomes D shaped. The nucleus may occupy a terminal end of the cell or lie along its length. Early spindle formation may be visible. These forms are found between days 1 to day 4 in *P falciprum* infections.

In stage three the erythrocyte becomes distorted. A staining difference between the male and female gametocytes is apparent (male stain pink while female stain faint blue with the usual stains). The male nucleus is noticeably larger than the female and more lobulated. The female cytoplasm has more ribosomes, endoplasmic reticulum and mitochondria.

In stage four erythrocytes is clearly deformed and the gametocyte is elongated. The male gametocytes stain red while the female stain violet blue. In the male pigment granules are scattered while in the female they are denser. In the male the kinetochores of each chromosomes are located over a nuclear pore. Osmophilic bodies are found in both but are more numerous in the female. These forms are found between day 6 and day 10 in *P falciparum* infections.

In stage five the gametocytes are clearly recognizable on light microscopy with the typical banana shaped female gametocytes. The subpellicular microtubules depolymerise but the membrane itself remains. The male gametocyte exhibit a dramatic reduction in ribosomal density. Very few mitochondria are retained and the nucleus enlarges with a kinetochore complex attached to the nuclear envelope. In the female gametocytes there are numerous mitochondria, ribosome's and osmophillic bodies. The nucleus is small with a transcription factory.

Stages other than five are not normally found in the peripheral blood. For reasons not yet understood stage 1 to IV are sequestered preferentially in the bone marrow and spleen. Stage V gametocytes only become infections to mosquito's after a further two days of circulation.

11. Infection of mosquito

In the mosquito's midgut, the gametocytes develop into gametes and fertilize each other, forming motile zygotes called ookinetes. It has been shown that up to 50% of the ookinetes may undergo apoptosis within the mighut. The reason for this behavior is unknown. While in the mosquito gut the parasites form thin cytoplasmic extensions to communicate with each other. These structures persist from the time of gametocyte activation until the zygote transforms into an ookinete. The function of these tubular structures remains to be discovered.[20]

The ookinetes penetrate and escape the midgut, then embed themselves onto the exterior of the gut membrane. As in the liver the parasite tends to invade a number of cells before choosing one to reside in. the reason for the behavior is not known. Here they divide many times to produce large number of tiny elongated sporozoites. These sporozoites migrate to the salivary glands of the mosquito where they are injected into the blood and subcutaneous tissue of the next host the mosquito bites.

The escape of the gametocytes from the erythrocytes has been until recently obscure. The parasitophorous vacuole membrane ruptures at multiple sites within less than a minute following ingestion. This process may be inhibited by cysteine protease inhibitors. After this rupture of the vacuole the subpellicular membrane begins to disintegrate. This process also can be inhibited by aspartic and the cysteine/ serine protease inhibitors. Approximately 15 minutes post-activation. The erythrocytes membrane rupture at a single breaking point a third process that can be interrupted by protease inhibitors.

Infection of the mosquito has noticeable effects on the host. The presence of the parasite induces apoptosis of the egg follicles.

12. Discussion

The pattern alternation of sexual and asexual reproduction which may seem confusing at first is a very common pattern in parasite species. The evolutionary advantages of this type of life cycle were recognized by Gregor Mendel.

Under favorable conditions asexual reproduction is superior to sexual as the parent is well adapted to its environment and its descendents share these genes. Transferring to a new host or in times of stress, sexual reproduction is generally superior as this produces a shuffling of genes which on average at a population level will produce individuals better adapted to the new environment.

Given that this parasite spends part of its life cycle in two different hosts it must use a proportion of its available resources within each host. The proportion utilized is currently unknown. Empirical estimates of this parameter are desirable for modeling of its life cycle.

Dormant Form

Plasmodium falciparum malaria

A report of *P. falciparum* malaria in a patient with sickle cell anemia four years after exposure to the parasite has been published . A second report that *P. falciparum* malaria had become symptomatic eight years after leaving an endemic area has also been published.[21]

A third case of an apparent recurrence nine years after leaving an endemic area of P. falciparum malaria has now been reported. A fourth case of recurrence in a patient with lung cancer has been reported. Two cases in pregnant woman both from Africa but who had not lived there for over a year have been reported.

A case of congenital malaria due to both *P. falciparum* and *P. malariae* has been reported in a child born to a woman from Ghana, a malaria endemic area, despite the mother having emigrated to Austria eighteen months before and never having returned. A second case of congenital malaria in twins due to *P. falciparum* has been reported. The mother had left Togo 14 months before the diagnosis, had not returned in the interim and was never diagnosed with malaria during pregnancy.[24,25]

It seems that at least occasionally *P. falciparum* has a dormant stage. If this is in fact the case, eradication or control of this organism may be more difficult than previously believed.[25,26]

13. Drug induced

Developmental arrest was induced by *in vitro* culture of *P. falciparum* in the presence of sub lethal concentration of artemisinin. The drug induced a subpopulation of ring stage into developmental arrest. At the molecular level this is associated with over- expression of heat shock and erythrocyte binding surface protein with the reduced expression of a cell-cycle regular and a DNA biosynthesis protein.

The schizont stage-infected erythrocyte in an experimental culture of *P. falciparum*, F32 was suppressed to a low level with the use of atovaquone. The parasite resumed growth several days after the drug was removed from the culture.[28]

14. Biological refuges

Macrophages containing merozoites dispersed on their cytoplasm. Called 'merophores', were observed in *P. vinkei petteri*- an organism that causes murine malaria. Similar merophores were found in the polymorph leukocytes and macrophages of other murine malaria parasite, *P. yoelii nigeriensis* and *P. chabudi chaaudi*. All these species unlike *P. falciparum* are known to produce hyponozoites that may cause a relapse. The finding of Landau *et al.* on the presence of malaria parasites inside lymphatics suggest a mechanism for the recrudescence and chronicity of malaria infections.[29,30,]

15. Evolution

As of 2007, DNA sequences are available from less than sixty species of *Plasmodium* and most of these are from species infecting either rodent or primate hosts. The evolutionary outline given here should be regarded as speculative, and subject to revision as more data becomes available.[31,32,]

The 'Apicomplexa (the phylum to which *Plasmodium* belong) are thought to have originated within the Dinofagellates -a large group of photosynthetic protists. It is thought that the ancestors of the Apicomplexa were originally prey organisms that evolved the ability to invade the intestinal cells and subsequently lost their photosynthetic ability. Many of the species within the Apicomplexa still possess plastids (the organelle in which photosynthesis occur in photosynthetic eukaryotes), and some that lack plastids nonetheless have evidence of plastid genes within their genomes. In the majority of such species, the plastids are not capable of photosynthesis. Their function is not known, but there is suggestive evidence that they may be involved in reproduction.[33]

Some extant dinoflagellates, however, can invade the bodies of jellyfish and continue to photosynthesise, which is possible because jellyfish bodies are almost transparent. In host organisms with opaque bodies, such an ability would most likely rapidly be lost. The 2008 description of a photosynthetic protist related to the Apicomplexa with a functional plastid supports this hypothesis.[32]

Current (2007) theory suggests that the genera *Plasmodium Hepatocystis* and *Haemoprotus* evolved from one or more *Leucoytozoon* species. Parasites of the genus *Leucocytozoon* infect white blood cells (Leukocytes) and liver and spleen cells, and are transmitted by 'black flies' (*Simulium* species) ----- a large genus related to the mosquitoes.

It is thought that *Leucocytozoon* evolved from a parasite that spread through the orofaecal route and which infected intestinal wall. At some point parasites evolved the ability to infect the liver. This pattern is seen in the genus *Cryptosporidium*, to which *Plasmodium* is distantly related. At some later point this ancestor developed the ability to infect blood cell and to survive and infect mosquitoes. Once vector transmission was firmly established, the previous orofecal route of transmission was lost.

Molecular evidence suggests that a reptile – specifically a squamte – was the first vertebrate host of *Plasmodium*. Birds were the second vertebrate hosts with mammals being the most recent group of vertebrates infected.

Leukocytes, hepatocytes and most spleen cells actively phagocytes particulate matter, which makes the parasite's entry into the cell easier. The mechanism of entry of *Plasmodium* species into erythrocytes is still very unclear, as it takes place in less than 30 seconds. It is not yet known if this mechanism evolved before mosquitoes became the main vectors for transmission of *Plasmodium*.[35]

The genus *Plasmodium* evolved (presumably from its *Leucocytozoon* ancestor) about 130 million years ago, a period that is coincidental with the rapid spread of the angiosperms (flowering plants). This expansion in the angiosperms is thought to be due to at least one gene duplication event. It seems probable that the increase in the number of flowers led to an increase in the number of mosquitoes and their contact with vertebrates.[36]

Mosquitoes evolved in what is now South America about 230 million years ago. There are over 3500 species recognized, but to date their evolution has not been well worked out, so a number of gaps in our knowledge of the evolution of *Plasmodium* remain. There is evidence of a recent expansion of *Anopheles gambiae* and *Anopheles arabiensis* populations in the late Pleistocene in Nigeria.[37]

The reason why a relatively limited number of mosquitoes should be such successful vectors of multiple diseases is not yet known. It has been shown that, among the most common disease – spreading mosquitoes, the symbiont bacterium *Wolbachia* are not normally present. It has been shown that infection with *Wolbachia* can reduce the ability of some viruses and *Plasmodium* to infect the mosquito, and that this effect is *Wolbachia*-strain specific.

16. Classification

Taxonomy

Plasmodium belong to the family plasmodium, order Haemosporidia and phylum Apicomplexa. There are currently 450 recognized species in this order. Many species of this order are undergoing reexamination of their taxonomy with DNA analysis. It seems likely that many of these species will be re-assigned after these studies have been completed. For this reason the entire order is outlined here.[38,39]

Order Haemoporida

Family Haemoproteidae

- Genus *Haemoproteus*
- Subgenus *Parahaemoproteus*

- Subgenus *Haemoproteus*

Family Garniidae

- Genus *Fallisia* Lainson, Landau & Shaw 1974
- Subgenus *Fallisia*
- Subgenus *Plasmodioides*
- Genus *Garnia*
- Genus *Progarnia*

Family Leucocytozoidae

- Genus *Leucocytozoon*
- Subgenus *Leucocytozoon*
- Subgenus *Akiba*

Family Plasmodiidae

- Genus *Bioccala*
- Genus *Billbraya*
- Genus *Dionisiu*
- Genus *Hepatocystis*
- Genus *Mesnilium*
- Genus *Nycteria*
- Genus *Plasmodium*
    - Subgenus *Asiamoeba* Telford 1988
    - Subgenus *Bennettinia* Valkiunas 1997
    - Subgenus *Carinamoeba* Garnham 1996
    - Subgenus *Giovannolaia* Corradetti, Garnham & Laird 1963
    - Subgenus *Haemamoebe* Grassi & Feletti 1890
    - Subgenus *Huffia* Garnham & Laird 1963
    - Subgenus *Lucertaemoba* Telford 1988
    - Subgenus *Laverania* Bray 1963
    - Subgenus *Novyella* Corradtti, Garnham & Laird 1963
    - Subgenus *Ophidiella* Garnham 1966
    - Subgenus *Plasmodium* Bray 1963 emend, Garnham 1964
    - Subgenus *paraplasmodium* Telford 1988
    - Subgenus *Sauramoeba* Garnham 1966
    - Subgenus *Vinekeia* Garnham 1964
- Genus *Polychromophilus*
- Genus *Ravella*
- Genus *Saurcytozoon*

The eleven 'Asian' species included here form a clade with *P.* vivax being clearly closely related as are *P. knowsell* and *P. coatneyi;* similarly *P. brazilium* and *P. malaria* are related. *P. hylobati* and *P. inui* are closely related. *P. gonderi* appear to be more closely related to *P. vivax* than *P. malaria.*

P. coatneyi and *P. inui* appear to be closely related to *P. vivax.*[38]

P. ovale is more closely related to *P. malaria* than to *P. vivax*.

Within the 'Asian' clade are three unnamed potential species. One infect each of the two chimpanzee subspecies included in the study *(Pan troglodytes troglodytes* and *pan troglodytes schweinfurthii)*. These appear to be related to the *P. vivax P. simium* clade.

Two unnamed potential species infect the bonbo *(Pan paniscus)* and these are related to the *P. malaria P. brazillium* calde.

17. Subgenera

The full taxonomic name of a species includes the subgenus but is often omitted. The full name indicates some features of the morphology and type of host species. Sixteen subgenera are currently recognized.

The avian species were discovered soon after the description of *P falciparum* and a variety of generic names were created. These were subsequently placed into the genus *Plasmodium* although some workers continued to use the genera *Laverinia* and *Proteosoma* for *P. falciparum* and the avian species respectively. The 5th and 6th Congresses of Malaria held at Istanbul (1953) and Lisbon (1958) recommended the creation and use of subgenera in this genus. *Laverinia* was applied to the species infecting human and *Haemamoeba* to those infecting lizard and birds. This proposal was not universally accepted. Bray in 1955 proposed a definition for the subgenus *Plasmodium* and a second for the subgenus *Laverinia* in 1958. Garnham described a third subgenus – *Vinckeia* – in 1964.[40]

18. Mammal infecting species

Two species in the subgenus *Laverania* are curreIntly recognized: *P. falciparum* and *P. reichenowi*. Three additional species – *Plasmodium billbrayi, Plasmodium billeollnisi* and *Plasmodium gaboni* - may also exist (based on molecular data) but a full description of these species have not yet been published. The presence of elongated gametocytes in several of the avian subgenus and in *Laverania* in addition to a number of clinical features suggested that these might be closely related. This is no longer thought to be the case.[41]

The type species is *Plasmodium falciparum.*

Species infecting monkeys and apes (the higher primate other than those in the subgenus *Laverania* are placed in the subgenus *Plasmodium.* The position of the recently described *Plasmodium Gor A* and *Plasmodium Gor B* has not yet been settled. The distinction between *P. falciparum* and *P. reichenowi* and the other species infection higher primates was based on the morphological findings but have since been confirmed by DNA analysis.[42,43]

The type speces is *Plasmodium malaria*

Parasites infecting other mammals including lower primates (lemurs and others) are classified in the subgenus *Vinckeia.* Vinckeia while previously considered to be something of a taxonomic 'rag has been recently shown – perhaps rather surprisingly – to form a coherent grouping.

The type species is *Plasmodium bubalis.*[44,45,46,47,48]

19. Bird infecting species

The remaining groupings are based on the morphology of the parasites. Revision to this system are likely to occur in the future as more species are subject to analysis of their DNA.

The four subgenera *Giovannolaia, Haemamoeba, Huffia* and *Novyella* were created by Corradetti *et al.* for the known avian malaria species. A fifth – *Bannettinia* – was created in 1997 by Valkiunas. The relationship between the subgenera are the matter of current investigation. Marinsen *et al.* 's recent (2006) paper outlines what is currently (2007) known. The subgenera *Haemamoeba, Huffia,* and *Bennettinia* appear to be monophyletic. *Novyella* appear to be well defined with occasional exceptions. The subgenus *Giovannolaia* need revision.[49,50]

P. juxtanucleare is currently (2007) the only known member of the subgenus *Bennettinia.*

Nyssorhynchus is an extinct subgenus of *Plasmodium.* It has one known member – *Plasmodium dominium*[51].

20. Reptile infecting species

Unlike the mammalian and bird malaria those species (more than 90 currently known) that infect reptiles have been more difficult to classify.

In 1966 Garnham classified those with large schizonts as *Sauramoeba,* those with small schizont as *Carinamoeba* and the single then known species infecting snakes *(Plasmodium wenyoni)* as Ophidiella. He was aware of the arbitrariness of this system and that it might not prove to be biologically valid. This scheme was used as the basis for the currently accepted system.[52]

These species have since been divided in to 8 genera –*Asiamoeba, Carinamoeba, Fallisia Garnia, Lacertamoeba,* and *Paraplasmodium* and *Sauramoeba.* Three of these genera *(Asiamoeba, Lacertamoeba* and *Plaraplasmodium)* were created by Telford in 1988. Another species *(Billbraya australis)* described in 1990 by Paperna and landau and is the only known species in this genus. This species may turn out to be another subgenus of lizard infecting *Plasmodium.*

With the exception of *P. elongatum* the exoerythrocytic stage occur in the endothelial cells and those of the macrophage - lymphoid system. The exoerthrocytic stage of *P. elongatum* parasite the blood forming celss.

The various subgenera are first distinguished on the basis of the morphology of the mature gametocytes. Those of subgenus *Haemamoeba* are round oval while those of the subgenera *Giovannolaia, Hiffia* and *Novyella* are elongated. These latter genera are distinguished on the basis of the size of the schizont: *Giovannolaia* and *Huffia* have large schizonts while those of *Novyella* are small.[52]

Species in the *subgenus Bennettinia* have the following characteristics:

The type species is *Plasmodium juxtanucleare.*

Species in the subgenus *Giovannolaia* have the following characteristics:

- Schizonts conyain plentiful cytoplasm, are larger than the host cell nucleus and frequently displace it. They are found only in mature erythrocytes.
- Gametocytes are elongated
- Exoerythrocytic schizony occur in the mononuclear phagocyte system.

The type species is *Plasmodium circumflexum.*

Species in the subgenus *Haeamoeba* have the following characteristics:

- Mature schizonts are larger than the host cell nucleus and commonly distplace it.
- Gametocytes are large, round, oval or irregular in shape and are substantially larger than the host nucleus.

The type species is *Plasmodium relictum*

Species in the subgenus *Huffia* have the following characteristics:

- Mature schizonts, while varying in shape and size, contain plentiful cytoplasm and are commonly found in immature erythrocytes.
- Gametocytes are elongated.

The type species is *Plasmodium elongated*

The type of spices subgenus *Novyella* have the following characteristics:

- Mature schizonts are either smaller than or only slightly larger than the host nucleus they contain scanty cytoplasm.
- Gametocytes are elongated. Sexual stage in this subgenus resemble those of *Haemoproteus.*
- Exoerythrocytic schizongony occur in the mononuclear phagocyte system[52]

The type species is *Plasmodium vaughni*

21. Malaria parasites

Malaria parasites are micro-organisms that belong to the genus *Plasmodium.* There are more than 100 species of *Plasmodium,* which can infect many animal species such as reptiles birds, and various mammals. Four species of *Plasmodium* have long been recognized to infect humans in nature. In addition there is one species that naturally infect macaques which has recently been recognized to be a cause of zoonotic malaria in humans. (There are some additional species which can, exceptionally or under experimental conditions, infect humans.)

- ***P. falciparum,*** which is found worldwide in tropical and subtropical. It is estimated that every year approximately I million people are killed by *P. falciparum,* especially in Africa where this species predominates. *P. falciparum,* can cause severe malaria because it multiples rapidly in the blood, and can thus cause severe blood loss (anemia). In addition, the infected parasites can clog small blood vessels. When this occur in the brain, cerebral malaria results, a complication that can be fatal.
- ***P. vivax,*** which is found mostly in Asia, Latin America, and in some parts of Africa. Because of the population densities especially in Asia it is probably the most prevalent human malaria parasite. *P. vivax* (as well as *P. ovale*), has dormant liver stages ("hypnozoites") that can activate and invade the blood ("relapse") several months or years after the infecting mosquito bite.

- ***P. ovale*** is found mostly in Africa (especially West Africa) and the island of the western pacific. It is biologically and morphologically very similar of *P vivax*. however, differently from *P. vivax,* it can infect individuals who are negative for the Duffy blood group, which is the case for many residents of sub-Saharan Africa. This explains the greater prevalence of *P. ovale* (rather than *P. vivax*) in most of Africa.
- ***P. malaria,*** found worldwide, is the only human malaria parasite species that has a quartan cycle (three-day cycle). (The three other species have a tertian, two-day cycle.) If untreated, *P. malaria* cause a long-lasting, chronic infection that in some cases can last a lifetime. In some chronically infected patients *P. malaria* can cause serious complications such as the nephritic syndrome.
- ***P. knowlesi*** is found throughout Southern Asia as a natural pathogen of long-tailed and pigtailed macaques. It has recently been shown to be a significant cause of zoonotic malaria in that region, particularly in Malaysia. *P. knowlesi* has a 24 –hour replication cycle and so can rapidly progress from an uncomplicated to a severe infection.

22. Cellular and molecular biology of *Plasmodium*

Members of the genus *Plasmodium* are eukaryotic microbes. Therefore, the cell and molecular biology of *Plasmodium* will be similar to other eukaryotes. A unique feature of the malaria parasite is its intracellular lifestyle. Because of its intracellular location the parasite has an intimate relationship with its host cell which can be described at the cellular and molecular levels. In particular, the parasite must enter the host cell, and once inside, it modifies the host cell. The molecular and cellular biology of host-parasite interactions involved in these two processes will be discussed.

23. Host cell invasion

Malaria parasites are members of the Apicomplexa. Apicomplexa are characterized by a set of organelles found in some stage of the parasite's life cycle. These organelles, collectively known as apical organelles because of their localization at one end of the parasite, are involved in interactions between the parasite and host. In particular, the apical organelles have been implicated in the process of host celll invasion. In the case of *Plasmodium,* three distinct invasive forms have been identified: sporozoite, merozoite, and ookinete (see *Plasmodium* Life Cycle). The following discussion focuses on the cellular biology of merozoites and erythrocyte invasion. Reference to other Apicomplexa and *Plasmodium* sporozoites will be made to illustrate common features.

Merozoites rapidly (approximately 20sec.) and specifically enter erythrocytes. This specificity is manifested both for erythrocytes as the preferred host cell type and for a particular host species, thus implying receptor – ligand interactions. Erythrocyte invasion is a complicated process which is only partially understood at the molecular and cellular levels.[53] Four distinct steps in the invasion process can be recognized:

1. Initial merozoites binding
2. Reorientation and erythrocyte deformation
3. Junction formation
4. Parasite entry

24. Merozoite surface proteins and host- parasite interaction

The initial interaction between the merozoite and the erythrocyte is probably a random collision and presumably involves reversible interactions between proteins on the merozoite surface and the host erythrocyte. Several merozoite surface proteins have been described. The best characterized is merozoite surface protein - 1 (MSP-1). Circumstantial evidence implicating MSP - I in erythrocyte invasion include its uniform distribution over the merozoite surface and the observation that antibodies against MSP-I inhibit invasion.[54] In addition, MSP-I does bind to band 3.[55] However, a role for MSP-I in invasion has not been definitively demonstrated. Similarly, the circumsporozite protein (CSP) probably plays a role in targeting sporozoites to hepatocytes by interacting with heparin sulfate proteoglycans . [56]

Another interacting aspect of MSP-I is the proteolytic processing that is coincident with merozoite maturation and invasion.[57] A primary processing occurs at the time of merozite maturation and result in the formation of several polypeptides held together in a non-covalent complex. A secondary processing occurs coincident with merozoite invasion at a site near the C-terminus. The non-covalent complex of MSP-I polypeptide fragments is shed from the merozoite surface following proteolysis and only a small C-terminal fragment is carried into the erythrocyte. This loss of the MSP-I complex may correlate with the loss of the 'fuzzy' coat during merozoite invasion. The C-terminal fragment is attached to the merozoite surface by a GPI anchor and consists of two EGF-like modules. EGF-like modules are found in a variety of protein and are usually implicated in protein-protein interactions. One possibility is that the secondary proteolytic processing functions to expose the EGF-like modules which strengthen the interactions between merozoite and erythrocyte. The importance of MSP-I and its processing are implied from the following observations:

- Vaccination with the EGF-like modules can protect against malaria, and
- Inhibition of the proeolytic processing blocks merozoite invasion.

The exact role(s) which MSP-I and its processing play in the merozoite invasion process are not known.

25. Reorientation and secretory organelles

After binding to erythrocyte, the parasite reorient itself so that the 'apical end' of the parasite is juxtaposed to the erythrocyte membrane. This merozoite reorientation also coincides with a transient erythrocyte deformation. Apical membrane antigen-I (AMA-I) has been implicated in this reorientation.[58] AMA-I is a transmembrane protein localized at the apical end of the merozoite and bind erythrocytes. Antibodies against AMA-I do not interfer with the initial contact between merozoite and erythrocytes thus suggesting that AMA-I is not involved in merozoite attachment. But antibodies against AMA-I prevent the reorientation of the merozoite and thereby block merozoite invasion.

specialized secretory organelles are located at the invasive stages of apicomplexan parasites. Three morphologically distinct apical organelles are detected by electron microscopy; mocronemes, rhoptries, and dense granules. Dense granules are not always included with the apical oganelles and probably represent a heterogeneous population of secretory vesicles.

The contents of the apical organelles are expelled as the parasite invades, thus suggesting that these organelles play some role in invasion. Experiments in *Toxoplasma gondii* indicate that the micronemes are expelled first and occur with initial contact between the parasite and host.[59] An increase in the cytoplasmic concentration of calcium is associated with microneme discharge.[60] as is typical of regulated secretion in other eukaryotes.

Dense granule contents are released after the parasite has completed its entry, and therefore, are usually implicated in the modification of the host cell. For RESA is localized to dense granules in merozoites and is transported to the host erythrocyte membrane shortly after merozoite invasion.[61] However, subtilisin-like proteases, which are implicated in the secondary proteolytic processing of MSP-I (discussed above), have also been localized to *Plasmodium* dense granules.[62,63] If MSP-I processing is catalyzed by these proteases, then at least some dense granules must be discharged at the time of invasion.

26. Specific interactions and junction formation

Following merozoite reorientation and microneme discharge a junction forms between the parasite and host cell. Presumably, microneme proteins are important for junction formation. Proteins localized to the micromenes include:

- EBA-175, a 175 kDa 'erythrocyte binding antigen *P. falciparum*
- DBP, Duffy-binding protein from *P. vivax* and *P. knowlesi*
- SSP2, *Plasmodium* sporozoite surface protein-2. Also known as TRAP (thrombospondin-related adhesive protein).
- Proteins with homology to SSP2/TRAP from *Toxoplasma* (MIC2), *Eimeria* (Etp100), and *Cryptosporidium*
- CTRP, circumsporozoite- and TRAP- related protein of *Plasmodium* found in the ookinete stage.

Of particular note are EBA-175 and DBP which recognize sialic acid residues of the glycohorins and the Duffy antigen, respectively. In other words, these parasite protein are probably involved in receptor-ligand interaction with proteins exposed on the erythrocyte surface. Disruption of the EBA-175 gene results in the parasite switchingfrom a sialic acid-dependentpathway to a sialic acid-independent pathway [64], indicating that there is some redundancy with regards to the receptor – ligand interactions.

Comparison of sequences of EBA-175 and DBP reveal conserved structural features. These include trans-membrane domains and receptor-binding domains.[65] The receptor-binding activity has been mapped to a domain in which the cysteine and aromatic amino acid residues are conserved between species. This putative binding domain is duplicated in EBA-175. The topography of the trans-membrane domain is consistent with the parasite ligands being integral membrane proteins with the receptor-binding domain exposed on the merozoite surface following microneme discharge.

The other microneme protein in the 'TRAP' family have also been implicated in locomotion and / or cell invasion.[66] All of these proteins have domains that are presumably involved in cell-cell adhesion, as N-terminal single sequences and trans-membrane domains at their C- terminal.

27. In summary

- An electron-dense junction forms between the apical end of the merozoite and host erythrocyte membrane immediately after reorientation.
- Tight junction formation and microneme release occur at about the same time
- Proteins localized to the micronemes bind to receptors on the erythrocyte surface

These observations suggest that the junction represents a strong connection between the erythrocyte and the merozoite which is mediated by receptor-ligand interaction. Junction formation may be initiated by microneme discharge which exposes the receptor-binding domains of parasite ligands. This mechanism for initiating a tight host-parasite interaction is probably similar in other invasive stages of apicomplexan parasites.

28. Parasite entry

Apicomplexan parasite actively invade host cells and entry is not due to uptake or phagocytosis by the host cell. This is particularly evident in the case of the erythrocyte which lacks phagocytic capability. Furthermore, the erythrocyte membrane has a 2-dimensional submembrane cytoskeleton which precludes endocytosis. Therefore, the impetus for the formation of the parasitophorous vacuole must come from the parasite.

Erythrocyte membrane proteins are redistributed at the time of junction formation so that the contact area is free of erythrocyte membrane proteins. A merozoite serine protease which cleaves erythrocyte band 3 has been described.[67]. Because of the pivotal role band 3 plays in the homeostasis of the submembrane skeleton, its degradation could result in a localized disruption of the cytoskeleton. An incipient parasitophorous vacular membrane (PVM) forms in the junction area. This membrane invagination is likely derived from both the host membrane and parasite component and expands as the parasite enters the erythrocyte. Connection between the rhoptries and nascent PVM are sometimes observed. In addition, the contents of the rhoptries are often lamellar (i.e. multilayered) membrane and some rhoptry proteins are localized to the PVM following invasion, suggesting that the rhoptries function in PVM formation.[68]

Ookinetes lack rhoptries and do not form a parasitophorous vacuole within the mosquito midgut epithelial cells. The ookinetes rapidly pass through the epithelial cells and cause extensive damage as they head toward the basal lamina.[69,70] Similarly, sporozoites can enter and exit hepatocytes without undergoing exoerythrocytic schizogony. Those parasites which do not undergo schzogony are free in the host cytoplasm, whereas those undergoing schizogony are enclosed within a PVM.[71] These observations suggest that the PVM is needed for intracellular development and is not necessary for the process of host cell invasion. As the incipient parasitophorous vacuole is being formed, the junction between the parasite and host becomes ring-like and the parasite appear to move through this annulus as it enters the expanding parasitophotous vacuole.

Apicomplexan parasite activity invade host cell and entry is not due to uptake or phagocytosis by the host cell. In addition, the zoites are often motile forms that crawl along the substratum by a type of motility referred to as 'gliding motility'. Gliding motility, like invasion, also involves the release of micronemal adhesions at the posterior end of the zoite. One difference between gliding motility and invasion is that the micronemes must be continuously released as the organism is moving. Thus gliding motility does not involve this relatively small moving junction, but a continuous formation of new junctions between the zoite and the substratum. In addition, the adhesins are cleaved from the surface of the zoite as the adhesion reach the posterior of the zotie and a trail of the adhesive molecules are left behind the moving zoite on the substratum. However, the mechanism of motility and invasion are quite similar and thus, during invasion the parasite literally crawls into the host cell through the moving junction. In addition, some apicomplexans use this type of motility to escape from cells and can traverse biological barriers by entering and exiting cells. Cytochalasins inhibit merozoite entry, but not attachment. This inhibition suggests that the force required for parasite invasion is based upon actin-myosin cytoskeletal elements. The ability of myosin to generate force is well characterized (eg.. muscle contraction). A myosin unique to the Apicomplexa has been identified and localized to the inner membrane complex.[72] This myosin is part of a motor complex which is linked to the adhesins. Members of the TRAP family and other adhesins have a conserved cytoplasmic domain. This cytoplamic domain is linked to short actin filaments via aldolase. The actin filaments and myosin are oriented in the space between the inner membrane complex and plasma membrane so that the myosin propels the actin filament toward the posterior of the zoite. The myosin is anchored into the inner membrane complex and does not move. Therefore, the transmembrane adhesins are pulled through the fluid lipid bilayer of the plasma membrane due to their association with the actin filament. Thus the complex of adhesins and actin filaments is transported towards the posterior of the cell. Since the adhesins are either complexes with receptor on the host cell or bound to the substratum, the net result is a forward motion of the zoite. When the adhesins reach the posterior end of the parasite they are proteolyitcally cleaved and shed from the zoite surface.

29. Summary

Merozoite invasion is a complex and ordered process. A tentative model of merozoite invasion includes:

1. Initial merozotie binding involves reversible interactions between merozotie surface proteins and the host erythrocyte. The exact roles of MSPI and other merozoite surface proteins are not known.
2. Reorientation by an unknown mechanism result in the apical end of the merozotie being juxtaposed to the erythrocyte membrane.
3. Discharge of the micronemes is coincident with the formation of a tight junction between the host and parasite. The tight junction is mediated by receptor-ligand interactions between erythrocyte surface proteins and integral parasite membrane proteins exposed by microneme discharge.
4. localized clearing of the erythrocyte submembrane cytoskeleton and formation of the incipient parasitophorous vacuole. PVM formation is correlated with the discharge of the rhoptries.
5. movement of the merozoite through the ring-shaped tight junction formed by the receptor/ligand complex. The force is generated by myosin motor associated with the trans-membrane parasite ligands moving along actin filaments within the parasite.
6. Closure of the PVM and erythrocyte membrane

Many proteins that are involved in the invasion process have been identified. However, much still remains to be learned about the cellular and molecular biology of merozoite invasion.[73,74]

30. Host erythrocyte modification

Once inside of the erythrocyte, the parasite undergoes a trophic phase followed by replicative phase. During this intra-erythrocytic period, the parasite modifies the host to make it a more suitable habitat. For example, the erythrocyte membrane becomes more permeable to small molecular weight metabolites, presumably reflecting the needs of an actively growing parasite.

Another modification of the host cell concerns cytoadherence of *P. falciparum*- infected erythrocyte to endothelial cells and the resulting sequestration of the mature parasite in capillaries and post-capillary veinules. This sequestration likely leads to microcirculatory alteration and metabolic dysfunctions which could be responsible for many of the manifestation of severe falciparum malaria. The cytoadherence to endothelial cells confers at least two advantages for the parasite: 1) a microaerophilic environment which is better suited for parasite metabolism, and 2) avoidance of the spleen and subsequent destruction.

31. Knobs and cytoadherence

A major structural alteration of the host erythrocyte are electron-dense protrusion, or 'knobs', on the erythrocyte membrane of *P. falciparum* cells. The knobs are induced by the parasite and several parasite proteins are associated with the knobs.[75] Two proteins which might participate in knobs formation are the knob-associated histidine rich protein (KAHRP) and erythrocyte membrane protein-2 (*Pf*EMP2), also called MESA. Neither KAHEP nor *Pf*EMP2 are exposed on the outer surface of the erythrocyte, but are localized to the cytoplasmic face of the host membrane. Their exact roles in knob formation are not known, but may involve reorganizing the submembrane cytoskeleton. The knobs are believed to play a role in the sequestration of infected erythrocytes since they are points of contact between the infected erythrocyte and vascular endothelial cells and parasite species which express knobs exhibit the highest levels of sequestration. In addition, disruption of the KAHRP results in loss of knobs and ability to cytoadhere under flow conditions.[76] A polmerophic protein, called *Pf*EMPI, has also been localized to the knobs and is exposed on the host erythrocyte surface. The translocation of *Pf*EMPI to the erythrocyte surface depends in part on another erythrocyte membrane associated protein called *Pf*EMP3.[77] *Pf*EMPI probably functions as a ligand which binds to receptors on host endothelial cells. Other proposed cytoadherence ligand include a modified band-3, called pfalhesin.[78] Seqestrin, rifins and clag9.[79]

*Pf*EMI is a member of the *var* gene family.[80] The 40-50 *var* gene exhibit a high degree of variability, but have a similar overall structure. *Pf*EMPI) has a large intracellular N- terminal domain, a transmembrane region and a C- terminal intracellular domain. The C- terminal region is conserved between members of the *var* family and is believed to anchor *Pf*EMPI to the erythrocyte submembrane cytoskeleton. In particular, this acidic C- terminal domain may interact with the basic KAHRP of the knob[81] as well as spectrin and actin.[82]

The extracellular domain is characterized by 1-5 copies of Duffy-binding (DBL) domains. These DBL domains are similar to the receptor-binding region of the ligand involved in merozoite invasion (discussed above). The DBL domain exhibit a conserved spacing of cystrine and hydrophobic residues, but otherwise show little homology analysis indicates that there are five distinct classes (designated as α,β,γ,δ........... and...ε.....) of DBL domains.[83] The first DBL is always the same type (designated α) and this is followed by a cysteine- rich interdomain region (CIDR). A variable number of DBL in various orders make up the rest of the extracellular domain of *Pf*EMP-I.

Possible Receptors Identified By in Vitro Binding Assays

- **CD36**
- Ig Superfamily
- **ICAMI**
- VCAMI
- PECAMI
- **Chondroitin sulfate A**
- Heparin sulfate
- Hyaluronic acid
- E- selectin
- Thrombospondin
- **Resetting Ligands**
- CR-I
- Blood group A Ag
- Glycosaminoglycan

Several possible endothelial receptors have been identified by testing the ability of infected erythrocytes to bind in static adherence assays.[84] One of the best characterized among these is CD36, an 88 kDa intergral membrane protein found on monocytes, platelets and endothelial cells infected erythrocytes from most parasite isolates bind to CD36 and the binding domain has been mapped to the CIDR of *Pf*EMPI. However, CD36 has not been detected on endothelial cells of the cerebral blood vessels and parasites from clinical isolates tend to adhere to both CD36 and intracellular adhesion molecule – 1 (ICAMI). ICAMI is a member of the immunoglobulin superfamily and functions in cell-cell adhesion. In addition, sequestration of infected erythrocytes and ICAMI expression has been co-localized in the brain.[85]

Chondroitin sulfate A (CSA) has been implicated in the cytoadhernce within the placenta and may contribute to the adverse effects of *P. falciparum* during pregnancy. The role of some the other potential receptors is not clear. For example, adherence to thrombospondin exhibits a low affinity and cannot support binding under flow condition. Binding to VCAMI, PECAMI and E- selectin appear to be rare and questions about their constrictive expression on endothelial cells have been raised. However, cytoadherence could involve multiple receptor/ligand interactions.

Resetting is another adhesive phenomenon exhibited by *P. falciparum*-infected erythrocytes. Infected erythrocytes from some parasite isolates will bind multiple uninfected erythrocytes and *Pf*EMPI appears to have a role in at least some resetting. Possible receptors include complement receptor-I (CRI), blood group A antigen, or glycosaminoglycan moieties on an unidentified proteoglycan.

The different types of DBL domains and CIDR (discussed above) bind to different endothelial cell receptors[86,87].For example, DBL, which comprises the first domain, bind to many of the receptors associated with resetting. The binding of the CIDR to CD36 may account for the abundance of this particular binding phenotype among parasite isolates.[88]

32. Antigenic variation

The encoding of the cytoadherence ligand by a highly polymorphic gene family presents a paradox in that receptor/ligand interactions are generally considered highly specific. Interestingly, selection for different cytoadherent phenotypes result in a concomitant change in the surface antigenic type.[89] Similarly, examination of clonal parasite lines revealed that change in the surface antigenic type correlated with difference in binding to CD36 and ICAMI. For example, the parental line (A4) adhered equally well to CD36 and ICAMI, whereas one of the A4-derived clones (C28) exhibited a marked preference for CD36.[90] Binding to ICAMI was then reselected by panning the infected erythrocytes on ICAMI. All three parasite clones (A4, C28, C28-I) exhibited distinct antigenic types as demonstrated by agglutination with hyper-immune sera.

The expression of a particular PfEMPI will result in a parasite with a distinct cytoadherent phenotype and this may also affect pathogenesis and disease outcome. For example, binding to ICAM-I is usually implicated in cerebral pathology. Therefore, parasites expressing a PfEMPI which binds to ICAMI may be more likely to cause cerebral malaria. In fact, higher levels of transcription of particular *var* genes are found in cases of severe malaria as compared to uncomplicated malaria.[91] Similarly, a higher proportion of isolates which bind to CSA are obtained from the placenta as compared to the peripheral circulation of either pregnant women or children.[92] Furthermore, placenta malaria is frequently associated with higher levels of transcription of a particular var gene which binds CSA .[93] This phenomenon is not restricted to the placenta in that, there is a dominant expression of particular *var* genes in the various tissue.[94] This tissue specific expression of particular *var* genes implies that different tissues are selecting out different parasite populations based on the particular PfEMPI being expressed on the surface of the infected erythrocyte. To CSA, CD36, or ICAM-I. infected erythrocyte were collected from the placenta, peripheral circulation of the mother, or peripheral circulation of the child. (designated as group 1-6) expressed in different tissues (brain, lung, heart and spleen) from 3 different patients. PM30 died of severe malaria anemia. PM32 was diagnosed with both cerebral malaria and severe anemia. PM55 was diagnosed with only cerebral malaria.

Although sequestration offers many advantages to the parasite, the expression of antigens on the surface of the infected erythrocyte provides a target for the host immune system. The parasite counters the host immune responses by expressing antigenically distinct *Pf*EMPI molecules on the erythrocyte surface. This allows the parasite to avoid clearance by the host immune system, but yet maintain the cetoadherent phenotype. This antigenic switching may occur as frequently as 2% per generation in the absence of immune pressure.[95] The molecular mechanism of antigenic switching is not known. Experimental evidence indicates that the mechanism is not associated with duplication into specific expression-linked sites as found in African trypanosomes. Only a single var gene is expressed at a time (i.e... allelic exclusion). The non-expressed genes are kept silent by protein which bind to the promoter region. A gene can become activated by repositioning to a particular location in the nucleus and is associated with chromatin modification. This expression spot can only accommodate a single active gene promoter. Thus the var promoter is sufficient for both the silencing and the monoclinic transcription of a PfEMPI allele. [96]

33. Summary

- The malaria parasite modifies the erythrocyte by exporting proteins into the host cell.
- One such modification is the expression of *Pf*EMPI on the erythrocyte surface which functions as cytoadherent ligand.
- The binding of this ligand to receptors on host endothelial cells promotes sequestration and allows the infected erythrocyte to avoid the spleen.
- Numerous *Pf*EMPI genes (i.e... the *var* gene family) provide the parasite with a means to vary the antigen expressed on the erythrocyte surface.
- This antigenic variation also correlates with different cytoadherent phenotypes.

34. References

[1] Chavatte J.M., Chiron F., Landau I. (March 2007). "Probable speciations by "host-vector ' fidelity"': 14 species of Plasmodium from magpies" (in French). *Parasite* 14 (1): 21-37.

[2] Gueriard P., Tavares J., Thiberge S.,et al. (October 2010). "Development of the malaria parasite in the skill if the mammalian host". *Proc. Natl. acad. Sci. U.S.A* 107 (43): 18640 – 5

[3] Manson-Bahr PEC, Bell DR, eds. (1987). *Manson's Tropical Diseases* London: Bailliere Tindall, ISBN 0-7020-1187-8

[4] Cogswell FB (January 1992). "The hypnozoite and relapse in primate malaria." *Clinical microbiology reviews* 5 (1): 26-35.

[5] Krotoski WA., Collin WE, Bray RS, *et al.* (November 1982). "Demonstration of hypnozoites in sporozites in sporozoite-transmitted plasmodium vivax infection." *The American journal of tropical medicine and hygiene* 31 (6): 1291-3.

[6] Greenwood BM, Fidock Da, Kyle DE, *et al* (April 2008). "Malaria: progress, perils, and prospects for eradication". *J. Clin. Onvest.* 118 (4): 1266-76.

[7] Tanomsing N, Imwong M, Pukittaykamee S. *et al.* (October 2007). "Genetic analysis of the dihydrofolate reductase-thymidylate synthase gene from geographically diverse isolates of plasmodium malaria". *Antimcrob, Agents Chemother.* 51 (10): 3523-30.

[8] Sturm, A; Amino, R; Van De Sand, C; Regen, T; Retzlaff, S; Rennenberg, A; Krueger, A; Pollok, JM; *et al.* (2006). "Manipulation of host hepatocytes by the malaria parasite for delivery into liver sinusoids". 313 (5791): 1287-1290.

[9] Baer, K; Klotz, C; Kappe, SH; Schnieder, T; Frevert, U; *et al.* (2007). "Release of hepatic *plasmodium yolii* merozoite into the pulmonary microvasculature". *Plos pathogen* 3 (11): e171. doi:10.1371/journal. Ppat. 0030171

[10] Leitgeb AM, Blomqvist K, Cho-Ngwa F, Samje M, Nde P, Titanji V, Wahlgren M. (2011). "Low Anticoagulant heparin disrupts *Plasmodium falciparum* rosettes in fresh clinical isolates". *Am J Trop Med Hyg* 84 (3): 390-396.

[11] Tamez PA, Liu H, Fernandez-Pol S, Haldar K, Wickrema A (October 2009). "Stage-specific susceptibility of human erythrocytes to plasmodium falicparum malaria infection". *Blood* 114 (17): 3652-5.

[12] Muehlenbachs A, Mutabingwa T.K., Fried M., Duffy P.E. (2007) An unusual presentation of placental malaria: A single persisting nidus of sequestered parasites. *Hum. Pathol.* 38 (3): 520-523,

[13] Robert V, Boudin C (2003). "Biology of man-mosquito *plasmodium* transmission". *Bull Soc Pathol Exot.* 96 (1): 6-20.

[14] Kitchen SF, Putnam P (1942). "Observation on the mechanism of the parasite cycle in falciparum malaria". *Am JTrop Med.* 22: 381-386

[15] Smalley MEm Sinden RE (1977). Plasmodium falciparum *gametocytes: their longevity and infectivity".* Parastology *74 (1): 1-8.*

[16] Field JW, Shute PG (1956) A morphological study of the erythrocytic parsites. Kuala Lumpur: government Press. The microscopic diagnostic of human malaria; p. 142

[17] Al-Olayana EM, Williamsb GT, Hurd H (2002. "Apoptosis in the malaria protozoan, *plasmodium berhei:* a possible mechanism for limiting intensity of infection in the mosquito". *Inter. J. parasitol* 32 (9): 1133-1143.

[18] Hurd H, Grant KM, Arambage Sc (2206). "Apoptosis-like death as a feature of malaria infection in mosquito". *Parasitology* 132 Suppl: S33-47.

[19] Sologub L, Kuehn A, Kern S, Przyborski J, Schillig R, Pradel G (2011) Malaria proteases mediate inside-out egress of gametocytes from red blood cell following parasite transmission to the mosquito. Cell microbiol. 1462-5822.

[20] Hopwood JA, Ahmed AM, Polwart A Williams GT, Hurd H. (2001). "malaria-induced apoptosis on mosquito ovaries: a mechanism to control vector egg production". *J. Exp. Biol.* 204 (Pt 16): 2773-2780.

[21] Greenwood, T.; *et al.* (2008). "Febrile *plasmodium falciparum* malaria four years after exposure in a man with sickle cell disease". *Clin Infect.* Dis. 47 (4): e39-e41.

[22] Szmitko, P. E.; Kohn, M L.; Simor, A. E. (2008). "*Plasmodium falciparum* malaria occurring eight years after leaving an endemic area". *Diagn. Microbi Infect. Dis.* 61 (1): 105-107.

[23] Theunissen, C.; Mutabingwa, TK; Fried, M; Duffy, PE; Van-Esbroeck, M; Van-Gomple, A, Van-Denende, j. (2009). "Falciparum malaria in patient 9 years after leaving malaria-endemic area". *Emerg Infect Dis.* 15 (1): 115-116

[24] Poilane I, Jeantils V, Carbillon L (October 2009). "[Pregnancy associated plasmodium falciparum malaria discovered fortuitously: report of two cases]" (in French). *Gynecol Obstet Fertil* 37 (10): 824-6.

[25] Zenz W, Trop M, Kollaritsch H, Reinthaler (2000) Congenital malaria due to *plasmodium falciparum* and *plasmodium malariae.* Wien Klin Wochenschr. 112 (10): 459-461.

[26] Romand S, Bouree P, Gelez J, Bader-Meunier B, Bisaro F, Dommergues Jp (1994) Congenital malaria. A case observed in twins born to an asymptomatic mother Presse Med 23 (17): 797-800

[27] Witkowski B, Lelievre J, Barragan MJ, *et al.* (May 2010). "Increased tolerance to artemisinin in plasmodium falciparum is mediated by a quiescence mechanism". *Antimcrob. Agents. Chemother.* 54 (5): 1872-7

[28] Thapar M.M., Gil J.P., Bjorkman A. (2005). *In vitro* recrudescence of *plasmodium falciparum* parasite were suppressed to dormant state both by atovaquone alone and in combination with proguanil. *Trans R Soc Trop Med Hyg* 99 (1): 62-70,

[29] Landau I, Cahbaud AG Mora-Silvera E. *et al.* (December 1999). "Survival of rodent malaria merozoite in the lymphatic network: potential role in chronicity of the infection." *Parasite (Paris, France)* 6 (4): 311-22.

[30] Gautret P. (2000). "The Landau and Chabaud's phenomenon". *Parasite* 7 (1): 57-58.

[31] Moore RB, Obornik M, Janouskovec J, *et al.* (February 2008). "A photosynthetic alveolate closely related to apicomplexan parasites". *Nature* 451 (7181): 959-963.

[32] Moore RB, Obornik M, Janouskovec J, *et al.* (February 2008). "A photosynthetic alveolate closely related to apicomplexan parasites". *Nature* 451 (7181): 959-63.
[33] Yotoko, KSC; C Elisei (2006-11). "Malaria parasites (Apicomplexa, Haematozoea) and their relationship with their hosts: is there an evolutionary cost for the specialization?". *Journal of Zoological Systematics and Evolutionary Research* 44 (4): 265-73
[34] Perkins SL, Schall JJ (October 2002). "A molecular phylogeny of malarial parsites recovered from cytochrome b gene sequences" *J. parasitol.* 88 (5): 972-8
[35] Yotoko, K.S.C; C Elisei (2006). "Malaria parasites (*Apicomplexa, Haematozoea)* and their relationship with their hosts: is there an evolutionary cost for the specialization?". *Zoo. Syst. Evol. Res.* 44 (4): 265
[36] Seethamchai S, Putapornitip C, Malaivijitnond S, Cui L, Jonwutiwes S. (2008). "Malaria and Hepatocystis species in wild macaques, southern Thailand". *Am J. Trop Med Hyg* 78 (4): 646-653.
[37] Leclerc M.C., Hugot J.P., Durand F. (2004). "Evolutionary relationships between 15 *plasmodium* species from new and old world primates (including humans): an 18S rDNA cladistic analysis". *Parasitology* 129 (6): 677-684
[38] Mitsui H, Arisue N, Sakihama N. *et al.* (January 2010). "Phylogeny of Asian primate malaria parasites inferred from apicoplast genome-encoded genes with special emphasis on the positions of Plasmodium vivax and P. fragile". *Gene* 450 (1-2): 32-8.
[39] Nishimoto Y, Arisue N, Kawai S, Escalante AA, Horii T, Tanabe K, Hashimoto T. (2008)."Evolution and phylogeny of the heterogeneous cytosolic SSU rRNA genes in the genes *Plasmodium*". *Mol Phylogenet Evol.* 47 (1): 45-53.
[40] Sawai H, Otani H, Arisue N, Palacpac N, de Oliveira Martins L, Pathirana S, Handunnetti S, Kawai S, Kishino H, *et al.* (2010). "Lineage-specific positive selection at the merozoite surface protein I (mspl) locus of *plasmodium vivax* and related simian malaria parsites". *Evol Biol.* 10 (1): 52.
[41] Escalante AA Cornejo OE, Freeland DE, Poe AC, Durrego E, Collins We, Lal AA. (2005). "Amonkey's tale: the origin of plasmodium vivax as a human malaria parasite". *Proc Natl Acad Sci USA* 102 (6): 1980-5.
[42] Kishore SP, Perkins Sl, Templeton TJ, Deitsh KW. (June 2009). "An unusual recent expansion of the C-terminal domain of RNA polymerase II in primate malaria parasites features a motif otherwise found only in mammalian polymerases". *J. Mol. Evol.* 68 (6): 706—14.
[43] Prugnolle F, Durand P, Neel C, Ollomo B, Ayala,FJ, Arnathau C, Etienne L, Mpoudi-Ngole E, Nkoghe D *et al* (2010). "African great apes are natural hosts of multiple related malaria species, including *plasmodium falciparum*". *Proc. Natl. Acad. Sci. USA* 107 (4): 1458-1463.
[44] Duval L, Fourment M, Nerrienet E, *et al* (June 2010). " African apes as reservoirs of plasmodium falciparum and the origin and diversification of the Laverania subgenus". *Proc. Natl. Acad. Sci. USA* 107 (23): 10561-6.
[45] Liu W, Li Y, Learn GH, Rudicell RS, Robertson JD, Keele, BF, Ndjango JB, Sanz CM, Morgan DB *et al* (2010). "Origin of the human malaria *plasmodium falciparum* in gorillas". *Nature* 467 (7314).
[46] Rich SM, Leendertz FH, Xu G, *et al* (September 2009). "The origin of malignant malaria". *Proc. Natl. Acad. Sci. U.S.A* 106 (35): 14902-7
[47] Ricklefs RE, Outlaw DC, (2010). "A molecular clock for malaria parasites". *Science* 329 (5988): 226-229.

[48] Sutherland CJ, Tanomsing N, Nolder D, Oguike M, Jennison C, Pukrirrayakamee S, Dolecek C, Hien TT, do Rosario VE, Arez AP, Pinto J Michon P, Escalante AA, Nosten F, Burke M, Lee R, Blaze M, Otto TD, Barnwell JW, Pain A, Williams J, White NJ, Day NP, Snounou G, Lockhart PJ, Chiodini Pl, Imwong M, Polley SD, (2010). "Two non-recombining sympatric forms of the human malaria parsite Iplasmodium *ovale* occur globally". *J Infect Dis* 201 (10): 1544-50.

[49] dos Santos LC, Curotto SM, de Moraes W, *et al.* (July 2009). "Detection of plasmodium sp, in capybara". *Vet parsitol* 163 (1-2): 248-51.

[50] Corradetti A,; Garnham P, C. C; Laird M. (1963). "New classification of the avian malaria parasites". *Parassitologia* 5: 1-4 ISSN 0048-2951.

[51] Martinesn ES, Waite JL, Schall JJ (April 2007). "Morphologically defined subgenera of plasmodium from avian hosts: test of monophyly by phylogenetic analysis of two mitochondrial genes". *Parasitology* 234 (Pt4): 483-90

[52] Telford, S. (1998). "A contribution to the systematic of the reptilian malaria parasites, family *Plasmodium (Apicomplexa: Haemosporing". Bulletin of the Flroida State Museum Biological Sciences* 34 (2): 65-96.

[53] Gratzer WB, Dluzewski AR (1993) The red blood cell and malaria parasite invasion. Semin Hematol 30, 232-247

[54] Holder AA, Blackman MJ, Borre M, Burghaus PA, Chappel JA, Keen JK, Ling IT, Ogun SA, Owen CA, Sinha KA (1994) Malaria parasite and erythrocyte invasion. biochem Soc Trans 22, 291-295.

[55] Goel VK, Li X, Liu SC, Chishti AH, Oh SS (2003) Band 3 is a host receptor binding merozite surface protein I during *Plasmodium falciparum* invasion of erythrocytes. Proc Natl Acad Sci 100, 5164-5169.

[56] Sinnis P, Sim BKL (1997) Cell invasion by the vertebrate stages of *plasmodium*. Tr Microbiol 5, 52-58.

[57] Cooper JA (1993) Merozoite surface antgen-1 of *Plasmodium*. Parasitol Today 9, 50-54.

[58] Mitchell GH, Thomas AW, Margos G, Dluzewski AR, Bannister LH (2004) Apical membrane antigen 1, a major malaria vaccine candidates, mediated the close attachment of invasive merzoites to host red blood cells. Infect. Immune. 72, 154-158.

[59] Carruthers VB, Sibley LD (1997) Sequential protein secretion from three distinct organelles of *Toxoplasma gondii* accompanies invasion of human fibroblasts. Eur. J Cell Biol 73, 114-123

[60] Carruthers VB, Sibley LD (1999) Mobilization of intracellular calcium stimulates microneme discharge in *Toxoplasma gondii*. Mol Microbilo 31, 421-428

[61] Culvenor JG, Day KP, Anders RF (1991) *P. falciparum* ring-infected erythrocyte surface antigen is released from merozoite dense granules after erythrocyte invasion. Infect immune 59, 1183-1187

[62] Blackman MJ, FuJioka H, Stafford WE, Sajid M, Clough B, Fleck SL, Aikawa m< Grainger M, Hackett F (1998) A subtilism-like protein in secretory organelles of *plasmodium falciparum* merozites. J Biol Chem 273, 23398-23409

[63] Barale JC, Blisnick T, Fujioka H, Alzari PM, Aikawa M, Braun,-Breton C, Langsley G (1999) *Plasmodium falciparum* subtilism-like protease 2, a merozite candidate for the merozoite surface pertein 1-42 maturase Proc Natl Acad Sci U S A 96, 6445-6450.

[64] Reed Mb, Caruana SR, Batchelor AH, Thompson JK, Carbb BS, Cowman AF (2000) Targeted disruption of an erythrocyte binding antigen in *plasmodium falciparum* is associated with a switch toward a sialic acid-independent pathway if invasion. proc Natl Acad Sci USA 97, 7509-7514.

[65] Adams JH, Sim BKL, Dolan SA, Fang XD, Kaslow DC, Miller LH (1992). A family of reythrocyte binding protein of malaria parasites. Proc Natl Acad USA 89, 7085-7089
[66] Tomley FM, Soldati DS (2001) Mix and match modules: structure and function of microneme proteins in apicomplexan parasites, trends Parasitol. 17, 81-88
[67] Braun-Breton C, Pereira da Silva LH (1993) Malaria proteases and red blood cell invasion. parasitol Today 9, 92-96.
[68] Sam-Yellowe TY (1996) Rhoptry organelles of the apicompexa: their role in host cell invasion and intercellular survival. Today 12, 308-316
[69] Han YS,Thompson J, Kafatos FC, Barillas-Mury C (2000) Molecular interactions between *Anopheles stephensi* midgut cells and *plasmodium berghei:* the time bomb theory of ookinete invasion of mosquitoes. EMBO J 19, 6030-6040
[70] Waller KL, Cooke BM, Nunomura W, Mohandas N, Coppel RL (1999) Mapping the binding domains involved in the interaction between the *Plasmodium falciparum* konb-associated histidine-rich protein (KAHRP) and the crtoadherence ligand *P. falciparum* erythrocyte membrane protein-I (PfEMPI). J Biol Chem 274, 23808-23813
[71] Mota MM, Pradel G, Vanderberg GP, Hafalla JCR, Frevert U, Nussenzweig RS, Nussenzweig V, Rofriguez A (2001) Migration of *Plasmodium* sporozites through cells before infection. Science 291, 141-144
[72] Kappe SHI, Buscaglia CA Bergman LW, Coppens I, Nussenzweig V (2004) Apicomplexan gliding motility and host cell invasion: overhauling the motor model. Trends in Parasitology 20,13-16.
[73] Iyer J, AC Gruner, L Renia, G Snounou and PR Preiser (2007) invasion of host cells by malaria parasite: a tale of two protein families. Molecular Microbiology 65:231-249.
[74] Baum J, Gilberger TW, Frischknecht F, Meissner M (2008). Host-cell invasion by malaria parasite: insights from *Plasmodium* and *Toxoplasma.* Trends in parasitology 24, 557-563.
[75] Deitsch KW, del Pinal A, Wellems TE (1996) membrane modifications in erythrocytes parasitized by *plasmodium falciprum.* Mol. Biochem Parasitol 76, 1-10
[76] Crabb BS, Cooke BM, Reeder JC, Waller RF, Caruana SR, Davern KM, Wickham ME, Brown GV, Coppel RL, Cowman AF (1997) Targeted gene disruption shows that knobs enable malaria-infected red cells to cytoadhere under physiological shear stress. Cell 98, 287-296.
[77] Waterkeyn JG, Wickham ME, Davern KM, Cooke BM Coppel RL, Reeder JC, Culvenor JG, Waller RF, Cowman AF (2000) Targeted mutagenesis of *Plasmodium falciparum* erythrocyte membrane protein 3 (PfEMP3) disrupts cytoadherence of malaria-infected red blood cells EMBO J 19, 2813-2823.
[78] Sherman IW, Eda S, Winograd E (2003) Cytoadherence and sequestration in *Plasmodium falciparum:* defining the ties that bind, microbes and infection 5, 897-909
[79] Craig A, Schert A (2001) Molecules on the surface of the *Plasmodium falciparum* infected erythrocyte and their role in malaria pathogenesis and immune evasion. Mol. Biochem. Parasitol. 115, 129-143.
[80] Deitsch KW, del Pinal A, Wellems TE (1999) intra-cluster recombination and var transcription switches in the antigenic variation *plasmodium falciparum.* Mol Biochem Parasitol 101, 107-116.
[81] Bannister LH, Mitchell GH, Butcher GA Dennis ED, Cohen S (1986). Structure and development of the surface coat of erythrocytic merozites of *plasmodium knowlesi.* Cell Tissue Res 245, 281-290

[82] Oh SS, Voigt S, Fisher D, Yi SJ, LeRoy PJ, Derick LH, Liu SC, Chishti Ah (2000) *Plamodium falciparum* erythrocyte membrane protein 1 is anchored to spectrin-actin junction and knob-associated histidine-rich protein the erythrocyte cytoskeleton. Mol Biochem Parasitol 100, 237-247
[83] Deitsch KW, del Pinal A, Wellems TE (1999) intra-cluster recombination and var transcription switches in the antigenic variation *plasmodium falciparum*. Mol Biochem Parasitol 101, 107-116.
[84] Beeson JG, Brown GV (2002). Pathogenesis of *Plasmodium falciparum* malaria: the roles of parasite adhesion and antigenic variation. Cell, Mol. Life Sci. 59,258-271
[85] Turner GDH, Morrison H, Jones M, Davis TEM, Looareesuwan S, Buley ID, Gatter KC, Newbold CI, Pukritaykamee S, Nagachinta B, White HJ, Berendt AR (1994) An immunohistochemical study of the pathology of fatal malaria – evidence for widespread endothelial activation and a potential role for intercellular adhesion molecule-I in cerebral sequestration. Am J Pathol 145, 1057-1069.
[86] Deitsch KW, del Pinal A, Wellems TE (1999) intra-cluster recombination and var transcription switches in the antigenic variation *plasmodium falciparum*. Mol Biochem Parasitol 101, 107-116.
[87] Craig A, Schert A (2001) Molecules on the surface of the *Plasmodium falciparum* infected erythrocyte and their role in malaria pathogenesis and immune evasion. Mol. Biochem. Parasitol. 115, 129-143.
[88] Sherman IW, Eda S, Winograd E (2003) Cytoadherence and sequestration in *Plasmodium falciparum:* defining the ties that bind, microbes and infection 5, 897-909
[89] Biggs BA, Anders RF, Dillon HE, Davern KM, Martins M, Petersen C, Brown GV (1992) Adherence of infected erythrocytes to venular endothelium selects for antigenic variants of *plasmodium falciparum* J Immunol 149, 2047-2054.
[90] Roberts DJ, Craig AG, Berendt AR, Pinches R, Nash G, Marsh K, Newbold CI (1992) Rapid switching to multiple antigenic and adhesive phenotpes in malaria. Nature 357, 689-692.
[91] Rottmann M, Lavstsen T, Mugasa JP, Kaestli M, Jensen ATR, Muller D, Theander T, Beck HP (2006) Differential expression of *var* gene groups is associated with morbidity caused by *Plasmodium falciparum* infection in Tanzanian children. Infect. Immune. 74, 3904-3911
[92] Beeson JG, Brown GV, Molneux Me, Mhango C, Dzinjalalala F, Rogerson SJ (1999) *Plasmodium falciparum* isolates from infected pregnant woman and children are associated with distinct adhesive and antigenic properties. J Infect Dis 180,464-472.
[93] Duffy EF, Caragounis A, Noviyanti R,. Kyriacou HM, Choong EK, Boysen K, Healer J, Rowe JA, Molyneux EM, Brown GV, Rogerson SJ (2006) Transcribed *var* genes associated with placental malaria in Malawian women. Infect. Immune. 74:487-4883.
[94] Montgomery J, Mphande FA, Berriman M, Pain A, Rogerson SJ, Taylor TE, Molyneux ME, Craig A (2007) Differential *var* genes expression in the organs of patients dying of falciparum malaria. Molecular Microbiology 65, 959-967.
[95] Scherf A, Hernandez-Rivas R, Buffet P, Bottius E, Benatar C, Pouvelle B, Gysin J, Lanzer M (1998) Antigenic variation in malaria: in situ switching, relaxed and mutually exclusive transcription of var genes during intra-erythrocytic development in *Plasmodium falciparum*. EMBO J 17, 5418-5426.
[96] Voss TS, Healer J, Marty AJ, Duffy MF, Thompson JK, Beeson JG, Reeder JC, Crabb BS, Cowman AF (2006) A *var* gene promoter controls allelic exclusion of virulence genes in *Plasmodium falciparum* Malaria. Nature 439: 1004-1008.

2

Malaria, a Pending Problem in Sub-Saharan Africa

Omolade O. Okwa
Department of Zoology, Parasitology Unit, Lagos State University (LASU), Lagos, Nigeria

1. Introduction

Human Malaria is still a serious problem in sub-Saharan Africa and the risk exists throughout the region. It is a real fact that most malaria cases and deaths occur in sub-Saharan Africa. This region has some of the poorest countries of the world with 90% of deaths occurring (approximately 3,000 deaths each day) [1]· The disease remains one of the leading causes of morbidity and mortality in the tropics. It is the most important and widespread of the tropical deadly diseases.

It exacts a heavy toll of illness and death on children and pregnant women [2].

In 2008, there were 247 million cases of malaria and nearly one million deaths - mainly among children living in sub-Saharan Africa [3]. A child dies every 45 second as a result of malaria, the disease accounts for 20% of all childhood deaths [3]. Malaria kills 3,000 children every day in sub-Saharan Africa—that is, a million a year [4].

In sub-Saharan Africa, many households, even children are familiar with malaria, where it has a reputation of causing teeth chattering chills, shakes and fever.

Specific population risk groups include:

- **Young children** in stable transmission areas who have not yet developed protective immunity against the most severe forms of the disease.
- **Non-immune pregnant women** are at risk as malaria causes high rates of miscarriage (up to 60% in *P. falciparum* infection) and maternal death rates of 10–50%.
- **Semi-immune pregnant women** in areas of high transmission. Malaria can result in miscarriage and low birth weight, especially during the first and second pregnancies. An estimated 200 000 infants die annually as a result of malaria infection during pregnancy.
- **Semi-immune HIV-infected pregnant women** in stable transmission areas are at increased risk of malaria during all pregnancies. Women with malaria infection of the placenta also have a higher risk of passing HIV infection to their newborns.
- **People with HIV/AIDS** are at increased risk of malaria disease when infected.
- **International travelers from non-endemic areas** are at high risk of malaria and its consequences because they lack immunity.
- **Immigrants from endemic areas and their children** living in non-endemic areas and returning to their home countries to visit friends and relatives are similarly at risk because of waning or absent immunity.

The following factors have made malaria a pending problem in sub-Saharan Africa.

2. The malaria parasite

Human Malaria is a parasitic disease caused by apicomplexan protozoan (single celled) coccidian. These parasites are haematozoans or haemosporinas of the family plasmodiidae. A contributing factor to the malaria problem in sub-Saharan Africa is the diversity of the parasite that infects humans. Four species infect man of which *Plasmodium falciparium* is the most virulent. The other species are *P. vivax, P. malariae* and *P. ovale. P. falciparium* and *P. vivax* are the most common [3].

In sub-Saharan Africa, *P. falciparium* poses the greatest threat because of its high level of mortality and the complications arising. *P. vivax* is worldwide in tropical and some temperate regions. *P. vivax* accounts for more than half of all malaria cases outside sub-Saharan Africa. *P. vivax* is unique in that a sporozoite injected into the blood stream may stay in hepatocytes as hyponozoites. *P. ovale* is mainly in found in tropical West Africa and *P. malariae* is found worldwide but with patchy distribution [3]. These malaria parasites can develop within, invade red blood cells (erythrocytes) and consume up to 75% - 80% of their haemoglobin as nutrient source [1].

For both *P. vivax* and *P. ovale,* clinical relapses may occur weeks to months after the first infection, even if the patient has left the malarious area. These new episodes arise from "dormant" liver forms (absent in *P. falciparum* and *P.malariae*), and special treatment - targeted at these liver stages – is mandatory for a complete cure [3].

3. Complications of malaria

P. falciparium causes severe complications as cerebral malaria, severe anaemia, acute renal failure, hypoglycemia and pulmonary infection. The two features that actually separate *P. falciparium* from the other human malaria are the ability to attack erythrocytes of all ages, causing high parasitaemia and enhanced growth and the capability to adhere to vascular endothelium through sequestration [2].

P. falciparium is a threat because of high level of mortality and spreading drug resistance. Cerebral malaria caused by *P. falciparium* is when infected blood cells obstruct blood vessels in the brain; other vital organs can also be damaged often leading to death of patient.

Malaria in pregnancy is widespread. Pregnant women are especially vulnerable because of iron deficiency, a special problem in malaria endemic areas .It endangers the health of women and prospects for the new born. Malaria causes anaemia and low birth weight babies. This is due to the loss of previously existing immunity. *P. falciparium* infects the Red Blood cells (RBC) that adheres to and accumulates in the placenta in pregnant women. Pregnancy exacerbates malaria through a nonspecific hormone-dependent depression of the Immune system. The protective antiplasmodial activity is suppressed at pregnancy, which has clinical consequences with important public health implications on pregnant women [2]. Malaria accounts for 6.5% of abortions, 15% of premature deliveries and 0.7% death in utero [3].

Malaria infection leads to increased morbidity and mortality and the delivery of premature infants with low birth weights due to intrauterine growth retardation (IUGR) that may have been as a result of placental parasitisation [2]. Malaria infection in pregnancy is significant in sub -Saharan Africa where its fatality as a result of virulent *P. falciparium* is a far greater problem than in most parts of the world [4].

Anaemia is another malaria complication that can lead to death. It occurs when *P. falciparium* disrupts the erythrocytes and so decreases the production of erythrocytes. The pathology associated with *P. falciparium* malaria is in particular due to adherence of infected red blood cells in the brain causing metabolic disturbances and organ dysfunction [5].

What of the devastating effect on children? Those children who succumb to the infection but survive are often left damaged. Recurrent infections can leave the child listless and with a poor appetite. It reduces social interaction, leading to poor development. Two percent of children who survive the cerebral form of the disease are left with learning difficulties and conditions such as spasticity and epilepsy [4].

4. The malaria vector

Malaria is transmitted by the *Anopheles* mosquito which carries infective sporozoites stage in its salivary glands which it injects into the human blood stream during a blood meal. Several *Anopheles* mosquitoes have been incriminated as the major malaria vectors. About 20 different *Anopheles* species are locally important around the world. The vector population in sub-Saharan Africa is uniquely effective, with the six species of the *Anopheles gambiae* complex being the most efficient vectors of human malaria in the region, and often considered the most important in the world [4]. *An. funestus* is also capable of producing very high inoculation rates in a wide range of geographic, seasonal, and ecological conditions. These vectors have proven effective in transmitting the malaria parasite to humans across the region, in rural and urban areas alike. *An. pharoensis* is also widely distributed in Africa, geographically and ecologically, and can maintain active transmission of malaria even in the absence of the main malaria vector.

All of the important vector species bite at night. They breed in still waters or shallow collections of freshwater like puddles, rice fields, and hoof prints. Transmission is more intense in places where the mosquito is relatively long-lived (so that the parasite has time to complete its development inside the mosquito) and where it prefers to bite humans rather than other animals. For example, the long lifespan and strong human-biting habit of the African vector species is the underlying reason why more than 85% of the world's malaria deaths are in sub-Saharan Africa [3]. Mosquito's habits therefore determine the geographic spread of the disease.

Malaria transmission is variable from one area to the other and this will impact on its epidemiology and control. In a study by Oyewole *et al* [7] in a coastal area of southern Nigeria in sub-Saharan Africa, several species of *Anopheles* mosquitoes occurred in sympatry. These species all combined to the transmission of malaria in the area. They were all competent vectors. For a mosquito to transmit malaria to man or other hosts the following points are crucial:

i. Vector capacity and competence:

Vectoral capacity has been used interchangeably to describe the ability of mosquitoes to serve as a disease vector. It is defined qualitatively and is influenced by such variables as vector density, longetivity and vector competence. Vectoral capacity takes into account environmental, behavioral, cellular and biochemical factors that influence the association between a vector, the pathogen transmitted by the vector and the vertebrate host to which the pathogen is transmitted [7].

Vector competence is a component of vectoral capacity and is governed by intrinsic and generic factors that influence the ability of a vector to transmit a pathogen. Susceptibility to sporozoite stage of *Plasmodium species* is an important component of vectoral competence.

Vectors competence, however differ from one species to another and from place to place. There are vector species complexes that vary in their behaviors, vectorial capacities and competence and these present a real problem to malaria control. The main factor governing the ability of *Anopheles* specie to act as malaria vector is the frequency with which it feeds on humans. The vectors associated with stable malaria are those which are strongly antropophagic, often feeding on humans to the exclusion of other hosts. Anopheline vectors of malaria consists of various behavior associated with their biting activities and hence transmission dynamics [6].

There is a considerable lack of information regarding vector habits, such as where *Anopheles* rest during the day, information that is critical for control efforts. Awolola *et al.* [8] reported that there is little information on sporozoite rates of *Anopheles* mosquitoes. This observation was the basis of several studies he carried out in Nigeria from 2003 – 2005. The paucity of data on species complexes and their bionomics hampers future vector control as an important component of malaria control.

Correct analysis of the distribution of specific malaria vectors is one of the prerequisites for meaningful epidemiological studies and for planning and monitoring of successful malaria control or eradication programmes. Control measures can only be effective if the abundance, behaviour and proportion of the vectors are known. The existence of species complexes containing morphologically cryptic sibling or isomorphic forms presents a major challenge to malaria control programmes as these require vector identification using molecular techniques. Meanwhile, the distribution of the molecular M (Mopti) and S (Savannah) forms of *An. gambiae s.s* is still being determined for much of the West African regions [6, 8]. The malaria problem in sub-Saharan Africa represents a peculiar case because the vectoral system is the most complex anywhere.

Beier [9] had suggested that malaria transmission dynamics is variable throughout Africa with huge variability in transmission patterns even within villages few kilometers apart. This vectoral system diversity impacts on malaria epidemiology and control. The *An. gambiae* complex is not the only vector in the field [6, 8]. Targeting only this species by whatever method is nonsense. The diversity of the epidemiological situation within sub-Saharan ecotypes presents differing malaria situation. Comprehensive knowledge of behaviour and heterogeneities that exist within, and among these vectors, will always be of benefit. Any strategy aiming at control will have to account for this heterogeneity.

ii. Host preference:

In some areas of sub-Saharan Africa people receive 200 to 300 infective bites per year [4]. This is another component of vectoral capacity and competence. The attractiveness of a blood meal host and the subsequent feeding success of a mosquito depend on characteristics such as host size, proximity to mosquito habitats, host abundance during mosquito host-seeking periods, and host defense mechanisms [7, 8].

There can also be differences in host attractiveness for those mosquito species that feed on humans, and it is not uncommon for some people to be more attractive to mosquitoes than others. Studies have shown that humans appear to exude different amounts of the volatile compounds that mosquitoes loves. Scientists are currently studying the reasons for the difference in attractiveness in order to assist development of repellent compounds for preventing blood feeding and attractants for mosquito traps [10,11].

Some mosquito species may never attack man. Different mosquito species have evolved to blood feed on various types of vertebrate hosts. Some mosquitoes prefer mammalian blood, while others would rather feed solely on birds. There are even mosquitoes specialized to feed on amphibians or reptiles. Opportunistic feeding mosquitoes will feed on any animal, depending on host availability during the host-seeking period [10].

Some *Anopheles* mosquitoes feed indoors and hence endophagic, while others feed outdoors hence exophagic. After blood feeding, some *Anopheles* mosquito may prefer to rest indoors hence are endophilic, while others prefer to rest outdoors hence exophilic. Some mosquito species search for hosts during daylight hours while others are active at dawn and dusk [10, 11]

The main factor governing the ability of *Anopheles* specie to act as malaria vector is the frequency with which it feeds on humans. The vectors associated with stable malaria are those which are strongly antropophagic, often feeding on humans to the exclusion of other hosts. Anopheline vectors of malaria consists of various behavior associated with their biting activities and hence transmission dynamics [6].

5. Human immunity

This is another important factor, especially among adults in areas of moderate or intense transmission conditions. Immunity is developed over years of exposure, and while it never gives complete protection, it does reduce the risk that malaria infection will cause severe disease. For this reason, most malaria deaths in sub-Saharan Africa occur in young children, whereas in areas with less transmission and low immunity, all age groups are at risk [3].

6. Climatic conditions

Transmission also depends on climatic conditions that may affect the abundance and survival of mosquitoes, such as rainfall patterns, temperature and humidity. In many places, transmission is seasonal, with the peak during and just after the rainy season. Malaria epidemics can occur when climate and other conditions suddenly favour transmission in areas where people have little or no immunity to malaria. They can also occur when people with low immunity move into areas with intense malaria transmission, for instance to find work, or as refugees [3].

7. Drug and vector resistances

Treatment and control of malaria have become more difficult because of drug and vector resistances. Growing resistance to antimalarial medicines has spread very rapidly, undermining malaria control efforts. Chloroquine was introduced in the 1950s. When resistance to the drug developed in the 1970s, (Fansidar) sulphadoxine-pyrimethamine (SP) was introduced. Resistance to these drugs is now so high as to render them "virtually useless [12]. These ineffective drugs continue to be used despite the spectacular levels of resistance, leading to increased treatment failure. There have also been reports of increasing multiple-drug resistance to drugs other than chloroquine, such as amodiaquine, mefloquine, rendering treatment of malaria even more problematic. Currently, the best available treatment, particularly for *P. falciparium* malaria, is artemisinin-based combination therapy (ACT) [3]. Artemisinin is part of a combination therapy that reduces or prevents the problem of drug resistance.

Artemisinin and its derivatives like Artesunate, artemether, arteether and dihydroartemisin are the more common drugs now in sub- Saharan Africa. This is not surprising as there is currently no evidence for clinically relevant Artemisinin resistance. Nevertheless, Chloroquine and SP continue to be used because they cost around 10 US cents per treatment, whilst artemisinin combination treatment (ACT) costs US$1.50 per treatment. This is estimated to be an annual cost of between US$100 million and US$200 million a year [4].

When treated with an artemisinin-based monotherapy, patients may discontinue treatment early following the rapid clearance of malaria symptoms. This results in partial treatment and patients still have persistent parasites in their blood. Without a second drug given as part of a combination (as is done with an ACT), these resistant parasites survive and can be passed on to a mosquito and then another person. Monotherapies are therefore the primary force behind the spread of artemisinin resistance [3]. The limitations of these group of drugs are the short duration of antimalarial activity and high recrudescence rate. However, there is low toxicity and they are highly potent and rapidly metabolized [10].

If resistance to artemisinin develops and spreads to other large geographical areas, as has happened before with chloroquine and (SP), the public health consequences could be dire, as no alternative antimalarial medicines will be available in the near future [3]. At least 300 to 500 million malaria episodes are treated annually in sub-Saharan Africa. Moreover, many communities engage in preventive and treatment practices outside what is provided by "official" programs.

Malaria vectors have shown resistance to numerous insecticides, including DDT, various organo-phosphates, and some carbamates. Mosquito control is being strengthened in many areas, but there are significant challenges, including:

- an increasing mosquito resistance to insecticides, including DDT and pyrethroids, particularly in Africa; and
- a lack of alternative, cost-effective and safe insecticides.

The development of new, alternative insecticides is an expensive and long-term endeavour. Detection of insecticide resistance should be an essential component of all national malaria control efforts to ensure that the most effective vector control methods are being used [3].

8. Socio economy aspects

Malaria was a serious obstacle to the colonization of Africa. It caused a lot of suffering and tragedy. Its effect was devastating. It interfered with human progress and development. The disease is still a serious impediment to economic and social development in sub- Saharan Africa.

The socio- economic aspects of a disease is a significant factor in the epidemiology and control of the disease. Malaria causes significant economic losses, and can decrease gross domestic product (GDP) by as much as 1.3% in countries with high levels of transmission. Over the long term, these aggregated annual losses have resulted in substantial differences in GDP between countries with and without malaria, particularly in Africa.

The health costs of malaria include both personal and public expenditures on prevention and treatment. In some heavy-burden countries, the disease accounts for:

- up to 40% of public health expenditures;
- 30% to 50% of inpatient hospital admissions;
- up to 60% of outpatient health clinic visits.

Malaria disproportionately affects poor people who cannot afford treatment or have limited access to health care, trapping families and communities in a downward spiral of poverty.

Malaria is the commonest cause of work and school absenteeism in the tropics. It is the commonest cause of outpatient attendance in sub-Saharan Africa. Economic costs due to malaria are enormous if quantified [13].

Socio economic consequences of diseases are better appreciated when expressed as loss of manpower. Poverty promotes malaria and malaria yields poverty. Socio economic cost can be measured in terms of absenteeism, drugs purchase, doctor's fee, transport, and opportunity cost of time spent waiting for treatment. In Africa alone, the estimated annual direct and indirect costs of malaria were US$800 million in 1987 and exceeded US$1800 million by 1995. Malaria undermines the health and welfare of families, endangers the survival and education of children, debilitates the active population and impoverishes individuals and countries. It is one of the most serious obstacles to mankind's effort to develop agriculture, settlement, development projects and irrigation

Knowledge, attitudes and practices are essential for control programmes. Without the rational concept of the cause of a disease, it is impossible to design control programmes. There still exist wrong misconceptions of malaria in sub Saharan Africa.

Women bear more brute of the disease than men in sub-Saharan Africa. They often tolerate symptoms of malaria until they are critically ill because of the perception that sick women are mean or lazy. Women are reproached when there are malaria epidemics for having failed as custodians of health. Women are increasingly been informed to help them recognize the symptoms of malaria in themselves and family members e.g., fever chills, headache. When children are sick from malaria, women usually bear the psychological effects. Severe convulsions, fever and other symptoms affecting children leave a psychological effect of fear and restlessness on the mothers [14].

9. Conclusion

Malaria in sub-Saharan Africa is a problem of dimensions unlike malaria seen anywhere else in the world today [13]. The magnitude of malaria is affected by a variety of factors, none of which addressed alone is likely to effect a resolution. It is further compounded by the generally poor social and economic conditions in sub-Saharan Africa.

Malaria could be brought under control in sub-Saharan Africa as it has been in Europe and America. Instead, it is being allowed to run out of control just like the AIDS epidemic because of the indifference of Western governments to the lives of the poorest people on the planet [15].

Poor people who represent most of the continent's malaria disease burden cannot afford to pay much more than what they currently pay for the old treatments, so costs must be subsidized by national governments with the help of international donors. What is missing is political will. Unless this situation changes, people will continue to die needlessly from taking drugs that no longer work.

Malaria has therefore remained a deadly scourge and pending problem in Africa and is a yet to be conquered disease.

10. References

[1] Anonymous. Africa malaria reports Executive summary. http://www.rbm.who.int. 2003.

[2] Okwa OO. The Status of Malaria among Pregnant Women: A Study in Lagos, Nigeria. African Journal of Reproductive Health : 2003; 7 (3): 77– 83

[3] WHO: Malaria fact sheet No 94 April 2010. http://www.who.int/mediacentre/factsheets/fs094/en/

[4] Mason B. Malaria appalling death toll in sub-Saharan Africa. http://www.wsws.org/articles/2003/may2003/mala-m14.shtml world socialist web site.international committee of the fourth international (ICFI); 2003

[5] Amajoh N, Odukoko JB, Monsanya ME. Preliminary investigations on malaria and anemia in the Atlantic coastal margin of Ibeju Lekki, Lagos Nigeria. Journal of Malaria in Africa and the Tropics. 2002; (1)17-22.

[6] Oyewole IO, Ibidapo CA, Okwa OO, Oduola AO, Adeoye GO, Okoh HI, Awolola TS (2010). Species Composition and Role of *Anopheles* Mosquitoes in Malaria Transmission along Badagry axis of Lagos Lagoon, Lagos, Nigeria. International Journal of Insect Science 2010; (2) 51–57

[7] Okwa OO, Carter V, Hurd H. Abundances, host preferences and infectivity rates of malaria vectors in Badagry Local government area of Lagos, Nigeria. Nigeria Journal of Parasitology. 2006; 27:41-48.

[8] Awolola TS, Oyewole IO, Koekemoer LL, Coetzee M. Identification of three members of the *Anopheles funestus* (*Diptera: Culicidae*) group and their role in malaria transmission in two ecological zones in Nigeria. Transactions of the Royal Society of Tropical Medicine and Hygiene. 2005; 99: 525-531.

[9] Beier JC. Malaria parasite development in mosquitoes. Annual Review of Entomology 1998; .43, 519-543.

[10] Richards SL, Ponnusamy L, Unnasch TR, Hassan HK, Apperson CS . Host-feeding patterns of *Aedes albopictus* (Skuse) (Diptera: Culicidae) in relation to the availability of human and domestic animals in suburban landscapes of Central North Carolina with notes on blood meal hosts of sympatric mosquito species. Journal of Medical Entomology 2006; 43 (3): 543-551.

[11] Richards SL, Anderson SL, CT Smartt. The female mosquito's quest for blood: Implications for disease cycles. University of Florida/IFAS Fact Sheet, ENY-855, IN-811. http://edis.ifas.ufl.edu/IN811.2009

[12] Krishna, S.O., Ursula, E., Joet, T; Uhlemann, A.C., Monnc, Webb R., Woodrow, C, Kun, J.F.J and Kremsner P.G. Transport processes in *Plasmodium falciparium* erythrocytes potential as new drug targets. International Journal of Parasitology. 2002; 32:1567-1573

[13] Gallup JL, Sachs JD. The economic burden of malaria. American Journal of Tropical Medicine and Hygiene. 2001; 64: 85-96.

[14] Okwa, O.O: Tropical parasitic diseases and women. Annals of African medicine 2007; 6 (4): 157-163.

[15] Anonymous: Malaria and development in Africa .A cross sectional approach. http://www.aaas.org/international/africa/malaria91/background.html.2010.

Part 2

Malaria Vector Research

3

Facing Malaria Parasite with Mosquito Symbionts

Guido Favia et al.*
School of Bioscience & Biotechnology, University of Camerino, Camerino (MC)
Italy

1. Introduction

Microbial symbiosis is an ubiquitous aspect of insect life and plays a fundamental role in the adaptation of insects to the most diverse environments. A very large proportion of insects are supposed to carry bacterial symbionts (Chaves et al., 2009). The variety of the relationships between symbionts and insects are very wide as well as biological function exerted by the symbionts and their localisation within the host. In fact, some are located within host cells while some others are outside. The genetic modification of microbial symbionts has been identified as novel tools to fight insect pests and vectors of infectious diseases. In this frame, in the last years, the use of manipulated symbiont has attracted a lot of attention for the potential application in the control of mosquito-borne diseases, with particular interest to malaria control.

Malaria still represents a major health problem with particular impact in the developing countries. Even though several control tools are employed for malaria control, such as bed nets, Anti-malarial drugs, insecticides and other vector control measures, the disease continue to exert a dramatic health burden on the world human populations. Consequently, new effective tools for malaria control are expected. Human malaria is transmitted by some mosquito species belonging to the genus *Anopheles* and methods aimed to control the malaria infection by blocking the transmission from mosquito to humans are particularly attractive.

Recently, quite a lot of attention has been addressed to the so-called Malaria Symbiotic Control (Favia et al., 2008). In fact, more generally, symbiotic microorganisms offer some possibilities for insect pest management strategies and two approaches are particular attractive: The first one implies the disruption of microbial symbionts required by insect pests. The second approach is the manipulation of microorganisms with major impacts on insect traits contributing to their "pest status" for example their capacity to act as vector for diseases like malaria and others. In particular, the paratransgenic approach looks feasible for malaria control.

Paratransgenesis is the genetic modification of insect symbionts to express anti-pathogen molecules within the vector to block pathogen transmission. In case of malaria infection,

---

*Irene Ricci, Patrizia Scuppa, Claudia Damiani, Paolo Rossi, Aida Capone, Chenoa De Freece, Matteo Valzano, Alessia Cappelli, Michela Mosca and Ulisse Ulissi

mosquitoes should be "forced" to host symbionts that have been previously manipulated to express effector molecules able to interfere with *Plasmodium* development, possibly blocking transmission.

In the frame of insect borne diseases, Chagas disease has already proven the feasibility of paratransgenesis in the control of the infection. Vectors of Chagas disease are obligate haematophagous triatomines that feed on vertebrate blood throughout their entire developmental cycle. These insects harbour populations of bacterial symbionts within their intestinal tract, which provide nutrients that insects do not acquire by the blood source. These symbionts have been isolated, cultured outside the host and genetically transformed to express molecules that render the insect refractory to the infection with *Trypanosoma cruzi*, the etiological agent of Chagas disease (Beard et al., 2001). Once reintroduced in the vector host, the paratransgenic insect vector showed refractoriness to parasite infection.

Thus, also on the basis of impulse related to these very exciting results in paratransgenic approach to control Chagas disease, since few years, some researches have been addressed to the identification microbial symbiont that could be implemented in the development of paratransgenic approach for malaria control.

In this chapter we will give an overview an update of the recent advance in symbiont based-malaria control.

2. Best symbiont candidates for malaria control

For malaria Symbiotic Control (SC), "good" candidates are those microbes residing within the mosquito, particularly those localised in the gut. In fact, malarial gametocytes, ingested by a feeding mosquito, must transform to gametes, fuse to form zygotes, and then, as ookinetes, migrate to the mosquito's midgut epithelium to develop as oocysts that release sporozoites to infect the mosquito's salivary glands. At the Oocysts stage of *Plasmodium*, the protozoan parasite causing the malaria infection, represents a favourable target for control method like paratransgenesis aimed to interrupt the disease transmission. In fact, in natural conditions, from thousands of gametocytes ingested by the mosquito vector in an infected blood meal, generally less than ten oocysts will develop.

As stated above, paratransgensis has been already proposed to control insect borne diseases. This is the case of *Rhodnius prolixus*, a triatomine commonly known as the kissing bug, vector of *Trypanosoma cruzi* the causative agent of the Chagas disease. *R. prolixus* harbours in its gut some bacteria that provide nutrients to the insect. These bacteria have been cultivate outside the host, modified to express specific anti-parasite effector molecules and reintroduced within the vector (Beard et al., 2001). These paratransgenic insects have shown to be unable to transmit the parasite. These evidences have posed the basis for the development of paratransgenic-related strategies, based on gut symbionts, to control insect borne diseases.

In the meanwhile they represent the cornerstone on which to base the development of SC of malaria infection.

The search of gut symbiont has been primarily addressed to the identification of bacteria residing in the mosquito gut. Some studies have described the structure of the bacterial community present in several mosquito species (Demaio et al., 1996; Pidiyar et al., 2002,

2004; Touré et al., 2000), pinpointing that different mosquito species harbour common bacterial genera (e.g. *Pseudomonas, Staphylococcus, Enterobacter, Escherichia*), some of which might be cultivated outside the vector and manipulated by the means of genetic tools that are already available.

Cultivability in cell-free media and applicability to genetic transformation are two of the fundamental prerequisite of a "good" symbiont to be applied in paratransgenesis control of insect vectors.

More recently, the application of advanced molecular techniques, led to the identification of bacterial species, never described before, has stable component of the microbiota associated to malaria vectors.

For example in the African malaria vector *Anopheles arabiensis* two new species have been recently described (Kämpfer et al., 2006a, 2006b). One was named *Janibacter anophelis* the other *Thorsellia anophelis* to remark the close relationship with the mosquito host. In particular, *T. anophelis* has been proposed in malaria paratransgenic control, since this bacterium, by the means of sequencing of major bands generated in Denaturing Gradient Gel Electrophoresis (DGGE) experiments, appears to be dominant in Kenyan populations of *Anopheles gambiae,* the main African malaria vector (Briones et al., 2008) and dominance is indeed one additional main features required for a symbiont to be employed in paratransgenesis.

The list of bacteria well adapted to malaria vectors midgut has been rapidly growing in the last few years. Among these bacteria two species have been recently described as particularly well adapted to *An. gambiae* midgut, *Pantoea stewartii* and *Elizabethkingia meningoseptica* (Lindh et al., 2008) and thus potentially useful for symbiotic control applications.

Recently, we have identified a Gram-negative α-proteobacteria as stably associated to different mosquito species with particular regards to some main malaria vector species (Favia et al., 2007, 2008; Damiani et al., 2008, 2010; Crotti et al., 2009) and its further microbiological and molecular characterization clearly indicate it as belonging to the genus *Asaia* (Ricci et al. 2011a).

The relationship between *Asaia* and mosquito is particularly intriguing in the view of paratransgenic applications since this bacterium localizes in the gut (Figure 1), in the salivary glands and in the reproductive organs of both male and female adult mosquitoes. These localizations are important since in the mosquito gut and salivary glands overlaps with that of *Plasmodium* thus supporting the use of *Asaia* for paratransgenic applications. The localization in the reproductive organs relates to vertical transmission routes that imply favourable means to introduce modified bacteria in the field (Damiani et al., 2010).

Furthermore, *Asaia* is easily cultivable in cell-free media, is detectable at all developmental stage of the mosquito and has high prevalence in mosquito populations. These characteristics have indicated *Asaia* as one of the potentially best bacterial symbiont of malaria vectors to develop paratransgenic protocols to control malaria infection.

Transformation of *Asaia* was originally achieved by a strain originally isolated from *Anopheles stephensi*, one of the major Asian malaria vector, and was attempted by using different plasmid vectors.

Among these, the plasmid pHM2 was the most efficient and transformed *Asaia* with high efficiency. The gene cassette coding for the green fluorescent protein (Gfp) was cloned into the plasmid vector pHM2 thus providing an efficiently detectable marker to trace mosquito body colonization. Transformed *Asaia* cells were found to efficiently express the protein and showed bright fluorescence useful for localization of the symbiotic cells in the insect body detectable by fluorescent confocal laser scanning microscopy (Figures 2 and 3). Furthermore, in laboratory, when we proposed fed mosquitoes by cotton pad soaked in a mixture of sugar and "green" bacteria, nearly 100% of the recipient populations resulted colonised by the modified *Asaia*.

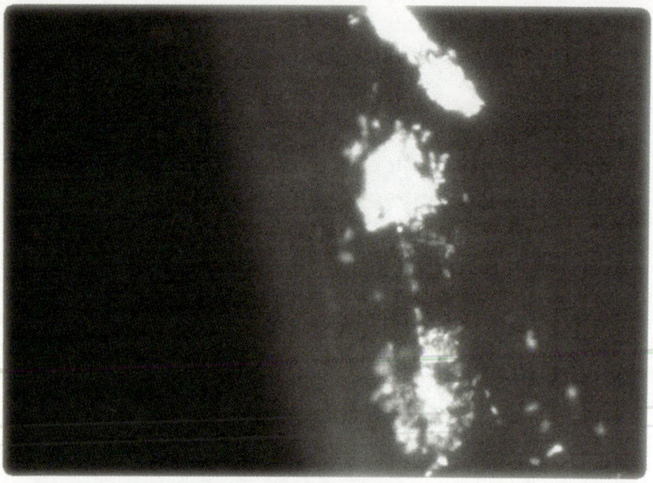

Fig. 1. *Asaia* bacteria in the gut of an adult *An. stephensi* mosquito.

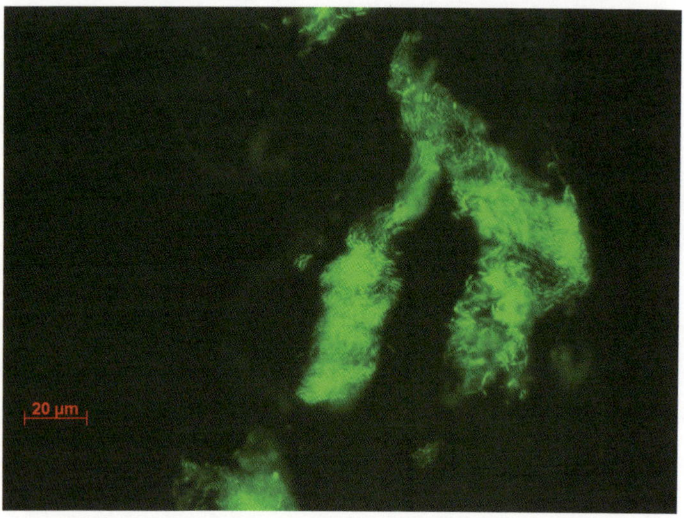

Fig. 2. *Asaia* strain expressing the green fluorescent protein in the midgut of an *Anopheles stephensi* female specimen.

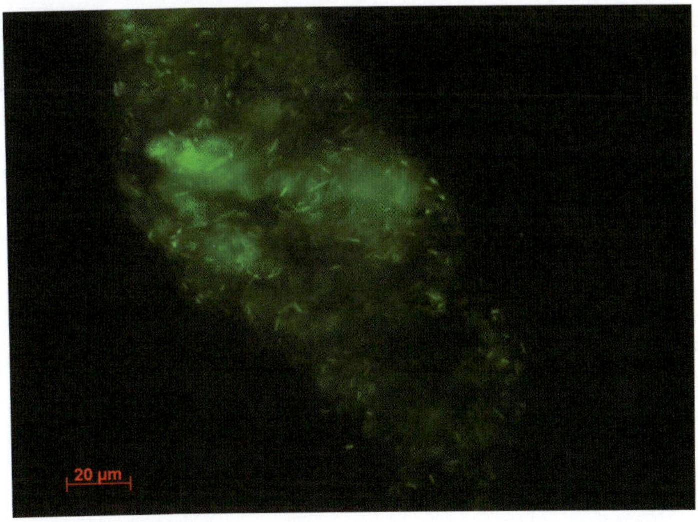

Fig. 3. *Asaia* strain expressing the green fluorescent protein in the midgut of an *An. stephensi* male specimen.

2.1 Effector molecules with anti-*Plasmodium* effects

Some molecules have proven to be effective in inhibiting the development of the malaria parasite within the mosquito vector and may be implemented in paratransgenic experiments aimed to block malaria transmission.

Among them has to be mentioned the small dodecapeptide SM1. This peptide is able to interfere with a binding protein of the lumen of the mosquito midgut and salivary glands that is required for *Plasmodium* invasion. This interference between SM1 and mosquito midgut results in the inhibition of parasite development (Ghosh et al., 2001). A second molecule to be mentioned is the snake venom phospholipase named PLA2 that is able to block *Plasmodium* development within the mosquito by the inhibition of the association between ookinetes and midgut surface (Zieler et al., 2001).

A third molecule is Scorpine an antimicrobial peptide isolated from the venom of the scorpion *Pandinus imperator*, with anti-bacterial activity and a potent inhibitory effect on the ookinete and gamete stages of the rodent malaria parasite *Plasmodium berghei* development (Conde et al., 2000).

Other effector molecules to be mentioned are two single chain antibodies called anti-PfNPNA1 and anti-Pbs 21 respectively.

The single-chain antibody PfNPNA-1 is based on a recombinant human monoclonal antibody that specifically recognizes the repeat region (Asn-Pro-Asn-Ala) of the *Plasmodium falciparum* surface circumsporozoite protein and agglutinates sporozoites (Chappel et al., 2004).

Pbs21 is an ookinete surface protein of *P. berghei*, a rodent's parasite, belonging to a class of sexual stage antigens able to induce in the vertebrate host a transmission-blocking immune response. The effectors of this transmission-blocking immunity are antibody molecules directed against particular protein epitopes (Spano et al., 1996). Anti-Pbs 21 may be used in paratransgenic experiment in the murine system to prove the feasibility of the approach.

Some studies have already shown the possibility to use mosquito guts bacteria to deliver anti-*Plasmodium* effector molecules within the mosquito vector (Riehle and Jacobs-Lorena 2005; Riehle et al., 2007).

In these studies are reported that *E. coli* bacteria expressing SM1 and PLA2, are able to partially inhibit the parasite development. Very recently, Bisi & Lampe (2011) described *Pantoea agglomerans* engineered to express and secrete anti-*Plasmodium* effector proteins. To this purpose, plasmids that included the pelB or hlyA secretion signals from the genes of related species were constructed and tested for their efficacy in secreting SM1, anti-Pbs21, and PLA2 in *P. agglomerans* and *E. coli*.

Very interestingly, *P. agglomerans* was able to secrete HlyA fusions of anti-Pbs21 and PLA2, and now ongoing experiments are evaluating these strains for anti-*Plasmodium* activity in infected mosquitoes.

It is worth to remind that parasites tend to have a heterogeneous genome that favours selection of individuals able to overcome barriers such as drugs or possibly effector gene products favouring the insurgence of resistant strains. Thus the possibility to release paratrasgenic mosquito carrying microbial symbionts modified to express several different molecules would circumvent the selection of resistant malaria strains.

The results cited above, represent a clear "proof of principle" about the applicability of paratransgenesis in malaria control.

In this context, the symbiotic bacterium *Asaia* previously described, may be very successfully implied.

We engineered *Asaia* strains that were transformed to produce fluorescent proteins; they showed a remarkable capacity to colonize the midgut, reproductive organs ad salivary glands of recipient mosquitoes (Favia et al., 2007; Damiani et al., 2008, 2010). These studies underline the possibility of using this bacterium to express anti-parasite molecules within the mosquito body, to inhibit the transmission of the parasite.

Furthermore, *Asaia* can be transmitted, vertically to the progeny (by maternal, paternal and trans-stadial routes) and horizontally between mosquito individuals by mating and co-feeding (Favia et al., 2007, 2008; Damiani et al., 2008, 2010).

As stated above, vertical transmission is important because it offers the chance of introducing engineered bacteria into mosquito populations in the field. In *An. gambiae* it has been proven that vertical transmission occurs by an egg-smearing mechanism, where the extracellular *Asaia* symbionts are smeared onto the egg surface, thus is quite likely that larvae, after emergence, are infected by the bacteria by feeding on them and on egg remnants (Damiani et al., 2010).

Larvae infection by bacteria in the breeding water, offers a way to spread recombinant bacteria in the field, moreover the vertical transmission of *Asaia* symbiont would allow the "passage" of recombinant symbionts through the generations.

Paternal transmission is also important because offers an alternative way to release engineered bacteria in the field in addition to their release in the larval breeding site to contaminate larvae and consequently adults by trans-stadial routes. Indeed, paternal transmission suggests the possibility of releasing not biting male mosquitoes that would be previously colonised with engineered bacteria (Damiani et al., 2010).

Ongoing studies are intended to modify *Asaia* to produce strains able to express and secrete anti-*Plasmodium* effector molecules and to test their ability in blocking malaria transmission.

2.1.1 Not only bacteria

It is worth to mention that not only bacteria symbiont may find application in paratransgenesis but several evidences indicate that virus, yeast and fungi may also be successfully use.

Ren and collaborators (2008) discovered, cloned and characterized the first known DNV (AgDNV) capable of infection and dissemination in *An. gambiae*. By the development of an AgDNV-based expression vector to express gene(s) of interest in *An. gambiae*, an exogenous gene (enhanced green fluorescent protein; EGFP) was expressed in *An. gambiae* mosquitoes. Wild-type and EGFP-transducing AgDNV virions were able to consistently infect *An. gambiae* larvae, expressed EGFP was detected in adult tissues such as midgut, fat body and ovaries and were transmitted to subsequent mosquito generations.

This work produced clear evidence that AgDNV could be used as part of a paratransgenic malaria control strategy by transduction of anti-*Plasmodium* effectors or insect-specific toxins in *Anopheles* mosquitoes.

In the last few months we have identified the yeast *Wickerhamomyces anomalus* as stably associated to some malaria vector species localising at the level of midgut and reproductive organs of the host (Ricci et al., 2011b, 2011c). This localization, the possibility to easily manipulate yeast and the chance to express effector molecules in a eukaryotic organism render *W. anomalus* a potential good candidate for paratransgenesis. Interestingly, very often we found in the midgut and reproductive organs of the mosquito a large number of *Asaia* bacteria in association with a relevant number of *W. anomalus*. This finding may support the idea to use synergistically these two symbionts to release different effector molecules in the mosquito.

We are now proceeding to achieve rapidly a stable transformation system to produce strains of *W. anomalus* able to express and delivery anti-*Plasmodium* peptides.

Very recently, Fang et al (2011) develop transgenic fungi that kill malaria parasite in the mosquito.

They used the fungus *Metarhizium anisopliae* to infect mosquitoes through the cuticle. Recombinant strains of *M. anisopliae* expressing three effector molecules (SM1, a single chain antibody called PfNPNA-1 and an antimicrobial peptide called scorpine) targeting sporozoites during their travel through the hemolymph to the salivary glands were used to infect mosquitoes that had a *Plasmodium*-infected blood meal eleven days before.

The reduction in sporozoite counts was relevant and even more when using *M. anisopliae* strain expressing scorpine and an [SM1](8): scorpine fusion protein (with the reduction in sporozoite counts of 98%). These experiments prove that *Metarhizium*-mediated inhibition of *Plasmodium* development could be an additional tool to contrast malaria development within the vector.

2.1.2 Not only paratransgenesis

Symbiont may be successfully implied in SC of mosquito vector even without their genetic manipulation. This would be the case of *W. anomalus*. In fact several strains of this yeast produce killer toxins with an antimicrobial effect on a wide spectrum of human pathogens (Séguy et al., 1998; Magliani et al., 2001), including insect-transmitted protozoan parasites such as *Leishmania* spp. (Savoia et al., 2002). Preliminary data seems to confirm that the *W. anomalus* strain isolated from *An. stephensi*, produces a killer toxin that is active against some yeast strains (Ricci et al. manuscript in preparation). We will soon test if this killer toxin is active against *Plasmodium* to verify the possibility to contrast malaria parasite development by the release of this natural killer within mosquito organs.

One mosquito symbiont that has been extensively studied is the alpha-proteobacterium *Wolbachia*, a very common cytoplasmic symbiont of the majority of insect species, crustaceans, mites, and filarial nematodes (Serbus et al., 2008). *Wolbachia* are maternally inherited bacteria that inducing cytoplasmic incompatibility in mosquitoes that they use to spread themselves through populations enhancing their transmission (Sinkins, 2004). This ability of self-spreading through mosquito populations attracted a lot of attention in the last few years and has been proposed as a gene drive system for mosquito genetic replacement, for the reduction of population size or for modulating population age structure to reduce disease transmission.

Interestingly, even though the very wide range of insect species naturally infected by *Wolbachia*, natural infection has never been detected in species belonging to the genus *Anopheles* (Ricci et al., 2002; Rasgon & Scott, 2004; Tiawsirisup et al., 2008). On the other hand cultured *Anopheles* cells can be infected (Jin et al., 2009), this has opened new possibility to study perspectives in the use of endosymbiont to control malaria infection.

An "over-replicating" strain of *Wolbachia pipientis* named wMelPop has recently been shown to induce immune upregulation and inhibition of pathogen transmission in *Aedes aegypti* the principal mosquito vector of dengue viruses, thus transient somatic infections of wMelPop were performed by intrathoracic inoculation in *An. gambiae*. As consequence of these inoculations, up-regulation of several specific immune genes was detected and some of these have shown a direct influence on the development of malaria parasites. Similar results have been achieved when using a stably infected *An. gambiae* cell line (Kambris et al., 2010).

Other studies have characterized somatic infections of two diverse *Wolbachia* strains (wMelPop and wAlbB) in *An. gambiae*. After infection, wMelPop was localized in fat body, head, sensory organs and other tissues but was not detected in midgut and ovaries, even though both *Wolbachia* strains inhibit *P. falciparum* oocyst in the mosquito midgut.

Even more interestingly, although not virulent in non-bloodfed mosquitoes, wMelPop was found to be virulent for around 12-24 hours post-bloodmeal. All these data strongly indicate that if stable transinfections would behave similarly to somatic infections, *Wolbachia* could potentially be used as part of a strategy to control malaria-transmitting mosquitoes (Hughes et al., 2010).

From this point of view, the "*Ae. aegypti* lesson", can be particularly important. Similar to *Anopheles*, *Ae. aegypti* has never been detected as naturally infected by *Wolbachia*, trans-infection of selected strains of *Wolbachia* in *Ae. aegypti* can block the development of dengue infection (Walker et al., 2011).

Very recently the wMel *Wolbachia* strain was introduced into *Ae. aegypti* from *Drosophila melanogaster* showing a successfully invasion two natural *Ae. aegypti* populations in Australia, reaching almost the fixation in a few months after the releases of wMel-infected *An. aegypti* adults (Hoffmann et al., 2011).

These findings demonstrate that *Wolbachia*-based strategies can be a successful approach to eliminate dengue infection and a similar approach may be developed to control malaria infection.

3. Future development and conclusion

The concept that manipulation of microbial symbionts may represent an important tool to contrast insect pests and insect vectors of infectious diseases is now widely accepted.

Recent studies have also pointed out that is possible to overcome many of the limitations that since some time ago represented strong limitation to this approach, including the difficulty to culture and transform many symbionts. As discussed in the previous paragraph, to date several symbionts of insect pests and vector borne diseases can be cultivated outside the host, manipulated to express specific factors and reintroduced within the host to produce *in situ* the effector molecules. A very informative example of advanced studies in genetic manipulation of insect symbionts is *Rhodococcus rhodnii*, a bacterial symbiont of the reduviid bug *Rhodnius prolixus*. This bacterium, if manipulated appropriately, can be reintroduced to the vector and inhibit the transmission of *Trypanosoma cruzi* that causes Chagas disease (Beard et al., 2001). Another example regards the bacterium *Alcaligenes*, a gut symbiont of the sharpshooter *Homalodisca coagulata*, the vector of Pierce's crop disease (Bextine et al., 2004).

Concerning malaria control, we have described some symbionts that can be cultured outside the mosquito and can be genetically modified to produce specific molecules that have proven to have an inhibitory effect on *Plasmodium* development. In the last 5 years our group has been focused in the study of symbiosis in mosquito vector. Our group as well as others research units, have indicated few microorganisms that possess a strong potential in the paratransgenic control of mosquito-borne diseases and in the very few last years, the number of parasite of medical and veterinary for which the paratransgenic approach has been proposed as one of the element of an integrated control strategy is increasing as demonstrated by study aimed to develop control method of *Leishmania* parasite (Hurwitz et al., 2011). However, even if the genetic modification of insect symbionts to inhibit parasite development, is clearly feasible and achievable in laboratories, many concerns need to be properly addressed before this approach can be applicable in the field. Even though the release of paratransgenic mosquito poses much less ethical and safety concerns that the release of genetically modified mosquitoes, for example the release of large-scale transgenic mosquitoes, would cause not only an increase of the nuisance but also the health risk related to other mosquito borne diseases (it is worth to remind that malaria vector mosquitoes may transmit other pathogens), the release into the field of modified symbionts needs to be approached with caution since particularly bacteria may spread very rapidly by horizontal transfer and colonize non target organisms with still unknown consequence. On the other hand is possible to argue that there is no reason to believe that any of the effector molecules identified to date will have any effects on non-target organisms (especially higher organisms) being specifically intended against *Plasmodium*. Still, it is necessary the release of paratransgenic mosquitoes must refer to previous experiences with different Genetically Modified Organisms (GMO) (i.e. GM plants) taking into account indications from different national and international authorities that have already established legal requirements for the safety of these products (Aguilera et al., 2011).

If scientific and ethical concerns have to be properly addressed it is also equally important to address concerns of public perception. First of all it is important to underline that no single approach can be successfully *per se* but only an integrated control program that will merge the benefits of different type of approaches would be effective in controlling malaria infection. This is true also for the paratransgenic approach.

It is important to involve residents of the malaria affected countries and their government in official way. In this context it is particularly important to widely release the results of safety tests regarding the use of paratransgenic mosquitoes without covering any possible risk associated to the use of such an approach pinpointing precisely the "real balance" between potential benefits and risks associated to the implementation of the paratransgenic strategy. Christopher Boete (2011) has just published the results of an important study about the use of transgenic mosquitoes as a potential approach to interrupt malaria transmission.

This study was performed through a questionnaire addressing questions related to the type of research, the location, the nationality and the perception of the public involvement by scientists. The results indicate that even if malaria researchers agree to interact with a non-scientific audience pinpointing that "*they remain quite reluctant to have their research project submitted in a jargon-free version to the evaluation and the prior-agreement by a group of non-specialists*". The study shows the importance of fostering structures and processes that could lead to an improved involvement of an unspecialized public in the debates linking scientific, technological and public health issues in Africa.

One more aspect that is very important to guarantee success to the paratransgenic approach is the capacity to integrate laboratory and field work bringing together competences from different disciplines and context to produce a variegate and efficient bulk of skills that will be more effective that the simple sum of independent competences.

Before any possible field applications, the next step in the assessment of the paratransgenic approach will take advantage by the so-called "semi-field" studies. They can be conducted in mosquito-proof greenhouses that have been termed "malaria spheres" by Knols and collaborators (2002). The green-houses consist in a space-limited ecosystem that recreates an ecological contest with plants, breeding sites etc in which is possible to perform the tests. These test will give important insights about the dynamic of transmission of a due symbiont, in fact releasing subsequent different small numbers of paratransgenic mosquitoes into a malaria sphere containing non-paratransgenic mosquito population it will be possible to determine to the minimum proportion of paratatransgenic insects that need to be introduced for the symbiont to spread over the whole population. Furthermore it will be possible to acquire information about the capacity of modified symbiont(s) to compete with the natural microbiota. Moreover, all the data acquired by semi-field studies would also provide valuable parameters for modelling experiments to assess the feasibility of introducing GM-symbionts under true field conditions.

Even though laboratory and field issues have still to be fully overcame, the fast and growing progress recently made in the field of the SC of insect pest and vectors of diseases, induces a relevant optimism that this approach may be applicable for field testing within the next decade thus offering a new weapon to the arsenal against malaria infection.

4. Acknowledgment

We wish to thank Luciano Pasqualini for his valuable technical support during the writing of the chapter. Our researches described in this chapter has been supported by the following agencies: agencies Firb-Ideas (grant RBID082MLZ) and Prin 2007 (grant 2007PK2HB7_002), both from the Italian Ministry of University and Research (MIUR), and by the EU-FP7 Capacities-Infrastructure 2008 (grant 228421) to G.F. P.R. benefited of travel grant from the COSTAction FA0701.

5. References

Aguilera, J., Gomes, A.R. & Nielsen K.M. (2011). Genetically modified microbial symbiont as arthropod pest controllers: risk assessment through the European legislations. *Journal of Applied Entomology,* (August 2011), pp. 494-502.

Beard, C.B., Dotsona, P.M., Pennington, S., Eichler, C., Cordon-Rosales, R. & Durvasular, V. (2001). Bacterial symbiosis and paratransgenic control of vector-borne Chagas disease. *Int. J. Parasitol,* (May 2001), pp. 621–627.

Bextine, B., Lauzon, C., Potter, S., Lampe, D. & Miller, T.A. (2004). Delivery of a genetically marked *Alcaligenes* sp. to the glassy-winged sharpshooter for use in a paratransgenic control strategy. *Curr Microbiol,* (May 2004), pp. 327-331.

Bisi, D.C. & Lampe, D.J. (2011). Secretion of anti-*Plasmodium* effector proteins from a natural *Pantoea agglomerans* isolate by using PelB and HlyA secretion signals. *Appl Environ Microbiol,* (July 2011), pp. 4669-4675.

Boete, C. (2011). Scientists and public involvement: a consultation on the relation between malaria, vector control and transgenic mosquitoes. *Trans R Soc Trop Med Hyg* (in press).

Briones, A.M., Shililu, J., Githure, J., Novak, R. & Raskin, L. (2008). *Thorsellia anophelis* is the dominant bacterium in a Kenyan population of adult *Anopheles gambiae* mosquitoes. ISME J, (November 2007), pp. 74-82.

Chaves, S., Neto, M. & Tenreiro, R. (2009). Insect-symbiont systems: from complex relationships to biotechnological applications. *Biotechnol.* (December 2009), pp. 1753–1765.

Chappel, J.A., Hollingdale, M.R. & Kang, A.S. (2004). IgG(4) Pf NPNA-1 a human anti-*Plasmodium falciparum* sporozoite monoclonal antibody cloned from a protected individual inhibits parasite invasion of hepatocytes. *Hum Antibodies,* (December 2004), pp. 91-96.

Conde, R., Zamudio, F.Z., Rodriguez, M.H. & Possani L.D. (2000). Scorpine, an anti-malaria and anti-bacterial agent purified from scorpion venom. *FEBS Lett*, (April 2000), pp. 165-168.

Crotti, E., Damiani, C., Pajoro, M., Gonella, E., Rizzi, A., Ricci, I., Negri, I., Scuppa, P., Rossi, P., Ballarini, P., Raddadi N., Marzorati,. M, Sacchi, L., Clementi E., Genchi, M., Mandrioli, M., Bandi, C., Favia,. G, Alma, A. & Daffonchio, D. (2009). *Asaia*, a versatile acetic acid bacterial symbiont, capable of cross-colonizing insects of phylogenetically distant genera and orders. *Environ. Microbiol*, (September 2009), pp. 3252-3264.

Damiani, C., Ricci, I., Crotti, E., Rossi, P., Rizzi, A., Scuppa, P., Esposito, F., Bandi, C., Daffonchio, D. & Favia, G. (2008). Paternal transmission of symbiotic bacteria in malaria vectors. *Curr. Biol*, (December 2008), pp. 1087-1088.

Damiani, C., Ricci, I., Crotti, E., Rossi, P., Rizzi, A., Scuppa, P., Capone, A., Ulissi, U., Epis, S., Genchi, M., Sagnon, N., Faye, I., Kang, A., Chouaia, B., Whitehorn, C., Moussa, G.W., Mandrioli, M., Esposito, F., Sacchi, L., Bandi, C., Daffonchio, D. & Favia, G. (2010). Mosquito-Bacteria Symbiosis: The Case of *Anopheles gambiae* and *Asaia*. *Microb Ecol*, (June 2010), pp. 644-654.

Demaio, J., Pumpuni, C.B., Kent, M. & Beier, J.C. (1996). The midgut bacterial flora of wild *Aedes triseriatus, Culex pipiens*, and *Psorophora columbiae* mosquitoes. *Am. J. Trop. Med. Hyg*, (February 1996), pp. 219-223.

Fang, W., Vega-Rodriguez, J., Ghosh, A.K., Jacobs-Lorena, M., Kang, A. & St Leger, R.J. (2011). Development of transgenic fungi that kill human malaria parasites in mosquitoes. *Science*, (February 2011), pp. 1074-1077.

Favia, G., Ricci, I., Damiani, C., Raddadi, N., Crotti, E., Marzorati, M., Rizzi, A., Urso, R., Brusetti, L., Borin, S., Mora, D., Scuppa, P., Pasqualini, L., Clementi, E., Genchi, M., Corona, S., Negri, I., Grandi, G., Alma, A., Kramer, L., Esposito, F., Bandi, C., Sacchi, L. & Daffonchio, D. (2007). Bacteria of the genus *Asaia* stably associate with *Anopheles stephensi*, an Asian malarial mosquito vector. *Proc. Natl. Sci. U S A*, (March 2007), pp. 9047-9051.

Favia, G., Ricci, I., Marzorati, M., Negri, I., Alma, A., Sacchi, L., Bandi, C., Daffonchio, D. (2008). Bacteria of the genus *Asaia*: a potential paratransgenic weapon against malaria, In:*Transgenesis and the Management of Vector-Borne Disease*, (Askoy, Serap Ed.), pp. 49-59, ISBN 978-0-387-78224-9, Yale University School of Public Health, New Haven,CT, USA.

Ghosh, A.K., Ribolla, P.E & Jacobs-Lorena, M. (2001). Targeting *Plasmodium* Ligands on Mosquito Salivary Glands and Midgut with a Phage Display Peptide Library. *Proc Natl Acad Sci U S A*, (November 2001), pp. 13278-13281.

Hoffmann, A.A., Montgomery, B.L., Popovici, J., Iturbe-Ormaetxe, I., Johnson, P.H., Muzzi, F., Greenfield, M., Durkan, M., Leong, Y.S., Dong, Y., Cook, H., Axford, J., Callahan, A.G., Kenny, N., Omodei, C., McGraw, E.A., Ryan, P.A., Ritchie, S.A., Turelli, M. & O'Neill, S.L. (2011). Successful establishment of *Wolbachia* in *Aedes* populations to suppress dengue transmission. *Nature*, (August 2011), pp. 454-457.

Hughes, G.L., Koga, R., Xue P., Fukatsu, T. & Rasgon, J.L. (2011). *Wolbachia* infections are virulent and inhibit the human malaria parasite *Plasmodium falciparum* in *Anopheles gambiae*. *PLoS Pathog*, (May 2011), pp. e1002043.

Hurwitz, I., Hillesland, H., Fieck, A., Das, P. & Durvasula R. (2011). The paratransgenic sand fly: a platform for control of *Leishmania* transmission. *Parasit Vectors*, (May 2011), pp. 82.

n, C., Ren, X. & Rasgon, J.L. (2009). The virulent *Wolbachia* strain wMelPop efficiently establishes somatic infections in the malaria vector *Anopheles gambiae. Appl Environ Microbiol,* (May 2009), pp. 3373-3376.

:ambris, Z., Blagborough, A.M., Pinto, S.B., Blagrove, M.S., Godfray, H.C., Sinden, R.E. & Sinkins S.P. (2010). *Wolbachia* stimulates immune gene expression and inhibits *Plasmodium* development in *Anopheles gambiae. PLoS Pathog,* (October 2010), pp. e1001143.

:ämpfer, P., Terenius, O., Lindh, J.M. & Faye. I. (2006). *Janibacter anophelis* sp. nov., isolated from the midgut of *Anopheles arabiensis. Int. J. Syst. Evol. Microbiol,* (February 2006), pp. 389-392.

Kämpfer, P., Lindh, J.M., Terenius, O., Haghdoost, S., Falsen, E., Busse, H.J. & Faye, I. *Thorsellia anophelis* gen. nov., sp. nov., a new member of the Gammaproteobacteria. *Int. J. Syst. Evol. Microbiol,* (February 2006), pp. 335-338.

Knols, B.G., Njiru, B.N., Mathenge, E.M., Mukabana, W.R., Beier, J.C., Killeen, G.F. (2002) MalariaSphere: a greenhouse-enclosed simulation of a natural *Anopheles gambiae* (Diptera: Culicidae) ecosystem in western Kenya. *Malar J,*(December 2002), pp.1-19.

Lindh, J.M., Borg-Karlson, A.K. & Faye, I. (2008). Transstadial and horizontal transfer of bacteria within a colony of *Anopheles gambiae* (Diptera: Culicidae) and oviposition response to bacteria-containing water. *Acta Trop,* (July 2008), pp. 242-250.

Magliani, W., Conti, S., Arseni, S., Frazzi, R., Salati A. & Polonelli L. (2001) Killer anti-idiotypes in the control of fungal infections. *Curr Opin Investig Drugs,* (April 2001), pp. 477-479.

Pidiyar, V., Kaznowski, A., Narayan, N.B., Patole, M. & Shouche, Y.S. (2002). *Aeromonas culicicola* sp. nov., from the midgut of *Culex quinquefasciatus. Int J Syst Evol Microbiol,* (September 2002), pp. 1723-1728.

Pidiyar, V.J., Jangid, K., Patole, M.S. & Shouche, Y.S. (2004). Studies on cultured and uncultured microbiota of wild *Culex quinquefasciatus* mosquito midgut based on 16s ribosomal RNA gene analysis. *The American Journal of Tropical Medicine and Hygiene,* (June 2004), pp. 597-603.

Rasgon, J.L. & Scott, T.W. (2004). Phylogenetic characterization of *Wolbachia* symbionts infecting *Cimex lectularius* L. and *Oeciacus vicarius* Horvath (Hemiptera: Cimicidae). *J Med Entomol,* (November 2004), pp. 1175-1178.

Ren, X., Hoiczyk, E., Rasgon, J.L. (2008) Viral paratransgenesis in the malaria vector *Anopheles gambiae. PLoS Pathog.,* (August 2008), e1000135.

Ricci, I., Cancrini, G., Gabrielli S., D'Amelio, S. & Favia G. (2002) Searching for *Wolbachia* (Rickettsiales: Rickettsiaceae) in mosquitoes (Diptera: Culicidae): large polymerase chain reaction survey and new identifications. *J Med Entomol,* (July 2002), pp. 562-567.

Ricci, I., Damiani, C., Rossi, P., Capone, A., Scuppa, P., Cappelli, A., Ulissi, U., Mosca, M., Valzano M., Epis, S., Crotti, E., Daffonchio, D., Alma, A., Sacchi L., Mandrioli M., Bandi C. & Favia, G. (2011). Mosquito symbioses: from basic research to the paratransgenic control of mosquito-borne diseases. *Journal of Applied Entomology,* (December 2010), pp. 487-493.

Ricci, I., Mosca, M., Valzano, M., Damiani, C., Scuppa, P., Rossi, P., Crotti, E., Cappelli, A., Ulissi, U., Capone, A., Esposito, F., Alma, A., Mandrioli, M., Sacchi, L., Bandi, C., Daffonchio, D. & Favia G. (2011). Different mosquito species host *Wickerhamomyces anomalus* (*Pichia anomala*): perspectives on vector-borne diseases symbiotic control. *Antonie Van Leeuwenhoek,* (January 2011), pp. 43-50.

Ricci, I., Damiani, C., Scuppa, P., Mosca, M., Crotti, E., Rossi, P., Rizzi, A., Capone, A. Gonella, E., Ballarini, P., Chouaia, B., Sagnon, N., Esposito, F., Alma, A., Mandrioli, M., Sacchi, L., Bandi, C., Daffonchio, D. & Favia, G. (2011). The Yeast *Wickerhamomyces Anomalus* (*Pichia Anomala*) Inhabits the Midgut and Reproductive System of the Asian Malaria Vector *Anopheles Stephensi*. *Environ Microbiol,* (April 2011), pp. 911-21.

Riehle, M.A. & Jacobs-Lorena, M. (2005). Using bacteria to express and display anti-parasite molecules in mosquitoes: current and future strategies. *Insect Biochem Mol Biol,* (July 2005), pp. 699-707.

Riehle, M.A., Moreira, C.K., Lampe. D., Lauzon. C. & Jacobs-Lorena, M. (2007). Using bacteria to express and display anti-*Plasmodium* molecules in the mosquito midgut. *Int. J. Parasitol,* (May 2007), pp. 595-603.

Savoia, D., Avanzini C., Conti, S., Magliani, V., Frazzi R. & Polonelli, L. (2002). In vitro leishmanicidal activity of a monoclonal antibody mimicking a yeast killer toxin. *J Eukaryot Microbiol,* (July 2002), pp. 319-323.

Séguy, N., Polonelli, L., Dei-Cas, E. & Cailliez J.C. (1998). Effect of a killer toxin of *Pichia anomala* to *Pneumocystis*. Perspectives in the control of pneumocystosis. *FEMS Immunol Med Microbiol,* (September 1998), pp.145-149.

Serbus, L.R., Casper-Lindley, C., Landmann F. & Sullivan, W. (2008) The genetics and cell biology of *Wolbachia*-host interactions. *Annu Rev Genet,* (December 2008), pp. 683-707.

Sinkins, S.P. (2004). *Wolbachia* and cytoplasmic incompatibility in mosquitoes. *Insect Biochem Mol Biol,* (July 2004), pp. 723-729.

Spano, F., Matsuoka, H., Ozawa, R., Chinzei, Y. & Sinden R.E. (1996). Epitope mapping on the ookinete surface antigen Pbs21 of *Plasmodium berghei*: identification of the site of binding of transmission-blocking monoclonal antibody 13.1. *Parassitologia,* (December 1996), pp. 559-563.

Tiawsirisup, S., Sripatranusorn, S., Oraveerakul. K. & Nuchprayoon S. (2008). Distribution of mosquito (Diptera: Culicidae) species and *Wolbachia* (Rickettsiales: Rickettsiaceae) infections during the bird immigration season in Pathumthani province, central Thailand. *Parasitol Res,* (March 2008), pp. 731-735.

Touré, A.M., Mackey, A.J., Wang, Z.X. & Beier, J.C., (2000). Bactericidal effects of sugar-fed antibiotics on resident midgut bacteria of newly emerged anopheline mosquitoes (Diptera: Culicidae). *J. Med. Entomol,* (March 2000), pp. 246-249.

Walker, T., Johnson, P.H., Moreira, L.A., Iturbe-Ormaetxe, I., Frentiu, F.D., McMeniman, C.J., Leong, Y.S., Dong, Y., Axford, J., Kriesner P., Lloyd, A.L., Ritchie, S.A., O'Neill, S.L. & Hoffmann A.A. (2011). The wMel *Wolbachia* strain blocks dengue and invades caged *Aedes aegypti* populations. *Nature,* (August 2011), pp. 450-453.

Zieler, H., Keister, D.B., Dvorak, J.A. & Ribeiro J.M.(2001) A Snake Venom Phospholipase a(2) Blocks Malaria Parasite Development in the Mosquito Midgut by Inhibiting Ookinete Association with the Midgut Surface. *J Exp Biol,* (December 2001), pp. 4157-4167.

4

Proteomics of *Anopheles gambiae*

V. Choumet
Institut Pasteur
France

1. Introduction

Mosquitoes are a family of around three and a half thousand species and belong to the order of Diptera. They are found throughout the world except in places permanently frozen. Three quarters of all mosquito species live in the humid tropics and subtropics, where the climate is warm and moist, well adapted to the development of all stages and allows adults survival. Mosquitoes are classified in three subfamilies (*Toxorhynchitinae, Anophelinae, Culicinae*). *Anopheles* mosquitoes are members of subfamily *Anophelinae*. Like all mosquitoes, its life cycle consists in four stages: egg, larva, pupa, and adult. Female mosquitoes lay 30-150 eggs every 2-3 days in water. *Anopheles* favors as breeding places, quiet water, like permanent or temporary ponds, or quite cove of rivers. Each egg is protected by an eggshell. Mosquitoes can develop from egg to adult in as little as 5 days but usually take 10–14 days in tropical conditions. *Anopheles* can be distinguished from other mosquitoes by their palps, which are as long as the proboscis. Most *Anopheles* mosquitoes are not exclusively anthropophilic or zoophilic. *Anopheles* mosquitoes are more frequent in tropical and subtropical countries but are also found in temperate climates. They are not found at altitudes above 2000-2500 m.

1.1 Pathogens transmitted by *Anopheles* mosquitoes

Anopheles mosquitoes are vectors of several pathogens. They can transmit O'nyong-nyong virus as well as parasitic nematodes that cause lymphatic filariasis. Of the approximately 460 known species of *Anopheles*, less than 100 can transmit human malaria in nature. The primary malaria vectors in Africa, *A. gambiae* and *A. funestus*, are strongly anthropophilic and, consequently, are two of the most efficient malaria vectors in the world.

Malaria is a parasitic disease that affects 200 million people worldwide and causes 1.5 to 2.7 million deaths per year. Of the 300–500 million clinical cases annually, nearly 90% are in the sub-Saharan countries of Africa where the malaria parasite, *Plasmodium falciparum*, is primarily transmitted by the mosquito *Anopheles gambiae*. The increasing resistance of the parasite to inexpensive drugs and the resistance of mosquitoes to insecticides have created an urgent need for innovative methods that block parasite transmission during its development within the insect. Strategies for the development of malaria vaccine candidates target the stages found within humans e.g. the asexual erythrocytic stages. However vaccine candidates have also been developed against both the sexual stages of malaria in the mosquito (reviewed in [1] and against the mosquito vector itself (reviewed in [2]). The

Anopheles mosquito not only carries the parasite from infected to uninfected people, but also plays a vital role in the parasite life cycle [3; 4]. The development of *Plasmodium* within the mosquito is a very complex process and represents a tight coevolved system in which genetic features of both vector and parasite characterize the potential of the parasite to develop and be transmitted. Identification of promising candidate antigens for a mosquito-based transmission blocking vaccine or interference requires a good knowledge of both partners and of proteins implied in cross-talk between them.

1.2 *Plasmodium* life cycle in mosquito

When a female *Anopheles* sucks the blood of an infected human host, it receives red blood cells (RBCs) containing different stages of erythrocytic cycle, including gametocytes. In its gut, all stages except the gametocytes are digested (Figure 1). These hatch out from RBCs into the lumen of host's midgut and become active to start the sexual cycle. After a process termed exflagellation, the male microgametes detach from the parent gametocyte.

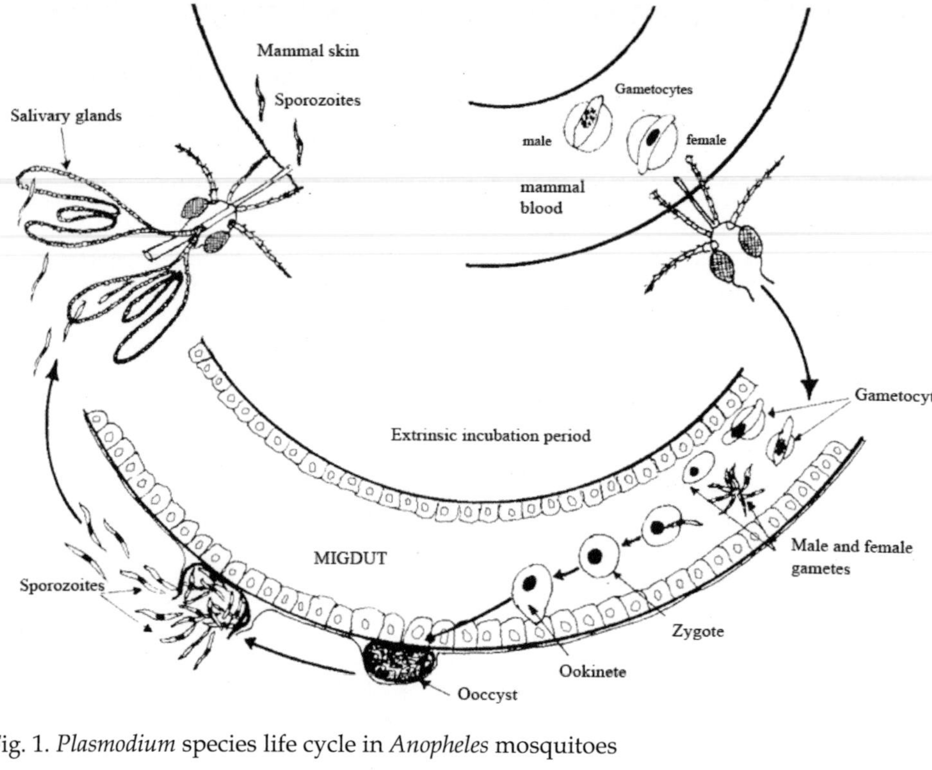

Fig. 1. *Plasmodium* species life cycle in *Anopheles* mosquitoes

The female, macrogametocytes undergo oogenesis and becomes a haploid macro-gamete. Zygotes are formed by fusion of male and female gametes. The zygotic stage of *Plasmodium* species develops to form ookinete. The ookinete passes through the epithelium of the midgut and forms an oocyst on the exterior wall of the midgut. The oocyst matures to form an enlarged structure, after which several nuclear divisions take place. Oocyst ruptures and releases hundreds of sporozoites. Eventually, these sporozoites migrate to the salivary gland of the female anopheles mosquito. The interval between the acquisition of an infectious agent by a vector and the vector's ability to transmit the agent to other susceptible vertebrate hosts is called the extrinsic incubation period. This parameter is dependent on host, parasite and environmental factors. Estimates are on the order of 10-14 days in areas of high malarial transmission [5].

During the successive stages of parasite development within the mosquito vector, it is faced to several barriers that are decisive for the fate of the parasite and the potential of its transmission. The proteome analysis of these barriers constitutes a first step to better understand the vector/pathogen interactions.

1.3 The genome of *Anopheles gambiae*

Anopheles gambiae sensus stricto. was selected for full genome sequencing from the 60 or so anopheline mosquito species that transmit malaria, largely because of the large number of malaria fatalities attributed to bites from this mosquito [6; 7]. At 278 Mb, *A. gambiae* genome is considerably larger than the genome size of *Drosophila melanogaster* [8](180 Mb), but smaller than the size of many other mosquito disease vectors such as *Aedes aegypti,* which at approximately 1376 million base pairs is about 5 times the size of the genome of the malaria vector [9]. The difference in size between *A. gambiae* and *D. melanogaster* is largely due to intergenic DNA. Despite evolutionarily diverging 250 million years ago, the two insects reveal remarkable similarities in their DNA sequences. However, there are also important differences in their genomes. Almost half of the genes in both insect genomes are presently identified as orthologs and show an average sequence identity of 56% [6]. This could be explained by successive adaptation of these insects to different life strategies and/or ecological niches, or to the evolutionary adaptation of pathogens to insect vectors or vice versa. Studies have led to the identification of mosquito genes that regulate malaria parasite infection in the mosquito ([10] and those involved in the ability to find and feed on blood of human hosts [11]. In *Aedes aegypti* genome, an increase in genes encoding odorant binding, cytochrome P450, and cuticle domains relative to *A. gambiae* suggests that members of these protein families support some of the biological differences between the two mosquito species [9].

With the genome of *A. gambiae* in hand, scientists possess molecular information to understand the biology of this arthropod vector better, and to possibly fight malaria transmission and other mosquito-borne human illnesses.

1.4 Genome versus proteome

Actually, DNA is a chemical instruction manual for everything a plant or animal does, while proteins are the dynamic components. DNA or mRNA sequences cannot sufficiently describe the structure, function and cellular location of proteins. Moreover, some important functional, post-translational modifications, such as glycosylation and phosphorylation, may not even be seen at the genome level. Hence, analysis of the human proteome revealed that it is much more complex than the human genome. While scientists are still deciphering the function of most of the 30,000 human genes, researchers estimate that each gene can give instructions for as many as 100 different proteins. On top of that, every organ has a different distribution of proteins, and the distribution may change frequently according to physiological modifications. The term "proteome" constitutes the total of proteins expressed by the genome. The technical improvements of the past decade have enhanced proteomic analyses and thereby enabled quantitative analysis of protein expression inside cells. The proteome of several *A. gambiae* organs were deciphered using various proteomic approaches and interesting insights in their function as well as in their putative interaction with pathogens were thereby gathered.

1.5 Proteomics methods

Thanks to the combination of developments in new instrumentation, fragmentation methods, availability of completed genome sequences and bioinformatics, there has been a shift from analysis of one protein at the time to more comprehensive proteome analyses. In the past decade, mass spectrometry (MS) has emerged as the dominant technology for in-depth characterization of the protein components of biological systems {12; 13; 14] but a number of other technologies, resources, and expertise are absolutely required to perform significant experiments. These include protein separation science (and protein biochemistry in general), genomics, and bioinformatics. Proteomics has evolved from 1D and 2D gel electrophoresis (1DE and 2DE)/MALDI TOF (Matrix Assisted Laser Desorption Ionization) MS to gel-free liquid chromatography (LC)-MS/MS (tandem mass spectrometry) approaches. Present-day 1D/2D LC-MS/MS workflows exhibit much higher sensitivity, speed, quantitative dynamic range and ease of use in comparison with gel-based resolving techniques. These various approaches are summarized in Figure 2.

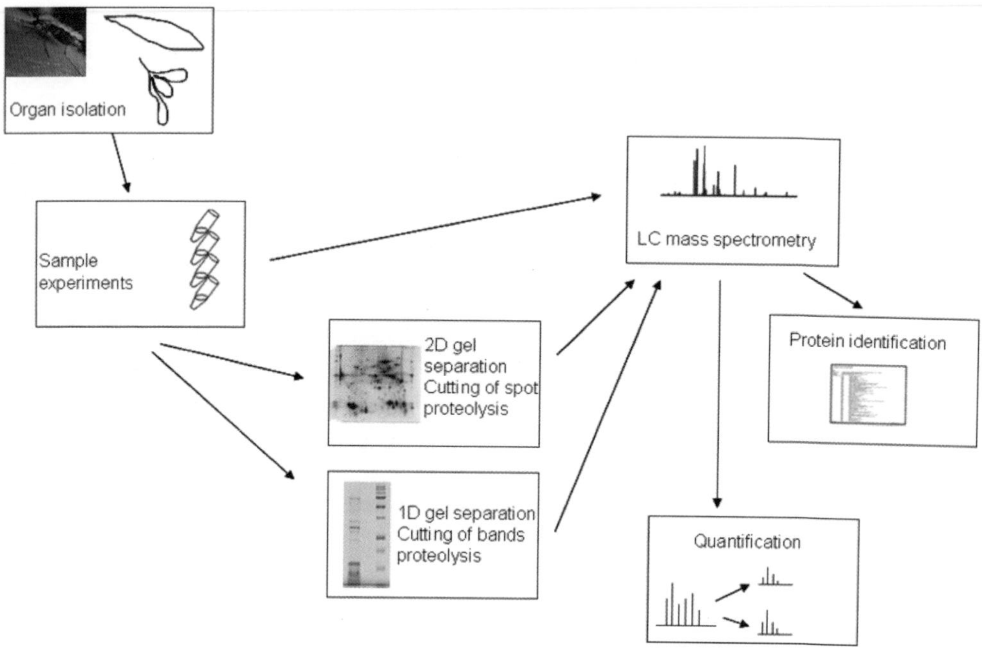

Fig. 2. Proteomic workflow

Beyond protein identification, there are a number of well-established options available for protein quantification. Difference gel electrophoresis (DIGE) following 2DE is one option. Various mass spectrometry based methods have been employed for quantitative analysis of protein expression in a complex protein mixture upon particular modification, such as prior to and after parasite infection. These quantitative approaches utilize the stable isotope-labelling techniques combined with mass spectrometry analysis, including isotope coded affinity tag (ICAT) [15; 16]), isobaric tag for relative and absolute quantitation (iTRAQ) [17], and stable isotope labelling of amino acids in cell culture (SILAC) [18; 19].

2. Proteomic analyses of *Anopheles gambiae*

During the last ten years, several approaches were followed to describe the protein content of *Anopheles gambiae*'s organs, hemolymph and saliva. The subsequent paragraphs will present protein data obtained from these various approaches.

2.1 The peritrophic matrix (PM) proteome

The peritrophic matrix (or peritrophic membrane) lines the gut of most insects at one or more stages of the life cycle [20]. This is the only region of the insect in contact with the "external" environment not covered by cuticle. It has important roles in the facilitation of the digestive processes in the gut and the protection of the insect from invasion by microorganisms and parasites. Since it poses a partial, natural barrier against parasite invasion of the midgut, it is speculated that modifications to the PM may lead to a complete barrier to infection. In agreement with this statement, it was showed that thickening of the PM by experimental manipulation resulted in decreased *Plasmodium* infectivity [21]. Within the blood mass, the *Plasmodium* gametes mate and develop into motile ookinetes, a process that takes 16–24 h depending on the *Plasmodium* species. To traverse the gut epithelium, the ookinetes must first cross the PM. For this purpose, the *Plasmodium* parasite secretes its own chitinase, which allows it to penetrate this chitin-containing structure [22]. Detailed characterization of the structure of the PM may help to find out new strategies to block the parasite at the midgut stage. The complete PM proteome of *A. gambiae* was determined using 1D-electrophoresis followed by LC-MS [23]. Out of the 209 proteins identified by mass spectrometry, 123 had predicted signal peptides, of which 17 also had predicted transmembrane domains and were therefore candidate midgut surface proteins that were coextracted from the gut during sample processing (Table 1). Among them were nine new chitin-binding peritrophic matrix proteins, expanding the list from three to twelve peritrophins. As expected, the number of proteins with signal peptides is relatively more abundant than those with transmembrane domains only. Based on their annotations, the proteins fell into different classes, with diverse putative functions ranging from immunity to blood digestion. Only 5% of the detected proteins were either known PM proteins or contained clear chitin binding domains (CBDs). Based on these results, the authors proposed a structural model of *A. gambiae* PM to explain the putative interactions among the proteins identified in their study. During the course of blood ingestion the PM is rapidly secreted by the distended midgut epithelium. The chitin fibrils are assembled into a wide cross-hatched pattern connected by peritrophins containing multiple CBDs. Between 0 and 24 h, the crosshatch is fully stretched and then slowly contracts like an accordion between 36 and 48 h post-blood feeding as blood digestion proceeds to completion. The various classes of peritrophins that have been identified by proteomic analysis were proposed to assemble together to produce a PM as well as perform several of its functions.

Peritrophic matrix	Protein/gene ID	Domain/motifs/Known/putative function/comments	Putatively secreted
	Protein with chitin binding domains (CBD)		
	AGAP006795	2 CBD	yes
	AGAP006796	1 CBD	yes
	AGAP009830	A CBD	yes
	AGAP010364	2 CBD	yes
	AGAP001819	1 CBD	yes
	AGAP010363	2 CBD	yes
	AGAP011616	3 CBD	yes
	AGAP006433	4-CBD	no
	AGAP006434	4-CBD	yes
	AGAP006432	2 CBD; immune-responsive gene	yes
	AGAP006414	1 CBD; mucin domain; chitinase	yes
	Proteins with no predicted CBD		
	AGAP006442	12.9 Conserved hypothetical protein; unknown function	yes
	AGAP004883	19.7 Conserved hypothetical protein; snake toxin-like protein folds/disulfide rich; unknown function	yes
	AGAP007860	33.8 Conserved hypothetical protein; putative protein binding motifs; unknown function	yes
	AGAP007612	92.2 Conserved hypothetical protein; snake toxin-like protein folds/disulfide rich; unknown function	yes
	AGAP002851	16.3 Conserved hypothetical protein; MD2-lipid recognition domain	yes
	AGAP001352	28.1 Conserved hypothetical protein; odorant/hormone binding domain	yes
	AGAP010132	52.1 Conserved hypothetical protein; CD36 scavenger receptor Class B domain	yes
	AGAP006398	31.2 Conserved hypothetical protein; galactose-like binding protein/lectin-like domain	no
	AGAP004916	35.0 Conserved hypothetical protein; Fibrillin/fibrinogen-like; globular domain; unknown function	yes

Table 1. PM proteins identified by 1D and LC-MS

The proteins of the PM may provide unique opportunities for the control of insect pests and vector borne diseases. Immunological control of blood and tissue-feeding insects by the effects of binding antibody to the proteins of the PM may be explored as well as other functional genetics approaches based on the understanding of the function of its components.

2.2 Hemolymph proteome

Insects employ an open circulatory system for the transport of nutrients, wastes, and signalling molecules throughout the body. The insect circulatory system also functions in thermoregulation, promoting ventilation through the tracheal system, and the circulation of humoral immune molecules and immune blood cells (hemocytes) that survey tissues for foreign entities. The primary organ driving hemolymph circulation in mosquitoes is a dorsal vessel that is subdivided into an abdominal heart and a thoracic aorta. Hemolymph plays a very important role in protecting against harmful microorganisms like *Plasmodium*. Two-dimensional SDS–PAGE and microsequencing or peptide mass fingerprinting was used to identify major proteins in the hemolymph of *A. gambiae* [24; 25]. They found about 280 protein spots in hemolymph and identified 28 spots, representing 26 individual proteins (Table 2). Most of these proteins have known or predicted functions in immunity. These include prophenoloxidase 2 subunit, two clip-domain serine proteases (CLIP B4 and A6), a thioester protein (TEP15), two serpins (SRPN2 and SRPN15), a cystatin and apolipophorin III (apoLPIII). Other proteins are implied, in iron transport like ferritin, or lipid biology. Many of the proteins have been found in hemolymph in other insects but one protein is novel: a new member of the MD-2-related lipid-recognition family. Fourteen spots were induced following bacterial injection but not by wounding. Three of the identified proteins increased in spot intensity or appeared de novo following bacterial injection: a phenoloxidase, and two chitinase-like proteins. A subset of proteins decreased following bacterial injections: these included the light and heavy chains of ferritin. Several proteins appeared in hemolymph following any wound or injection. These included two isoforms of phosphoglycerate mutase (PGM), triose phosphate isomerase (TPI), an actin, glutathione S transferase S1-1, and adenylate kinase. Most of these are metabolic enzymes lacking signal peptides that are likely to be released as a result of damage to muscles and other tissues by injury. The map obtained is a useful tool for examining changes in hemolymph proteins following blood feeding and infection by parasites.

Interestingly, antibodies raised against hemolymph proteins were shown to decrease mosquito infection by *Plasmodium vivax* [26]. These antibodies are directed against 11 different antigens, 6 of which were specific of the hemolymph and four were common to midgut and ovary. Identification of these antigens by mass spectrometry could lead to the development of blocking vaccines against malaria.

2.3 Proteomics of salivary glands and saliva

Mosquito saliva and salivary glands are central to the interaction between parasite, vector and mammalian host. Sporozoite maturation in the mosquito salivary glands before its transmission to vertebrates is a key stage for the effective transmission to humans since it increases the sporozoite's ability to infect vertebrate hepatocytes [27; 28]. Additionally, sporozoites are injected into the vertebrate skin with nanoliter volumes of saliva. Saliva is a complex biologically active solution, contains a large number of biomolecules responsible for antihemostatic activity, which assist hematophagous arthropods during the feeding process [29].

Hemolymph	Protein/gene ID	Domain/motifs/Known/putative function/comments	Putatively secreted
Constitutevely expressed proteins	agCP2491	OBP9, odorant binding protein	yes
	agCP1503	apoLP-III, Apolipophorin IIII	yes
	agCP1469	Ferritin, heavy	yes
	agCP1261	Ferritin, light chain	yes
	agCP5831	AgLLP1, lipocalin-like protein	yes
	agCP10937	D7H1, salivary D-7 like protein	yes
	agCP3566	TEP15, thioester protein	yes
	agCP9948	AgH-1, hemolymph glycoprotein family	yes
	agCP9547	ML3, ML-domain protein	yes
	AF007166	CLIPA6, Clip domain serine protease	yes
	agCP9254	CLIPB4, clip domain serine protease	yes
	agCp3768	Srpn15, putative haplotype of Srpn9 Serpin	yes
	ebiP6959	Srpn2, Serpin	yes
	agCP1375	chitinase	no
	agCP1985	Cystatin	yes
	ebiP1964	aldo/keto reductase	no
	AF004915	PPO2, prophenoloxidase subunit	no
	AF513639	GST-S1-2, glutathione S transferase	no
Proteins modulated			
appearing after any injection	BM624855	GST-SI-I, glutathione S transferase	no
	agCP12756	Phosphoglycerate mutase	no
	agCP12096	Triosephosphate isomerase	no
	BM622046	Adenylate cyclise	no
appearing or altered after bacterial injury	AY496420	BR-1, chitinase-like	yes
	AY496421	BR-2, chitinase-like	yes
	AJ010195	PO6, phenoloxidase	no

Table 2. Proteins identified in *Anopheles gambiae* hemolymph

Following SDS-PAGE of *A. gambiae* salivary proteins, under denaturing non-reducing conditions and Edman sequencing, 12 saliva proteins were identified [30]. Among these proteins were *A. gambiae* D7-related proteins 1-3, similar to *Aedes aegypti* D7. The D7 proteins are among the most abundant salivary proteins in adult female mosquitoes and sand flies [31]. D7 sequences were identified in *Culex quinquefasciatus, An. arabiensis, An. stephensi, An. darlingi* mosquitoes and *Lutzomyia longipalpis* and *Phlebotomus papatasi* sand flies.

The other identified proteins were GSG6, hypothetical protein 8 (CB1), similar to hypothetical protein 9 (bB2) and herein called HP 9-like, SG1-like 2, putative 5′ nucleotidase and SG1. Edman degradation for other bands was reported to be unsuccessful, either because the protein's amino terminus was blocked, or because PTH-amino acids could not be reliably identified.

A proteomic analysis of salivary glands from female *A. gambiae* mosquitoes was carried out [32]. Salivary gland extracts were hydrolyzed with trypsin using a 1-DE in-gel and an in solution digestion and analyzed by LC-MS/MS. This led to identification of 69 unique proteins, 57 of which were novel. A large proportion of the identified proteins were involved in protein, carbohydrate and nucleic acid metabolism, transport or energy pathways. Almost 25% of the proteins could be not be ascribed any biological function. A subcellular localization was assigned to each protein either based on the literature or the presence of particular domains/motifs. The majority of the proteins were classified as extracellular proteins. D7 family proteins, apyrases and proteins of the salivary gland-like (SGlike) family were the commonest extracellular proteins. Proteins involved in translation and protein folding were the predominant cytoplasmic proteins with a small number of proteins classified as nuclear, vesicular or lysosomal proteins. Approximately 40% of proteins could not be assigned any specific localization because of lack of any distinctive features and lack of homology to other known proteins.

To further describe *A. gambiae* salivary gland and saliva contents, several techniques: 1-DE, 2-DE and LC-MS/ MS were combined to characterize the protein content of 8 year-old and 21 year-old mosquito salivary glands [33]. Overall, this study has identified five saliva proteins and 122 more proteins from the salivary glands, including the first proteomic description for 89 of these salivary gland proteins. Proteomic analysis of 8 year-old blood-fed mosquitoes allowed the identification of 55 proteins. LC-MS/ MS and 2-DE-MS identified a similar number of proteins and both appear more effective than 1-DE-MS. Thirty percent of the proteins identified are secreted (Table 3).

2D-E profiles suggested that several secreted proteins may present sequence divergence or be extensively processed and/or post-translationally modified in *A. gambiae* salivary glands.

Since the invasion and sporozoite maturation take place during the process of salivary glands ageing, the effect of salivary gland age on salivary component composition was examined. LC MS/MS profiling of young *versus* old salivary gland proteomes suggests that there is an over-representation of proteins involved in signalling and proteins related to the immune response in the proteins from older mosquitoes.

A comparative proteomic analysis of salivary gland samples from infected or *Plasmodium berghei*-free mosquitoes was performed using the iTRAQ labeling.

The expression levels of five secreted proteins were altered when the parasite was present. The levels of GSG6, apyrase, D7 related-1 protein precursor and D7 precursor allergen AED A2 are decreased whereas the level of gVAG is increased in infected salivary glands. Apyrase, GSG6 and D7 precursor allergen AED A2 were shown to be implied in blood feeding [34; 35; 36]. In addition, GSG6 was found to be a serological indicator of exposure to Afrotropical malaria vectors [37].

Secreted salivary gland proteins	Protein/gene ID	Domain/motifs/Known/putative function/comments
	GI:18389879	30 kDa protein, anti-platelet
	AGAP011971-PA	Alpha-amylase, carbohydrate digestion
	AGAP008278-PA	Apyrase, anti-aggregation
	AGAP008284-PA	D7 precursor allergen AED A2
	AGAP008282-PA	D7 related-1 protein precursor, anti-inflammatory
	AGAP008283-PA	D7 related-2 protein precursor, anti-inflammatory
	AGAP008281-PA	D7 related-3 protein precursor, anti-inflammatory
	AGAP008280-PA	D7 related-4 protein precursor, anti-inflammatory
	GI:4127305	D7 related-5 protein precursor
	AGAP004334-PA	GSG3
	AGAP000150-PA	GSG5 precursor
	AGAP008216-PA	GSG6, implied in blood-feeding
	AGAP008307-PA	GSG7
	AGAP008306-PA	Guanine nucleotide releasing factor
	AGAP006494-PA	putative gVAG protein precursor, implied in defense
	AGAP003168-PA	Hypothetical 10 kDa protein
	AGAP006821-PA	Hypothetical 10.2 kDa protein
	AGAP001903-PA	Hypothetical 8.8 kDa protein
	AGAP006340-PA	Lysozyme precursor
	AGAP004038-PA	Maltase, carbohydrate digestion
	AGAP000607-PA	Putative 5′ nucleotidase precursor, anti-platelet
	AGAP006507-PA	putative Salivary protein SG
	AGAP000175-PA	Salivary D3 protein
	AGAP012335-PA	Salivary gland 1-like 3 protein
		SG3

Table 3. List of *Anopheles gambiae* salivary proteins possessing a signal peptide and detected by proteomic approaches ([30; 32; 33]

The D7 short proteins bind serotonin with high affinity, as well as histamine and norepinephrine, thus antagonizing the vasoconstrictor, platelet-aggregating, and pain-inducing level of these factors [38]. gVAG is a defense-related protein [39]. These observations suggest an important role of these proteins in the interaction between *A. gambiae, Plasmodium* and the mammalian host and a putative modulation of the feeding behaviour of the parasitized mosquito.

2.4 *Anopheles gambiae* head proteome

Many of the most dangerous pathogens have been shown to manipulate the behaviour of their vectors, such as feeding behaviour, in ways that enhance the contact with the vertebrate host and consequently favour pathogen transmission {40]. Several studies with different systems support the idea that parasites indeed increase the probing and feeding rate of their vectors by a variety of mechanisms [40].

In the *Plasmodium-Anopheles* interaction, facts showing that *Plasmodium* spp. influence the behaviour of their mosquito vectors, *Anopheles* spp. have accumulated [41; 42; 43; 44; 45; 46]. In this system, an altered behaviour of the vector has been shown when sporozoites have invaded the salivary glands [43; 45; 46]. For instance, malaria parasites were shown to manipulate their mosquito vectors in two different ways and in a stage-dependent mode: when the sporozoites are ready to be transmitted to the vertebrate hosts, the parasite increases the biting rate of its vector [45; 46]. In contrast, at the oocyst stage and yet not transmissible to the vertebrate host, the parasite decreases the contact between vector and vertebrate host by decreasing the natural host-seeking behaviour of the insect [46]. Moreover, it was recently shown that the presence of the parasite extends the oviposition cycle of the mosquito, thereby enhancing malaria transmission [47]. Interestingly, few studies have been undertaken to demonstrate the existence of a general manipulative mechanism by which the parasite manipulate the host central nervous system. A 2-D DIGE coupled with MS was used to analyse and compare the head proteome of *A. gambiae* infected with *Plasmodium berghei* with that of uninfected mosquitoes [48]. This approach allowed detecting modulations of 12 protein spots in the head of mosquitoes infected with sporozoites. After their identification by MS, these proteins were functionally classified as belonging to metabolic, synaptic, molecular chaperone, signalling and cytoskeletal groups. These results indicate an altered energy metabolism in the head of sporozoite-infected mosquitoes. Some of the up-/down-regulated proteins identified, such as synapse-associated protein, 14-3-3 protein and calmodulin, have previously been shown to play critical roles in the CNS of both invertebrates and vertebrates. Interestingly, two proteins revealed in the study have been demonstrated to be involved in behavioural modifications in other host–parasite systems. Tropomyosin has been shown to be involved in the behavioural manipulation of crustacean gammarids by acanthocephalans [49], while phosphoglycerate mutase was involved in cricket behavioural manipulation induced by hairworms [50]. Furthermore, a heat shock response (HSP 20) and a variation of cytoarchitecture (tropomyosins) have been shown. Discovery of these proteins demonstrates potential molecular mechanisms that trigger behavioural modifications and offers new insights into the study of close interactions between *Plasmodium* and its *Anopheles* vector.

2.5 Proteome of the eggshell

Insect eggshells offer the embryo protection from physical and biological damages and assure their survival. Most current knowledge of insect eggshell morphology and composition are based on studies of *Drosophila melanogaster* [51; 52]. Mosquito eggshells show notable diversity in physical properties and structure, presumably resulting from adaptation to the large variety of environments exploited by these insects.

In contrast to *Aedes* mosquitoes, which are highly resistant to desiccation allowing embryos to survive for months in dry conditions [53], eggshells of the human malaria vector, *A. gambiae* are more permeable, restricting their survival and development to humid environments [54]. Greater knowledge of the proteins that comprise eggshells is required to understand these differences and how they contribute to successful mosquito reproductive strategies. A mass spectrometry/proteomics approach was used to identify 44 proteins as putative components of the eggshell (Table 4) [55]. Among the identified molecules are two vitelline membrane proteins and a group of seven putative chorion proteins. Enzymes with peroxidase, laccase and phenoloxidase activities, expected to be involved in cross-linking reactions that stabilize the eggshell structure, were also identified. Seven odorant binding proteins were found in association with the mosquito eggshell, although their role has yet to be demonstrated.

Eggshell	Protein/gene ID	Domain/motifs/Known/putative function/comments
	Odorant binding proteins	
	AGAP000641	OBP34/37
	AGAP000642	OBP35
	AGAP000643	OBP36
	AGAP002025	OBP11
	AGAP011647	OBP1
	AGAP010648	OBP44
	AGAP002189	OBP13
	Enzymes	
	AGAP004038	chorion peroxidase
	AGAP006176	Laccase 2
	AGAP005959	Yellow-g2-dopachrome conversion enzyme
	AGAP004978	Prophenoloxidase 9
	AGAP003233	Peroxidase
	AGAP007020	Thioredoxin
	Vitelline membrane components	
	AGAP002134	Vitelline membrane component
	AGAP008696	Vitelline membrane component
	Putative chorion components	
	AGAP00655	Putative chorion protein
	AGAP006555	Putative chorion protein
	AGAP006553	Putative chorion protein
	AGAP006554	Putative chorion protein
	AGAP006549	Putative chorion protein
	AGAP006556	Putative chorion protein
	AGAP006550	Putative chorion protein
	Others	
	AGAP006524	Unknown
	AGAP006563	Unknown
	AGAP003149	Unknown
	AGAP010147	Unknown
	AGAP004182	Unknown
	AGAP006527	Unknown
	AGAP003047	Schistosoma mansoni egg protein
	AGAP004969	Ionotropic glutamate receptor

	AGAP010252	Ribosomal protein L14
	AGAP002306	Ribosomal protein L4
	AGAP002830	c-1-Tetrahydrofolate synthase
	AGAP012261	Unknown
	AGAP005802	Unknown
	AGAP005061	Unknown
	AGAP000547	Unknown
	AGAP006584	Unknown
	AGAP005338	Unknown
	AGAP003911	Unknown
	AGAP004887	Ribosomal protein S17
	AGAP000672	Unknown
	AGAP007758	Unknown
	AGAP006805	Unknown

Table 4. Proteome of *Anopheles gambiae* eggshell

2.6 Functional genomics approaches

Genomics, transcriptomics and proteomics studies have been complemented by studies using RNAi for gene silencing. RNAi allows characterization of genes *in vivo* which can later be targeted for transmission blocking studies. Boisson et al. [56] demonstrated the role of the gene AgApy, which encodes an apyrase, in the probing behaviour of *A. gambiae*. An RNAi-mediated gene silencing approach has also been used to assess the potential involvement of 10 selected *A. gambiae* salivary gland genes in regulating mosquito blood-feeding capacity [36]. Silencing of several salivary gland transcripts; D7L2, anophelin, peroxidase, 5'nucleotidase and SG2 precursor, produced a significantly lowered blood-feeding phenotype and increased probing time, confirming that these genes could play an important role in blood-feeding.

3. Conclusion

In a recent publication, the results of an extensive qualitative proteomic analysis of *Anopheles gambiae* to better understand gene structures and their functions were presented [57]. In their manuscript, the authors reported validation of existing genes, correction of existing gene models, identification of novel genes, identification of novel splice variants, confirmation of splice sites and assignment of translational start sites based on high-resolution mass spectrometry-derived data. A total of 2,682 peptides were identified that could not be mapped onto existing VectorBase annotations. This study emphasizes on the interest of proteomic tools to complement other approaches for genome annotation.

Dissecting the molecular basis of the interplay between vector and pathogen is essential for vector-borne disease transmission. Deciphering the proteome of the main mosquito barriers for parasite development and transmission may pave the way to novel disease control mechanisms.

4. References

[1] Crompton P.D., Pierce S.K. & Miller L.H. (2010) Advances and challenges in malaria vaccine development. *J Clin Invest* 120, 12 (Dec 2010), pp. 4168-4178, 1558-8238.

[2] Lavazec C. & Bourgouin C. (2008). Mosquito-based transmission blocking vaccines for interrupting Plasmodium development. *Microbes Infect* 10, 8 (Jul 2008), pp. 845-849, 1286-4579.

[3] Vlachou D., Schlegelmilch T., Christophides G.K. & Kafatos F.C. (2005) Functional genomic analysis of midgut epithelial responses in Anopheles during *Plasmodium* invasion. *Curr Biol* 15, 13 (Jul 2005), pp. 1185-1195, 0960-9822.

[4] Aly A.S., Vaughan A.M. & Kappe S.H. (2009) Malaria parasite development in the mosquito and infection of the mammalian host. *Annu Rev Microbiol* 63, pp. 195-221, 1545-3251.

[5] Killeen G.F., McKenzie F.E., Foy B.D., Schieffelin C., Billingsley P.F. & Beier J.C. (2000) A simplified model for predicting malaria entomologic inoculation rates based on entomologic and parasitologic parameters relevant to control. *Am J Trop Med Hyg.* 62, 5 (May 2000), pp. 535-44, 0002-9637.

[6] Zdobnov E.M., von Mering C., Letunic I., Torrents D., Suyama M., Copley R.R., et al. (2002) Comparative genome and proteome analysis of *Anopheles gambiae* and *Drosophila melanogaster*. *Science* 298, 5591 (Oct 2002), pp 149-59, 1095-9203.

[7] Holt R.A., Subramanian G.M., Halpern A., Sutton G.G., Charlab R., Nusskern D.R., et al. (2002). The genome sequence of the malaria mosquito *Anopheles gambiae. Science.* 298, 5591 (Oct 2002):129-49, 0036-8075.

[8] Adams M.D., Celniker S.E., Holt R.A., Evans C.A., Evans C.A, Gocayne J.D, et al. (2000) *The genome sequence of Drosophila melanogaster. Science.* 287, 5461 (Mar 2000), pp 2185-2195, 0036-8075.

[9] Nene V., Wortman J.R., Lawson D., Haas B., Kodira C., Tu ZJ., et al. (2007) Genome sequence of Aedes aegypti, a major arbovirus vector. *Science.* 316, 5832 (Jun 2007), pp. 1718-23, 1095-9203.

[10] Riehle M.M., Markianos K., Niaré O., Xu J., Li J., Touré A.M., Podiougou B., Oduol F., Diawara S., Diallo M., Coulibaly B., Ouatara A., Kruglyak L., Traoré S.F. & Vernick K.D. (2006) Natural malaria infection in Anopheles gambiae is regulated by a single genomic control region. *Science.* 312, 5773 (Apr 2006), pp. 577-579,1095-9203.

[11] Kwon H.W., Lu T., Rutzler M. & Zwiebel L.J. (2006) Olfactory responses in a gustatory organ of the malaria vector mosquito Anopheles gambiae. *Proc Natl Acad Sci* U S A 103, 6 (Sep 2006), pp. 13526-13531, 0027-8424.

[12] Gingras, A. C., Aebersold, R. & Raught, B. (2005) Advances in protein complex analysis using mass spectrometry. *J Physiol* 563 Pt1 (Dec 2004), 11-21, 0022-3751.

[13] Mayer D., Baginsky S. & Schwemmle M. (2005) Isolation of viral ribonucleoprotein complexes from infected cells by tandem affinity purification. *Proteomics* 5, 17 (Nov 2005), pp. 4483-4487. 1615-9853.

[14] Jorba N., Juarez S., Torreira E., Gastaminza P., Zamarreno N., Albar J.P. & Ortin J. (2008) Analysis of the interaction of influenza virus polymerase complex with human cell factors (2008) *Proteomics* 8, 10 (May 2008), p. 2077-2088, 1615-9861.

[15] Gygi S.P., Rist B., Gerber S.A., Turecek F., Gelb M.H. & Aebersold R. (1999) Quantitative analysis of complex protein mixtures using isotope-coded affinity tags (1999) *Nat. Biotechnol.* 17, 10 (Oct 1999), pp. 994-999, 1087-0156.

[16] Guaragna A., Amoresano A., Pinto V., Monti G., Mastrobuoni G., Marino G. & Palumbo G. (2008) Synthesis and proteomic activity evaluation of a new isotope-coded affinity tagging (ICAT) reagent. *Bioconjug. Chem.* 19, 5 (May 2008), pp. 1095-2104, 1520-4812.

[17] Ross P.L., Huang Y.L.N., Marchese J.N., Williamson B., Parker K., Hattan S., et al. (2004) Multiplexed protein quantitation in Saccharomyces cerevisiae using amine-reactive isobaric tagging reagents. *Mol. Cell. Proteomics* 3, 12 (Dec 2004), pp. 1154-1169, 1535-9476.

[18] Ong S.E., Blagoev B., Kratchmarova I., Kristensen D.B., Steen H., Pandey A. & Mann M. (2002) Stable isotope labeling by amino acids in cell culture, SILAC, as a simple and accurate approach to expression proteomics. *Mol. Cell. Proteomics* 1, 5 (May 2002), p. 376-386, 1535-9476.

[19] Mann M. (2006) Functional and quantitative proteomics using SILAC *Nat. Rev. Mol. Cell Biol.* 7, 12 (Dec 2006), pp. 952-958, 1471-0072.

[20] Tellam R.L., Wijffels G. & Willadsen P. (1999) Peritrophic matrix proteins. *Insect Biochem Mol Biol* 29, 2 (Feb 1999), pp. 87-101, 0965-1748.

[21] Billingsley P.F. & Rudin W. (1992) The role of the mosquito peritrophic membrane in bloodmeal digestion and infectivity of Plasmodium species. *J Parasitol* 78, 3 (Jun 1992), pp. 430-440, 0022-3395.

[22] Huber M., Cabib E. & Miller L.H. (1991) Malaria parasite chitinase and penetration of the mosquito peritrophic membrane. *Proc Natl Acad Sci* U S A 88, 7 (Apr 1991), pp. 2807-2810, 0027-8424.

[23]] Dinglasan R.R., Devenport M., Florens L., Johnson J.R., McHugh C.A., Donnelly-Doman M., Carucci D.J., Yates J.R. 3rd & Jacobs-Lorena M. (2009) The *Anopheles gambiae* adult midgut peritrophic matrix proteome. *Insect Biochem Mol Biol* 39, 2 (Feb 2009), pp. 125-134, 1879-0240.

[24] Pinto S.B., Lombardo F., Koutsos A.C., Waterhouse R.M., McKay K., An C., Ramakrishnan C., Kafatos F.C. & Michel K. (2009) Discovery of *Plasmodium* modulators by genome-wide analysis of circulating hemocytes in Anopheles gambiae. *Proc Natl Acad Sci* U S A 106, 50 (Dec 2009), pp. 21270-21275, 1091-6490.

[25] Paskewitz S.M. & Shi L. (2005) The hemolymph proteome of Anopheles gambiae. *Insect Biochem Mol Biol* 35, 8 (Aug 2005), pp. 815-824, 0965-1748.

[26] Kumari A., Gakhar S.K. & Hooda V. (2009) Antibodies raised against hemolymph of *Anopheles culicifacies* reduce the fecundity and malaria parasite development. *J Vector Borne Dis* 46, 4 (Dec 2009), pp. 255-260,0972-9062.

[27] Kappe S.H., Gardner M.J., Brown SM, Ross J, Matuschewski K., Ribeiro J.M., Adams J.H., Quackenbush J., Cho J., Carucci D.J., Hoffman S.L. & Nussenzweig V. (2001) Exploring the transcriptome of the malaria sporozoite stage. *Proc Natl Acad Sci* U S A 98, 17 (Aug 2001), pp. 9895-9900, 0027-8424.

[28] Kappe S.H., Buscaglia C.A. & Nussenzweig V. (2004) *Plasmodium* sporozoite molecular cell biology. *Annu Rev Cell Dev Biol* 20, pp. 29-59, 1081-0706.

[29] Ribeiro JM, Francischetti IM. (2003) Role of arthropod saliva in blood feeding: sialome and post-sialome perspectives. Annu Rev Entomol 48 (Jun 2003), pp.73-88, 0066-4170.

[30] Francischetti, I. M., Valenzuela, J. G., Pham, V. M. , Garfield, M. K., Ribeiro, J. M. (2002) Toward a catalog for the transcripts and proteins (sialome) from the salivary gland of the malaria vector *Anopheles gambiae. J Exp Biol* 205 Pt16 (Jul 2002), 2429-2451, 0022-0949.

[31] Valenzuela, J. G., Charlab, R., Gonzalez, E. C., de Miranda-Santos, I. K., Marinotti, O., Francischetti, I. M., Ribeiro, J. M. (2002) The D7 family of salivary proteins in blood sucking diptera. *Insect Mol Biol* 11, 2 (Apr 2002), 149-155, 0962-1075

[32] Kalume D.E., Okulate M., Zhong J., Reddy R., Suresh S., Deshpande N., Kumar N. & Pandey A. (2005) A proteomic analysis of salivary glands of female *Anopheles gambiae* mosquito. *Proteomics* 5, 14 (Sep 2005), pp. 3765-3777, 1615-9853

[33] Choumet V., Carmi-Leroy A., Laurent C., Lenormand P., Rousselle J.C., Namane A., Roth C. & Brey P.T. (2007) The salivary glands and saliva of *Anopheles gambiae* as an essential step in the *Plasmodium* life cycle: a global proteomic study. *Proteomics* 7, 18 (Sep 2007), pp.3384-94, 1615-9853.

[34] Champagne D.E. (2005) Antihemostatic molecules from saliva of blood-feeding arthropods. *Pathophysiol Haemost Thromb* 34, 4-5, pp. 221-227, 1424-8832

[35] Lombardo F., Ronca R., Rizzo C, Mestres-Simòn M., Lanfrancotti A., Currà C., Fiorentino G., Bourgouin C., Ribeiro J.M., Petrarca V., Ponzi M., Coluzzi M. & Arcà B. (2009) The *Anopheles gambiae* salivary protein gSG6: an anopheline-specific protein with a blood-feeding role. I*nsect Biochem Mol Biol* 39, 7 (Jul 2009), pp. 457-466, 1879-0240.

[36] Das S., Radtke A., Choi Y. J., Mendes A. M., Valenzuela J. G., Dimopoulos G. (2010) Transcriptomic and functional analysis of the *Anopheles gambiae* salivary gland in relation to blood feeding. BMC Genomics 11 (Oct 2010), 566, 1471-2164.

[37] Rizzo C., Ronca R, Fiorentino G., Mangano V.D., Sirima S.B, Nèbiè I., Petrarca V., Modiano D. & Arcà B. (2011) Wide cross-reactivity between *Anopheles gambiae* and *Anopheles funestus* SG6 salivary proteins supports exploitation of gSG6 as a marker of human exposure to major malaria vectors in tropical Africa (2011) *Malar J* 10, 206 (Jul 2011), pp. 1475-2875, 1475-2875.

[38] Calvo, E., Mans, B. J., Ribeiro, J. M., Andersen, J. F. (2009) Multifunctionality and mechanism of ligand binding in a mosquito antiinflammatory protein. *Proc. Natl. Acad. Sci. USA* 2009, 106, 3728-3733.

[39] Dong Y., Aguilar R., Xi Z., Warr E., Mongin E. & Dimopoulos G. (2006) *Anopheles gambiae* immune responses to human and rodent *Plasmodium* parasite species. *PLoS Pathog* 2, 6 (Jun 2006), pp. e52, 1553-7374.

[40] Hurd H. (2003) Manipulation of medically important insect vectors by their parasites. *Annu Rev Entomol* 48, pp. 141-161. 0066-4170

[41] Rossignol P.A., Ribeiro J.M. & Spielman A. (1984) Increased intradermal probing time in sporozoite-infected mosquitoes. *Am J Trop Med Hyg* 33, 1 (Jan 1984), pp. 17-20, 0002-9637.

[42] Rossignol P.A., Ribeiro J.M. & Spielman A. (1986) Increased biting rate and reduced fertility in sporozoite-infected mosquitoes. *Am J Trop Med Hyg* 35, 2, pp. 277-279. 0002-9637

[43] Wekesa J.W., Copeland R.S. & Mwangi R.W. (1992) Effect of *Plasmodium falciparum* on blood feeding behavior of naturally infected *Anopheles* mosquitoes in western Kenya. *Am J Trop Med Hyg* 47, 4 (Oct 1992), pp. 484-488, 0002-9637.

[44] Koella J.C. & Packer M.J. (1996) Malaria parasites enhance blood-feeding of their naturally infected *vector Anopheles punctulatus. Parasitology* 113 (Pt 2), pp. 105-109, 0031-1820

[45] Koella J.C., Sorensen F.L. & Anderson R.A. (1998) The malaria parasite, *Plasmodium falciparum,* increases the frequency of multiple feeding of its mosquito vector, *Anopheles gambiae. Proc Biol Sci* 265, 1398 (May 1998), pp: 763-768, 0962-8452.

[46] Anderson R.A., Koella J.C. & Hurd H. (1999) The effect of Plasmodium yoelii nigeriensis infection on the feeding persistence of *Anopheles stephensi* Liston throughout the sporogonic cycle. *Proc Biol Sci* 266, 1430 (Sep 1999), pp. 1729-1733, 0962-8452.

[47] Charlwood JD, Tomás EV.Do developing malaria parasites manipulate their mosquito host? Evidence from infected *Anopheles funestus* (Giles) from Mozambique (2011) *Trans R Soc Trop Med Hyg* 105, 6 (Jun 2011), pp. 352-354, 1878-3503.

[48] Lefevre T., Thomas F., Schwartz A., Levashina E., Blandin S., Brizard JP, Le Bourligu L., Demettre E., Renaud F & Biron D.G. (2007) Malaria *Plasmodium* agent induces alteration in the head proteome of their *Anopheles* mosquito host. *Proteomics* 7, 11 (Jun 2007), pp: 1908-1915, 1615-9853.

[49] Biron D.G., Marché L., Ponton F., Loxdale H.D., Galéotti N., Renault L., Joly C., Thomas F. (2005) Behavioural manipulation in a grasshopper harbouring hairworm: a proteomics approach. *Proc Biol Sci* 272, 1577 (Oct 2005), pp. 2117-2126, 0962-8452.

[50] Ponton F., Lefevre T., Lebarbenchon C., Thomas F., Loxdale H.D., Marché L., Renault L., Perrot-Minnot M.J. & Biron DG. (2006) Do distantly related parasites rely on the same proximate factors to alter the behaviour of their hosts? *Proc Biol Sci* 273, 1603 (Nov 2006), pp. 2869-2877, 0962-8452.

[51] Waring G.L. (2000) Morphogenesis of the eggshell in *Drosophila. Int Rev Cytol* 198, pp. 67-108. 0074-7696.

[52] Cavaliere V., Bernardi F., Romani P., Duchi S. & Gargiulo G. (2008) Building up the *Drosophila* eggshell: first of all the eggshell genes must be transcribed. *Dev Dyn* 237, 8 (Aug 2008), pp. 2061-2072, 1058-8388.

[53] Sota T. & Mogi, M. (1992) Interspecific variation in desiccation survival time of *Aedes* (Stegomyia) mosquito eggs is correlated with habitat and egg size. *Oecologia* 90, pp. 353–358.

[54] Beier J.C., Copeland R., Oyaro C., Masinya A., Odago W.O., Oduor S., Koech D.K. & Roberts C.R. (1990) *Anopheles gambiae* complex egg-stage survival in dry soil from larval development sites in western Kenya. *J Am Mosq Control Assoc* 6, 1 (Mar 1990), pp. 105-109, 8756-971X.

[55] Amenya D.A., Chou W., Li J., Yan G., Gershon P.D., James A.A. & Marinotti O. (2010) Proteomics reveals novel components of the *Anopheles gambiae* eggshell. *J Insect Physiol* 56, 10 (Oct 2010), pp: 1414-1419, 1879-1611.

[56] Boisson B., Jacques J.C., Choumet V., Martin E., Xu J., Vernick K. & Bourgouin C. (2006) Gene silencing in mosquito salivary glands by RNAi. *FEBS Lett* 580, 8 (Apr 2006), pp. 1988-1992, 0014-5793.Calvo E., Mans B.J., Andersen J.F. & Ribeiro J.M. (2006) Function and evolution of a mosquito salivary protein family. *J Biol Chem* 281, 4 (Jan 2006), pp. 1935-1942, 0021-9258.

[57] Chaerkady R., Kelkar D.S., Muthusamy B., Kandasamy K., Dwivedi S.B., Sahasrabuddhe N.A., et al. (2011) A proteogenomic analysis of *Anopheles gambiae* using high-resolution Fourier transform mass spectrometry. Genome Res. 2011 Jul 27.

Part 3

Malaria Parasite Research

5

Recent Advances in Studies on Avian Malaria Parasites

Alfonso Marzal
University of Extremadura
Spain

1. Introduction

In 1902, Sir Ronald Ross was awarded the Nobel Prize in Medicine for his discovery of the mosquito transmission of malaria. This finding was achieved working with avian malaria and its vector, giving him a control over his experimental subjects difficult to attain with human models. Since then, malaria parasites of birds have played an essential role as a model in human malaria studies. Important advances in medical parasitology such of the study of the life cycle, development of chemotherapy, and cultivation *in vitro* have initially been developed using bird haemosporidian models. Significant anti-malarial compounds such as plasmochin, primaquine and atebrin were evaluated in bird model. In the same way bird parasites were used for drug testing and for further malaria-associated experiments. Nowadays, research on bird malaria is at the very peak since scientists have realized the benefits of using studies on avian malaria to answer ecological, behavioural and evolutionary questions. This review will highlight the importance of studies on avian malaria, showing the results of some recent investigations on this topic and describing new applications of avian malaria researches that could be useful for conservation and health policies in 21th century.

2. Studies on avian malaria parasites

Haemosporidians (Sporozoa: Haemosporida) are one of the most well known groups of parasitic protists. They include the agents of malaria, one of the most lethal human diseases. But the systematic and ecological diversity of malaria parasites is much larger. Systematic parasitologists have erected more than 500 described species belonging to 15 genera within the order Haemosporidia (Phylum Apicomplexa) that infect squamate reptiles, turtles, birds, and mammals, and use at least seven families of dipteran vectors (Levine, 1988; Martinsen et al., 2008). These parasites are distributed in every terrestrial habitat on all the warm continents.

Bird haemosporidians are the largest group of haemosporidians by number of species. Avian malaria and related haemosporidians are widespread, abundant and diverse and are easily sampled without disrupting the host populations. In addition, experimental studies on bird malaria usually present bigger samples sizes than primate or human studies, achieving a high degree of precision and confidence in the outcome of the study. More than

200 parasite species of the genera *Plasmodium, Haemoproteus* and *Leucocytozoon* have been morphologically described among the 4.000 bird species investigated worldwide (Valkiūnas, 2005). All these characteristics turn bird blood parasites into an excellent model for the study of host–parasite interactions.

The term "malaria parasites" has been a controversial issue among parasitologists, ecologists and evolutionary researchers (Pérez-Tris et al., 2005; Valkiūnas et al., 2005). The debate stems from the incomplete knowledge of the phylogenetic relationships and pathogenicity of non human malaria parasites. The life cycles of *Plasmodium, Haemoproteus* and *Leucocytozoon* are similar, but they differ in important aspects. Looking at these differences in vectors, life cycles and epidemiology of these organisms, the traditional view accepts only *Plasmodium* species as being the true malaria parasites (Valkiūnas et al., 2005). The presence of both erythrocytic schizonts and gametocytes in infections with *Plasmodium* is a key difference from *Haemoproteus* and *Leucocytozoon* (these two latter undergo schizogony only in fixed non-circulating cells in the host) which is important for the identification, pathogenicity and experimental transmission of *Plasmodium*. Species of *Plasmodium* can be transmitted from infected to uninfected hosts by simple blood inoculation, while *Leucocytozoon* and *Haemoproteus* need an arthropod vector. These vectors are different among the three genera: blood-sucking mosquitoes are the main vectors of avian *Plasmodium*, whereas biting midges and hippoboscid flies are the vectors of *Haemoproteus* and simuliid flies transmit *Leucocytozoon*. The number of merozoites produced in schizonts also differs among haemosporidians. Some species of *Leucocytozoon* and *Haemoproteus* form megalozhizonts in host tissues that yield millions of merozoites, species of *Plasmodium* form smaller tissue schizonts that produce tens to hundreds of merozoites (Atkinson & van Riper, 1991).

However, based on recent molecular genetic studies describing the phylogeny of the group, other authors include other genera, particularly *Haemoproteus*, among the malaria parasites (Pérez-Tris et al., 2005). Since the introduction of polymerase chain reaction-based methods for parasite identification (Bensch et al., 2000), research in avian malaria has boosted. Also, the publication of genetic database of these parasites based on mitochondrial cytochrome b lineages (Bensch et al., 2009) has provide a valuable tool for cooperation between research groups and benefit the understanding of the ecology, evolution and taxonomy. In consequence, the number of scientific publications on this topic has remarkably increased in last decade (Figure 1). In this chapter I summarize some of the most recent advances in the study of malaria of birds, stating the solutions that avian malaria offers to human malaria research.

2.1 Importance of studies on avian malaria

Only five years later than Charles Louis Alphonse Laveran discovered the human malaria, in 1885 the Russian physiologist and protistologist Vassily Danilewsky found intraerythrocytic parasites in the blood of amphibians, birds and reptiles. He described in great detail the morphology of the various forms he observed, becoming aware of the fact that parasites from birds resembled the malaria parasites described by Laveran, Marchiafava and Celli. Intrigued and highly motivated with such similarities, he developed many ecological, anatomical and pathological investigations on infected birds, showing that the haemosporidiosis was accompanied by anemia, enlargement and whitening of the spleen and liver, and an accumulation of pigment. He also noticed some seasonality in parasitemia, where the presence of blood parasites in birds was higher during warm seasons. In 1888, he published a monograph in Russian on bird Haemosporidia, identifying and describing the main characters of the three main genera. But it was not until his three volume book *La Parasitologie Comparée du Sang* had been published in French in 1889 that this information became widely available. This monograph drew Laveran's attention and he studied with interest Danielewsky's results. In 1891, Laveran urged physicians to enter the domain of naturalists and to research bird malaria (Sá, 2010, Valkiūnas, 2005). This example clearly illustrates that human and avian malaria researches are intimately linked.

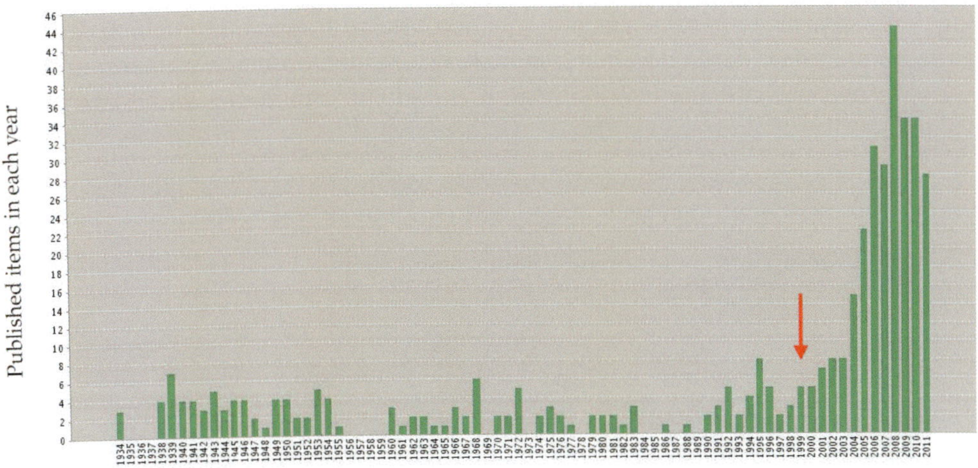

Fig. 1. Increase in number of articles published within the framework of "avian malaria" and "bird malaria" over the period 1934 – 2011. The figure is based on a literature search in the ISI-Web of Science (Thomson, September 2011). Arrow shows publication of Bensch et al. (2000).

As we have seen, from its origin research on bird malaria parasites has played an important role as human malaria research. Experiments with avian malaria contributed a great deal to our understanding of the life cycle of the human malaria parasite. In addition, the fundamental studies on chemotherapy of malaria were carried out with birds, and resulted in the discovery of two very well known synthetic drugs, plasmochin and atebrin. The most remarkable scientific advance linking avian and human malaria was done by Sir Ronald Ross (Figure 2), a British officer in the Indian Medical Service. Because malaria was a devastating health problem in India, he began to study its cause in 1890. For a long time malaria was thought to be spread by odours, and vapours produced in swamps were blamed as the origin of malaria infection. But Laveran verified the presence of pigmented bodies of parasites in the blood of malaria infected patients, suggesting an alternative cause. In that time, Ross believed that malaria was caused by an intestinal infection, following numerous failed attempts to infect human "volunteers" with water contaminated with malarial mosquitoes and larvae. In 1894, Sir Patrick Manson informed to Ross about Laveran's observation and suggested that mosquitoes, and not the water, were responsible for transmitting these parasites to humans. Ross began to breed mosquitoes for experimental research on malaria inoculation in humans. Finally, in 1897, he managed to get mosquitoes to feed on malarial patients and found evidences of the parasite within the stomach cavities of *Anopheles* mosquitoes. But during these researches on human models he found many frustrating obstacles, including a transfer within the Service prevented further work with human "volunteers", and his malaria research seemed to aim to an ending point. He still had, however, access to laboratory facilities. And he remembered that in 1894 Manson had suggested to him the idea of using malaria parasites of birds in his investigations. Ross then turned his attention to avian malaria parasites, giving him a control over his experiment subjects difficult to attain with human models. Working with caged birds, Ross confirmed the transmissive way of spreading of malaria, revealing the further development of the avian malaria parasite in the body of the mosquito. He followed the parasites *Plasmodium relictum* from an infected bird into the stomach of a *Culex* mosquito which had fed on the bird and from there to the mosquito's salivary glands. The bite of this mosquito then transmitted the malaria parasite to another bird. For this discover, Ross was awarded the Nobel Prize in 1902. At this point, it should be stressed that the first out of the four Nobel Prizes bestowed to malaria researches was awarded on investigations on avian malaria.

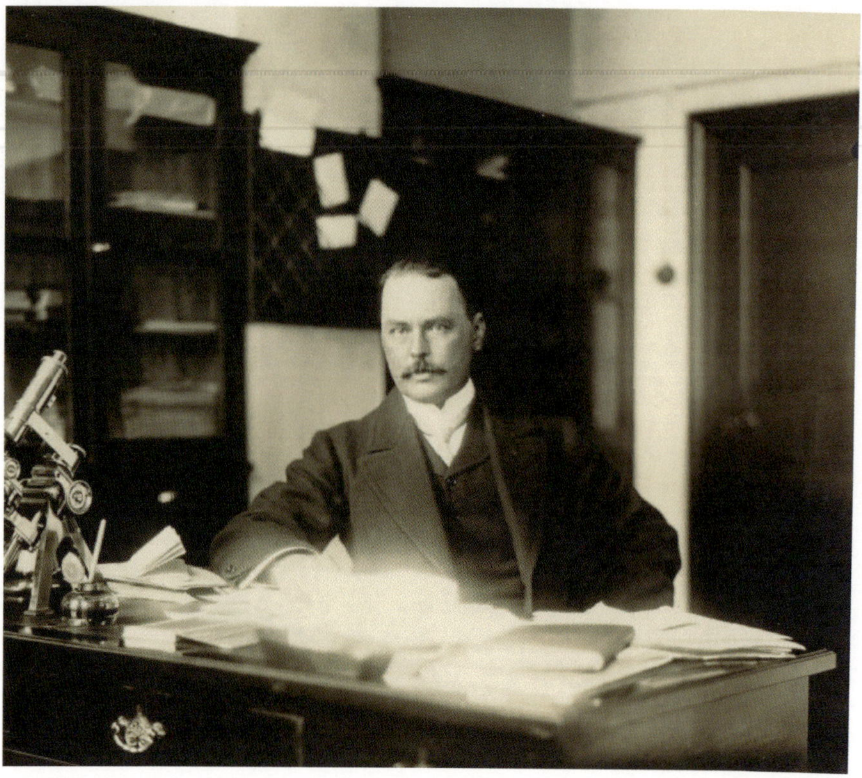

Fig. 2. Sir Ronald Ross (1857 - 1932), in 1904 at the Liverpool School of Tropical Medicine.

Malaria has shaped the course of wars for millennia. In many conflicts, more troops were lled by malaria than in combat. In World War I, British, French and German armies were nmobilized in Macedonia for 3 years by malaria. In this area, nearly 80 percent of French oops were hospitalized with malaria and 25.000 British soldiers were sent home with hronic malaria. German soldiers also suffered from the shortage of quinine, hampered his nissions on East Africa, Balkans and Turkey. In this and other conflicts, avian malaria esearch has played a decisive role. In his book "War and disease", Slater (2009) highlighted he importance of avian investigations for biomedical research on malaria in the twentieth entury. In 1910's German company Bayern invested many resources in the development of ynthetic anti-malaria drugs. With this purpose, Wilhelm Roehl, a former assistant of Paul Ehrlich, joined the Bayer research group. Roehl believed that malaria research was hindered by the lack of good model system for research. He noticed that treatments against human malaria were also effective against avian malaria, but nobody had tested the reverse: to discover a new effective anti-malaria substance in birds that later proved effective on human malaria. And he did it. With his discover of synthetic compound plasmochin, Roehl was successful extending his finding from the bird to human malaria (Slater, 2009). Some years ater, avian malaria research also played a major role in the World War II. During the first years of operations in the South West Pacific, the losses caused by malaria disease among the Allies greatly exceeded the number of battle casualties. In response to such situation, governments from United States and Britain started research and development programs to discover new anti-malarial drugs. Thousands of new anti-malarial drugs synthesized during the war, such as sulphadiazine group of drugs and amino-quinolines, were tested in first instance on malaria infected birds. And only those with high activity and low toxicity were then tested in humans (Fairley, 1947; Sweeney, 2000). It is clear that without this valuable information from bird malaria, the use of anti-malaria drugs by man would have been greatly curtailed.

Ross and Roehl's studies represent the peak achievement of discoveries in avian malaria research. However, the list of contributions of avian malaria investigations to human malaria research is striking. The formation of chemical therapy (Wasielewsky, 1904; Sergent and Sergent, 1921), the first cultivation methods of the tissue and erythrocytic stages *in vitro* (Ball & Chao, 1961; Trager, 1947), and first steps in the development of antimalarial vaccines (McGhee et al., 1977) were first successfully achieved on the model of bird malaria parasites. Moreover, avian malaria was the most extensively model for tests of blood schizonticides, allowing the examination of new anti-malaria compounds in different birds, such as chicken, canaries, pigeon and ducks. With the implantation of the rodent malaria models, avian malaria research in Medicine fall into disuse. After the discovery of the rodent malaria parasite in 1950 and experimental inoculation of the three-striped night monkey with human malaria in 1966, the interest in research of medical parasitologists on bird haemosporidians decreased. At present, the low cost and easily availability of models of bird *Plasmodium* spp. have not lost their practical importance, primarily in immunological, genetic, biochemical and ecological investigations (Valkiūnas, 2005). Nowadays, there are increasing evidences that *Plasmodium facilparum* have become resistant to almost every anti-malarial drug. Moreover, in some endemic areas of the world some *P. facilparum* isolates have developed multi-resistance to most available anti-malarial, especially to those in the aminoquinoline group (chloroquine, amodiaquine and mefloquine). Even recently it has been reported some causes of malaria resistance to the up to now effective combination of artemisinin derivatives with other antimalarials. Since History shows that once resistance emerges, it can swiftly travel around the world, these resistances constitute an enormous threat to the malaria control programs, making the development of new anti-malarial drugs urgent (Krettli et al., 2009). Once again, animal models for anti-malarial screening, like avian models, become important in the fight against human malaria. In recent times it has been suggested that avian malaria models would be especially important in places where there are no *Anopheles* mosquitoes raised indoors available to infect with mammalian malaria (Krettli, 2009). Also, they would be very useful in testing of new prophylactic compounds able to inhibit sporozoite development. For instance, a Brazilian medicinal plant species (*Ampelozizyphus amazonicus*) has successfully been examined demonstrating its prophylactic activity when tested *in vivo* against sporozoite-induced infections in an avian model (Krettli et al., 2001). In addition, the avian malaria *P. gallinaceum* is very useful in studying the activity of compounds (e.g. primaquine) aiming to cure the late relapse caused by *P. vivax* (Krettli et al., 2009).

By the other hand, the widespread geographic distribution of avian malaria parasites and their broad range of host species make them excellent models for exploring the ecological and evolutionary dynamics of host-parasite associations, including human malaria parasites (Fallon et al., 2005). Issues such as conservation of endemic fauna (Atkinson et al., 2000), speciation (Perez-Tris et al., 2007), co-evolution (Charleston and Perkins, 2002; Mu et al., 2005), life history tradeoffs (Jovani, 2002), the evolution of virulence (Bell et al., 2006; Schall, 2002), sexual selection (Spencer et al., 2005), and competition and community structure (Fallon et al., 2004; Paul et al., 2002) have been studied in last ten years in avian malaria models.

In 21th century, Emerging Infectious Diseases are on the major threat to animal biodiversity and human health. Millions of organisms have experience, and likely will suffer the devastating effects of the rapid increase of these of new and existing infectious diseases. Recently it has been proposed that climate change could alter the equilibrium between parasites and host, potentially resulting in an epidemic. Wild bird populations are widely infected with *Plasmodium* and related haemosporidians, providing very precious information for the study of environmental threats such as climate change (Huijben et al., 2007). However, the factors favouring malaria outbreaks go beyond the basic biological elements and include ecological as well as socio-economic factors (Wilson, 2001). Since vectors populations and reproductive biology of malaria parasites are affected by climate change at a global scale, the resulting increase in malaria transmission should also be evident in birds. In human malaria studies it is very difficult to know if the change in parasite prevalence is due to socio-ecological factors or to the effect of climate change. But these confounding effects are irrelevant in the context of parasites that infect wild animals. Recently, Garamszegi (2010) compiled data on avian malaria and analyzed 43 surveys covering a time span from the 1940s to the present. Together, the surveys provided data on more than 3,000 bird species that had been screened for malaria in different regions. He found that avian malaria has nearly tripled in the last 70 years, in parallel with increasing global temperatures. And the most dramatic increases took place during the past 20 years. This avian study will be very valuable to improve our understanding of the effect of climate change on malaria in humans.

Summarizing, research on bird malaria parasites has played an important role in human malaria research. The practical importance of bird haemosporidians should not be underestimated. For many years, they represent a stimulus for the development of medical parasitology. Notable advances in malaria research such as development of chemotherapies and vaccines, cultivation in vitro and study of life cycles, as well as other evolutionary, genetic and immunological investigations, have been possible thanks to avian models. Far from loosing validity, studies on avian malaria represent a formidable model for researchers, providing valuable tools to face new health and environmental challenges in 21th century.

2.2 Pathogenicity of avian malaria parasites

Malaria parasites are supposed to have strong negative effects on host fitness because this group of intra-cellular parasites causes dramatic reductions in the efficiency of metabolism (Chen et al., 2001). The infection begins with the bite of an insect inserting sporozoite stages from its saliva into the blood stream of the host. Then the development of extraerthrocytic meronts starts by asexual division inside internal organs for several generations (a minimum of two generations) until penetration into erythrocytes gives rise to gametocytes. This extraerythrocytic step is very important in order to improve the initial infectious source. Once intensity of infection has increased, a few merozoites penetrate into red blood cells to initiate the erythrocytic cycle producing macro- and microgametocytes by sexuall division (Valkiūnas, 2005; Wakelin, 1996). After a period of growth there is production of new erythrocytic meronts (schizonts). The infected cells then burst, releasing merozoites that will infect red blood cells, so that a high proportion of available erythrocytes may become infected. Erythrocytic cytoplasm and hemoglobin is digested by the parasite to obtain amino acids, but the haem is stored in the form of an insoluble pigment. When infected red blood cells burst, pigment and other metabolic products are released into the circulation, inducing the characteristic fever and other symptoms of illness (Wakelin, 1996). During the exo-erythrocytic meronts stage there are pathological changes such as blocking of brain capillaries and capillaries of other vital organs thereby producing anoxia, death of cells and necrosis of tissues (i.e. liver and spleen). The most severe pathology happens in the blood stage, when destructions of host blood cells provoke acute anemia. Other consequences of malarial parasites infections include development of pneumonia-like symptoms and excessive enlargement of the spleen and liver that eventually causes rupture (Valkiūnas, 2005).

Previously blood parasites were considered low pathogenicity organisms (Weatherhead & Bennett 1992; Bennett et al. 1993) in spite of them causing disease and death in captive birds. Other studies demonstrated subtle but important effects of hematozoan parasites on the life history of their avian hosts (Allander & Bennett 1994; Dufva 1996; Korpimäki et al. 1993, 1995; Rätti et al. 1993). However, some researchers did not find detrimental effect of these parasites (Fallis & Desser 1977; Dufva & Allander 1995; Dawson & Bortolloti 2000). Therefore, there are no clear conclusions about parasite pathogenicity and about regulation of their host populations. The main problem of most of these studies is the lack of experimentation. The demonstration of effects of parasites requires an empirical approach, where experimental manipulation of natural blood parasite loads may reveal their harmful effects (Keymer & Read 1991; Knowles et al. 2010; Merino et al. 2000). In this sense, two have been the most successful methodologies employed for experimental approaches to test fo fitness effects of avian malaria infection: i) direct inoculation of a parasite on uninfectec individuals, and ii) experimental removal of parasites through medication.

The experimentally removal of parasites by anti-malaria medication has been a popula methodology to test the fitness consequences of avian malaria infection. Following this procedure, Merino et al. (2000) reduced through medication the intensity of infection by *Haemoproteus majoris* and the prevalence of infection by *Leucocytozoon majoris* in blue tits *Cyanistes caeruleus*. Medicated females then devoted more resources to parental care and consequently, increased their reproductive success. This experimental reduction of parasite load revealed the causality in the association of natural infection levels with life-history variables.

But clutch size, one of the most important reproductive patterns in birds, could also be affected by malarial parasites. In addition, if malarial parasites have early effects on the reproductive cycle then they could have disproportionately large effects on seasonal reproductive success. In this line, Marzal et al. (2005) studied the effect of *Haemoproteus* spp. on the reproductive success of migratory house martin *Delichon urbica*. At the beginning of the breeding season they experimentally reduced levels and intensity of *Haemoproteus* infection, by randomly treating birds with an anti-malarial drug (primaquine). The results showed that clutch size was on average 18% larger in treated birds, while these differences increasing to 39% at hatching and 42% at fledging. These findings demonstrated that malarial parasites can have dramatic effects on clutch size and other demographic variables, potentially influencing the evolution of clutch size, but also the population dynamics of heavily infected populations of birds.

In the same year, Tomás et al. (2005) studied the role of blood parasites as a potential source of physiological stress for avian hosts in the wild. Through a medication, they reduced the intensity of infection by *Haemoproteus majoris* and the prevalence of infection by *Leucocytozoon majoris* in female blue tits *Cyanistes caeruleus*. They showed an increase in stress proteins (heat shock proteins) in control females in compare to medicated ones, reporting the first experimental evidence relating blood parasite infection to the physiological stress response in a wild avian population.

Because intensity of blood parasite infection varies during infection, the dynamics of infection could have been the cause of difficulties for detecting their fitness effects in wild populations of birds. During the brief acute stage of a haemosporidian infection, parasites usually appear in the blood at high density and hosts can suffer marked mortality (Atkinson & van Riper, 1991; Valkiūnas, 2005). However, in individuals that survive the acute stage, long-term chronic infections develop, in which parasites persist at low density and are thought to be controlled by acquired immunity (Atkinson & van Riper, 1991). Recently, two studies have shown the negative effects of this malaria chronic infection to their avian hosts. Martínez de la Puente et al. (2010) have experimentally demonstrated long-term direct survival costs of chronic *Haemoproteus* infection in wild birds. They medicated males and females blue tits *Cyanistes caeruleus* with primaquine. This anti-malaria drug reduced the intensity of *Haemoproteus* infection in females, but not in males, showing a sex-specific effect of medication on *Haemoproteus* intensity, probably due to sex effects on drug kinetics. Medicated females, but not males, showed increased local surviving until the next breeding season compared to control birds. In addition, Knowles et al. (2010) have illustrated that chronic avian malaria infections can have significant effects on host fitness and may thus constitute an important selection pressure in wild bird populations. They used the anti-malarial drug Malarone™ to test experimentally for fitness effects of chronic malaria infection in blue tits *Cyanistes caeruleus*. The recently developed molecular methodology quantitative PCR revealed that medication caused a reduction in *Plasmodium* infection intensity, leading to a higher hatching success, provisioning rates and fledging success.

On the other hand, experimental inoculation of avian malaria parasites from infected donors has also been widely used by researchers to study the harmful effects of parasitic infection. Atkinson et al. (1988) were among the first researches experimentally demonstrating the detrimental effects of *Haemoproteus* infection in birds. With a sporozoite-induced experimental infection of *Haemoproteus meleagridis*, they showed the pathological effects of such infection in domestic turkeys. Some years later, Garvin et al. (2003) studied the pathogenicity of *Haemoproteus danilewsky* in captive blue jays *Cyanocitta cristata*. By mean of an intraperitoneally inoculation of 3.000 – 4.000 sporozoites of *H. danilewsky* obtained from *Culicoides edeni* (Diptera: Ceratopogonidae), they showed sublethal pathologic changes in the liver, lung and spleen of birds. Also, Valkiūnas et al. (2006a) infected nestling blackcaps *Sylvia atricapilla* by inoculation in their pectoral muscle with 45 sporozoites of *Haemoproteus belopolskyi* developed in the experimentally infected biting midge *Culicoides impunctatus*. When compared with controls, they showed that experimentally infected birds suffered from a significant weight loss, indicating a short-term influence of the infection on the birds' body mass. Some years later Palinauskas et al. (2008, 2009) carried out some experimental inoculations on captive passerines to test for the susceptibility of different hosts to the same malaria parasite. They evaluated the effects of *Plasmodium relictum* (lineage P-SGS1), which is a host generalist, to five species of passerine birds. They demonstrated that the same parasite lineage can cause malaria of different severity even in phylogenetically closed related bird species.

Studies based on microscopic examination of thin blood smears have revealed that parasitized birds may frequently carry several different parasites (Palinauskas et al., 2005; Valkiūnas, 2005). In addition, recent advances in methods of genotyping have shown that the number of avian malaria species is much higher than can be distinguished by traditional methods (Bensch et al., 2004), revealing coinfections by different parasite lineages or genera (Hellgren, 2005; Pérez-Tris & Bensch, 2005). For example, a recent study combining molecular and traditional methods found this mixed infections in more than 43 percent of the examined birds (Valkiūnas et al., 2006b). But besides this abundance, the effects of simultaneous infections of avian malaria parasites are largely unknown.

Although antagonistic effects between parasites have been described in some studies (Fenwick, 1980; Juhl & Permins, 2002), some others have found synergetic effects between two malaria parasites infecting simultaneously (Taylor et al., 1998; Zehtindjiev et al., 2008). In this sense, theory predicts that multiple infections could be especially injurious for hosts, leading to anaemia, loss of body mass and reduced survival (Graham et al., 2005; Davidar & Morton, 2006). Such effects of malaria double infections have been poorly investigated and the reported results are inconclusive. For instance, Sanz et al. (2001) found no relationship between primary reproductive parameters and the number of blood parasite species infecting female pied flycatchers *Ficedula hypoleuca*. On the other hand, Evans & Otter (1998) showed a lethal combined effect of infections with *Haemoproteus* and *Leucocytozoon* in juvenile snowy owls *Nyctea scandiaca*, although both parasite species on their own were not considered to be pathogenic. In 2008, Marzal et al. investigated the effects of single and double malaria infections on survival, body condition and reproductive success in house martins, using the performance of uninfected individuals as a reference. They expected to observe a trend in pathogenic consequences from uninfected to single-infected to double-infected birds. Their finding showed that the infection with malaria parasites had detrimental effects on house martins, as shown by the decreased survival prospects of double- and single-infected individuals. The negative effects of infection were detectable in reduced body condition of double-infected house martins, but not in single-infected ones. But surprisingly and contrary to their predictions, individuals harboring a double infection invested more in current reproduction, despite being in poor physical condition. More recently, Palinauskas et al. (2011) have shown that co-infections of *Plasmodium relictum* and *Plasmodium ashfordi* are highly virulent and act synergistically during primary infections in some but not all passerine birds (Palinauskas et al., 2011).

At the same time, however, in many of these above studies is quite frequent to find infected individuals that seem do not suffer from detrimental effect of blood parasites (e.g. no negative effect on survival and/or reproductive success). The question arising from here is why not all infected birds experience the pathological effect of malaria. Of course these differences could be explained by a sampling bias in these studies. In this sense, only relatively healthy specimens (uninfected birds or with low intensity of infection) are active and can be caught in mist nets or stationary traps, whereas bird weak due to heavy parasitemias are undersampled because they are inactive (Valkiūnas, 2005). Nowadays ecologists and evolutionary biologists are investigating how host organisms do defend themselves against parasites, dividing host defenses into two conceptually different components: resistance and tolerance. Following this line, once infected, hosts can resist the assault by minimizing the success of enemy harass directly attacking parasites and thereby reducing parasite loads. Or alternatively, they can tolerate the parasite limiting the injury caused by a given parasite burden and minimizing the fitness impact of enemy attacks (Råberg et al., 2009; Svensson & Råberg, 2010). Recent evidence indicates that some native Hawaiian birds have developed some tolerance to malaria (Freed et al. 2005). This could lead to an increase of reservoirs of the disease, which in turn increases the risk of transmission to rarer species that are vulnerable to avian malaria. Whatever it is, it seems that pathogen burden and health are not always well correlated. Further experimental studies with the aim of quantifying both tolerance and resistance are needed for a better understanding of these co-evolutionary dynamics in host-parasite interactions.

To recapitulate, traditional studies on pathogenicity of avian malaria on wild populations of birds initially showed the negative consequences of the infection of this group of haemosporidian parasites. These and new detrimental effects were later confirmed by empirical studies, either by means of experimental inoculation of the parasites on uninfected birds or by removal of infection after an anti-malarial medication. Nowadays, new advances in molecular methodologies combined with traditional microscopy will throw light for understanding the way in which parasites impose selection on hosts.

2.3 Malaria parasites as geographical markers in migratory birds

Migratory birds have suffered a worldwide dramatic decrease in numbers in the past several decades (Terborgh, 1989). In 2010, BirdLife International found that population of 45% of Europe's common birds and more than 80% of Australia's wading species have declined. The exact reason for the birds' decline is a mystery, but scientists have begun to point out the possible basis for such downward trend. Several reasons have emerged as the greatest threats to their survival, mainly associated to disruption, fragmentation and destruction of breeding habitats, stopover sites and wintering grounds. This data are warning to us that environmental degradation is having a huge impact on all biodiversity, not only in birds. This deterioration of the environment contributes to health threats worldwide. Environmental degradation can have a significant impact on human health, ranging from death caused by cancer due to air pollution to psychological problems resulting from noise. Thus, a better understanding of the causes of the destruction of natural habitats and ecosystems can help to inform environmental policy design.

Migratory bird species can provide us with this information. They are excellent indicators of large-scale ecosystem health and landscape integrity. Moreover, because of the large distances they travel and sensitivity to minor ecological changes at sites across their established routes, migratory species are most likely to be affected by climate change and offer a hint into how ecosystems are changing. Since migratory individuals spend different periods of their annual cycle in widely separated and ecologically disparate locations, only the knowledge of the migratory connectivity could help us to identify the specific threats on the wintering location, stopover sites and breeding grounds of endangered migratory bird populations. Unfortunately, our current understanding of the migration routes and wintering areas of many migratory bird species is still limited. To solve this problem, researchers have employed several methods to determine migratory patterns and know the wintering areas with varying success. In recent times it has been suggested that parasites, specifically avian malaria and related haemosporidians, can be used as geographical markers in migratory birds. In this section I evaluate the studies that have been developed in the last ten years in this field, exploring several lines of research that might be worth following in the future.

In the beginning, researchers attempted to band birds by attaching a small, individually numbered, metal or plastic tag to their legs or wings in their breeding grounds and then recapture them on the wintering quarters. This technique has been used since 1899, and it has provided the most information about migration routes, stopover sites and wintering grounds for birds. Unfortunately, most ringed animals are never seen again and the number of rings recovered from sub-Saharan Africa is very low (Sillet & Holmes, 2002). Alternatively, morphological variations can be used to directly track migratory birds, but the validity of this technique is limited to species with geographically segregated morphotypes (Webster et al., 2002). In recent years, satellite telemetry has been the most important advance in the field, allowing for a scale-independent tracking of individuals birds anywhere in the world. However, the current size and weight of even smaller satellite tags is too large (> 18 g) to allow its use in small birds, which represent the vast majority of migratory birds (Webster et al., 2002).

While all these traditional capture-recapture and new techniques have been relatively inefficient for linking wintering and breeding habitats, other new advances in molecular ecology and stable isotope composition of animal tissues have provided promising results. Given that isotopic ratio in the local environments are incorporated into plants during nutrient uptake and then passed through local food chains, the isotopic composition of animal tissues reflects that of the local environment where those tissues were grown (Hobson et al., 2001). Then, isotopic markers have a great potential for identifying the source area where, for example, a migratory bird has moulted their feather during winter. However, some limitations should be considered such as variation in isotopic signatures with diet, altitude and trophic levels (Hobson et al., 2004; Hobson 2005; Wassenaar & Hobson, 2000).

In 2002, Webster et al. proposed several genetic approaches to determine the geographical origins of bird sampled at particular sites. This technique is useful when genetic markers are specific to particular populations or subsets of populations. Unfortunately, birds are usually widespread dispersal and none or very weak genetic differentiation among population can be found when analyzing bird DNA. However, they also suggested an exciting and powerful genetic approach to measuring connectivity: to use the genes from organisms that birds carry (e.g. parasites) rather than genes from the birds themselves. Following this line, avian malaria parasites can provide valuable information about wintering or breeding sites since these vector-borne parasites can be transmitted only in the area where they coexist with the host. Moreover, new advances in amplifying and sequencing DNA from avian malaria has allowed the identification of different parasite lineages, providing information about parasite-transmission area at a finer scale.

The first approach to the use of avian malaria as geographical markers was even before than Webster's proposal. By microscopy scanning of blood smears, Rintamäki et al. (1998) showed differences in time of main occurrence of *Haemoproteus* and *Leucocytozoon* infection of migrating willow warblers *Phylloscopus trochilus* at a stopover sites. They suggested that these differences could indicate that the birds had become infected in different areas. Some years later, Waldenström et al. (2002) used molecular techniques to study the phylogeny of avian haemosporidian parasites in a number of African resident and European migratory songbird species. They showed three clades of avian malaria which transmission seems to occur solely in Africa, and two *Haemoproteus* clades that appeared to be transmitted both in wintering and breeding grounds.

After these promising results, Fallon et al. (2006) were not successful in the use of malaria parasites as geographical markers in migratory birds. They tested the hypothesis that malaria parasites could provide sufficient geographical signal to track population movements of black-throated blue warblers *Dendroica caerulescens* between breeding and wintering habitats in North America. They screened and genetically typed malaria parasites from more than 1.000 individual, showing that parasite lineages were geographically widespread and did not provide site-specific information.

More recently, Pagenkopp et al. (2008) analysed liver tissue and blood trying to determine whether haemosporidian parasite lineages detected significant geographic structure in common yellowthroats *Geothlypis trichas*. They compared *Plasmodium* lineages infecting birds showing some geographical structure, where some lineages seems to be more geographically specific than others, allowing some discrimination of origin. However, they concluded stating that this variation was not enough for their use as a marker of migratory connectivity.

Yohannes et al. (2008) combined the study of the composition of stable isotopes in winter moulted feathers and the analyses of malaria parasites to track whether great reed warblers *Acrocephalus arundinaceus* wintering in different areas showed differences in blood parasite infection. They found marked differences in isotopic signatures when comparing infected and non-infected birds, showing that birds infected with malaria have moulted in different geographical areas than the non-infected birds. But they found no significant relationship between feather isotope value and malaria type, indicating that parasite composition was not related to moulting area.

By analysing the spatial and temporal differences in the blood parasite fauna of three species of warblers during the spring migration in Bulgaria, Shurulinkov and Ilieva (2009) illustrated spatial differences in the prevalence and composition of blood parasite fauna in two species. They argued that these differences found between sites could be explained with the different origin of the migrants at different migration stopover sites.

Finally, von Rönn has recently shown (2010) an association between stables isotopes composition in feathers moulted in the African winter quarters and the diversity and prevalence of malaria parasites in barn swallows *Hirundo rustica*. Hence, individuals wintering in different areas become infected with different *Plasmodium* parasites.

Summarizing, understanding the factors operating on environmental degradation could help us to identify the specific threats and predict ecological responses to changes in habitat quantity and quality. Since they spend different periods of their annual cycle in disparate locations, migratory birds are excellent bioindicators to estimate the environmental quality of diverse areas. In recent years, avian malaria parasites have been used to provide an excellent tool to track bird populations during migration, but the outcomes from these studies are not enough to complete our knowledge on migratory routes. Future researches with more migratory bird species combining multiple markers will provide vital information to preventing the decline and extinction of many organisms.

2.4 Malaria parasites and avian invasion

The total cost of Global nature destruction is estimated $ 4,500 billion annually (The Economics of Ecosystems and Biodiversity [TEEB], 2010). Most of this biodiversity loss is provoked by intentional and unintentional introductions of non-indigenous species becoming invaders in new ecosystems. These invasive species are a greater threat to native biodiversity than pollution, harvest, and diseases combined. Also, invasive species can have substantial impacts on ecological systems, gene pools, and the disease environments for livestock, crops, and humans (Allendorf & Lundquist, 2003; Mack et al., 2000; Mooney & Cleland, 2001). Hence, understanding the causes of invasion success can help us to predict effects of species introductions and to design interventions.

Despite the economic importance of invasive species and the efforts from government organizations as well as conservation groups to understand biological invasions, the mechanisms that allow one species to become invasive are still poorly understood. Since many introduced species fail to establish or to spread significantly, but many others become successful colonizers, we questionnaire what makes a species a successful invader. Scientists have proposed several mechanisms to explain invasive, including species-based mechanisms (i.e. competition) and ecosystem-based mechanisms (i.e. availability of resources). Parasites and other pathogens have been proposed to play an important role on the invasive process, facilitating colonization and spread of their hosts in new continents and islands. Based on the analysis of traits of invasive species, two main hypotheses have been proposed to explain the mechanisms conferring invasiveness to the organisms. According to the *Enemy Release Hypothesis*, non-native species become successfully established because they are freed from their co-evolved pathogens, parasites and predators (Torchin et al., 2002; Colautti et al., 2004). Because parasites can reduce host population abundance, density and spread (Anderson & May, 1978), this decrease in parasite pressure may allow introduced species to decrease their investment in defenses and maximize their capital in growth and reproduction, thus increasing their competitive ability and displace native species (Bloosey and Nötzold, 1995). Alternatively, the *Novel Weapon Hypotheses* proposes that introduced species possess allelopathic chemicals, parasites, and pathogens against which the introduced species but not the natives have evolved defenses (Callaway & Ridenour, 2004; Prenter et al., 2004). Consequently, individuals and populations in their native areas can be seriously damaged by the pathogens brought with invaders.

Novel weapons have played a role in many human invasions. In his war against Incas, apart from steel armaments and horses, Pizarro relied on another powerful weapon: germs. Smallpox, brought to the Americas by the Spanish, had spread south from Panama well ahead of Pizarro´s troops, becoming an epidemic with devastating consequence for the native people. As well as other endemic European diseases such as measles, influenza, typhus and bubonic plague, smallpox played a decisive role in European conquests. These novel weapons spread quickly in America, from tribe to tribe, killing an estimated 95% of the indigenous population far in advance of the European themselves (Diamond, 1997).

In last centuries, several bird species have been successfully introduced and become invaders in many parts of the world (Blackburn et al., 2009). Despite the large amount of information on the distribution, ecology, and evolution of birds could provide excellent opportunities for examining the factors that facilitate invasions, their biological invasions have received relatively little attention in compare to other organisms. Just recently some researchers have focused on avian species addressing important questions about the factors that facilitate invasions. In this line, malaria and related haemosporidian parasites have been proposed to play a major role on the successful colonization of exotic bird species. Next I present two of the most dramatic examples of the fatal consequences of introduction of birds, and a review of the latest scientific contributions explaining the importance of malaria parasites in avian invasions.

The Hawaiian Islands are some of the most isolated landmasses in the world, with approximately 70 million years of isolation for avian population (Mac et al., 1998). This isolation allowed the evolution of its species into endemism. Nowadays, many exotic bird species invaded Hawaiian forests displacing local species. This invasion seems to be prompted by a powerful allied: avian malaria. The introduction of avian malaria (*Plasmodium relictum*) and its active vector *Culex quinquefasciatus* in the Hawaiian Island of Maui in 1826 provided an excellent model system for studying the effect of exotic disease on naïve host populations. As an outcome of this fatal introduction, the mortality of resident birds increased up to 90% and many native species were extinct (Jarvi et al., 2001; Van Riper et al., 1986). This enormous mortality can be result of the long isolation period, where the Hawaiian bird populations did not have a close evolutionary history with avian malaria parasites. As a consequence of this lack of co-evolution, the relatively benign malaria parasites in the introduced exotic birds were highly virulent when infecting the naïve Hawaiian birds (Atkinson et al., 1995). Those exotic birds not only provided the original pathway for the introduction of avian malaria into the islands, but now they continue to contribute to its impact. Most of this foreign birds are malaria-resistant and do not suffer from its detrimental effects. However, they maintain low-level infections and act as reservoirs for this disease. Therefore, mosquitoes can feed on these low-infected birds and pass this novel pathogen on the naïve native species. As a consequence of this parasite pressure, many native birds can no longer breed in their historical breeding forests at lower elevations and are forced to breed in higher elevations grounds, which are free from mosquitoes but where food and cover may be scarce. By the other hand, in avian malaria studies, as well as in other organisms, the highest mortalities rates among the hosts are usually found to be associated to mixed infection with two or more malaria species (Marzal et al., 2008; Tang et al., 2010). However, this seems not to be the case in mortality induced by malaria in native Hawaiian birds. Despite thousands of shorebirds and ducks migrating to Hawaii and exotic bird released in last two centuries can have harbored hundreds of novel parasites, only the parasite lineage GRW4 from *P. relictum* seems to be the cause of the high mortality of many species of Hawaiian passerines (Beadell et al., 2007), showing the dramatic effects that a single novel malaria parasites can provoke in naïve hosts.

A similar situation reported in Hawaii is currently studied in New Zealand (Tompkins & Poulin, 2006). In the earliest years of 20th century it was first postulated the connection between the extinction of New Zealand native birds and imported fauna through the exotic protozoa carried by these foreign birds (Doré, 1918). Exotic birds could act as reservoirs for these parasites and exacerbated disease problems for native avifauna. In addition, four different exotic species of mosquitoes were successfully established in New Zealand from 19th century, being *Culex quinquefasciatus*, the primary vector of avian malaria in Hawaii, among them (Laird, 1995). The increasing distribution of this vector could enhance the incidence of avian malaria, probably boosting the parasitemia in infected species, increasing its host range in areas where *Plasmodium* is already present, and/or increasing its geographical range in New Zealand (Tompkins & Poulin, 2006). It seems plausible that malaria parasites could tip the scale in alien bird species favor when competing with local birds. And the situation is not promising: the impact of blood parasites on New Zealand birds and the colonization of exotic avifauna are likely to increase in the near future.

New Zealand and Hawaii Islands represent two of the most well known examples of Novel Weapon Hypothesis, where parasitism and species invasions interact to influence natural communities. But the opposite scenario is also possible in invasions of exotic birds. The Enemy Release Hypothesis is recently summoned as an explanation of the success of introduced bird species when arriving in a non-native region (MacLeod et al., 2005; Shwartz et al., 2009). It suggests that flourishing colonizers are successful because they have left behind their natural coevolved predators or pathogens. In consequence, successful colonizers do not have to invest in anti-parasite or anti-predators defenses and can reallocate resources into other important biological functions (e.g. reproduction and growth). In this sense, Shwartz et al. (2009) have shown that the release from predators facilitated the reproductive success and therefore the invasiveness of parakeets (*Psittacula krameri*) in new regions.

Because of their deleterious effects on their host populations described above, removing weak individuals from wild populations (Valkiūnas 2005) or reducing hosts ´reproductive output (Marzal et al. 2005; Merino et al. 2000), avian blood parasites have been considered an interesting model to test the Enemy Release Hypothesis. Ishtiaq et al. (2006) were the first to study the avian blood parasites as a model to test this evolutionary hypothesis. They assessed the prevalence and distribution of malaria parasite lineages in the common myna *Acridotheres tristis*, a common passerine native to southern Asia that has been introduced to many parts of the world. Their results showed that not all comparisons of introduced populations to the native populations were consistent with the predicted Enemy Release Hypothesis. Moreover, they found some evidences of Novel Weapon Hypothesis, where common mynas carried parasite lineages from native to introduced locations. These mixed results could partially be due to the difficulty to differentiate between parasites that are native and introduced, because *Haemoproteus* and *Plasmodium* lineages infecting common mynas often did not show regional or host specificity.

Lima et al. (2010) also tested two predictions of the Enemy Release Hypothesis by comparing the presence and intensity of avian malaria parasites among house sparrows (*Passer domesticus*) and native birds from Brazil, as well as comparison with European house sparrows. Their results supported the hypothesis. According to their predictions, they found that native birds from Brazil presented significantly higher parasite prevalence. Also, they found that house sparrows native to Europe exhibited higher parasite prevalence than introduced house sparrows from Brazil, suggesting that sparrows from Brazil might have experienced a parasitic release during the process of introduction.

Just recently, an international team formed by 27 researchers has presented the most extensive study of the geographic distribution of a species rich group of parasites in a globally distributed vertebrate in the wild (Marzal et al., 2011). They examined these two important hypotheses (Enemy Release Hypothesis and Novel Weapon Hypothesis) to assess the role of avian malaria in the global spread of a common invasive bird. By analyzing prevalence and genetic diversity of malaria parasites in 58 localities on 6 continents, they showed that house sparrows did not retain their native parasites in newly colonized regions. In addition, house sparrows in non-native regions were exposed to a lower diversity and prevalence of haemosporidian infections than in their native range. They conclude that, since the house sparrows lost their native parasite when colonizing new regions, the release from these natural enemies may have facilitated its global invasion in the last two centuries.

To conclude, two points should be highlighted. First one, anthropogenic factors are almost always involved in biological invasions. Human introduction of animals to new geographical regions is usually accompanied by detrimental effects on native communities. Important and severe policies such as strict border control biosecurity regimes and controlled human traffic to remote populations or endangered species are necessary to prevent accidental or deliberate introductions. And second one, our current knowledge relevant to the disease effects of biological invasions is still poor. The allocation of resources in the research of biological invasions is essential to address this gap and design interventions, but mostly policies goes in the wrong way: current annual environmental, economic, and health-related costs of invasive species exceed the resources invested in the research of preventing biological invasions.

3. Conclusion

Investigations of avian malaria have contributed significantly to the knowledge on biology and ecology of malaria parasites of other vertebrates, including human malaria. For almost 100 years, bird malaria parasites have been widely used as an experimental model in many laboratories for discovering and testing of new chemotherapies, development of anti-malarial vaccines and cultivation in vitro of tissues and erythrocytic stages, helping save millions of human lives. In addition, the widespread geographic distribution of avian malaria parasites and their broad range of host species made them excellent models for exploring the ecological and evolutionary dynamics of host-parasite associations. Nowadays, far from being outdated, research on avian malaria is essential to fence new health and environmental challenges in this time of unprecedented global change. Climate change, the introduction of invasive species, urbanization, deforestation of natural environments and the loss of biodiversity are all implicated in increasing the spread of infectious pathogens such as malaria. Current and new advances in avian malaria research will be crucial to help predict and prevent outbreaks that could affect avifauna, humans and other wildlife worldwide in 21th century.

4. Acknowledgment

The author conveys thanks for the invitation to write this review. The author also is grateful to Laszlo Z. Garamszegi and F. de Lope for helpful suggestions regarding the manuscript. Spanish Ministry of Education and Science (CGL2009-08976) and Junta of Extremadura (PRI08A116 and GRU10143) provided funding for this research.

5. References

Allander, K. & Bennett, G. F. (1994). Prevalence and intensity of hematozoan infections in a population of great tits *Parus major* from Gotland, Sweden. *Journal of Avian Biology*, Vol. 25, pp. 69-74

Allendorf, F. W. & Lundquist, L. L. (2003). Introduction: population biology, evolution, and control of invasive species. *Conservation Biology*, Vol. 17, pp. 24-30

Anderson, R. M. & May, R. M. (1978). Regulation and stability of host-parasite population interactions: I. Regulatory processes. *Journal of Animal Ecology*, Vol. 47, pp. 219–247

Atkinson, C.T.; Forrester, D. J. & Greiner, E. C. (1988). Pathogenicity *of Haemoproteus meleagridis* (Haemosporina: Haemoproteidae) in experimentallyinfected domestic turkeys. *Journal of Parasitology*, Vol. 74, pp. 228-239

Atkinson, C. T. & Van Riper III, C. (1991). Pathogenicity and epizootiology of avian haematozoa: *Plasmodium*, *Leucocytozoon* and *Haemoproteus*. In *Bird-Parasite interacctions*, J. E. Loye & M. Zuk (Eds.), 19-48, Oxford University Press, ISBN 978-0198577386, Oxford, UK

Atkinson, C. T.; Woods K. L.; Dusek, R. J.; Sileo, L. S. & Iko, W. M. (1995).Wildlife disease and conservation in Hawaii: Pathogenicity of avian malaria (*Plasmodium relictum*) in experimentally infected Iiwi (*Vestiaria coccinea*). *Parasitology*, Vol. 111, pp. S59-S69

Atkinson, C.T.; Dusek, R.J.; Woods, K.L. & Iko, W.M. (2000). Pathogenicity of avian malaria in experimentally-infected Hawaii Amakihi. *Journal of Wildlife Diseases*, Vol. 36, pp. 197–204

Ball, G. H. & Chao, J. (1961). Infectivity to canaries of sporozoites of *Plasmodium relictum* developing in vitro. *The Journal of Parasitology*, Vol. 47, pp. 787-790

Beadell, J. S.; Ishtiaq, F.; Covas, R.; Melo, M.; Warren, B. H.; Atkinson, C. T., Bensch, S., Graves, B. R., Jhala, J. V., Peirce, M. A.; Rahmani, A. R.; Fonseca, D. M. & Fleischer, R. C. (2006). Global phylogeographic limits of Hawaii's avian malaria. *Proceedings of the Royal Society of London* B, Vol. 273, pp. 2935–2944

Bell, A.S.; de Roode, J.C.; Sim, D. & Read, A.F. (2006). Within-host competition in genetically diverse malaria infections: parasite virulence and competitive success. *Evolution*, Vol. 60, pp. 1358–1371

Bennett, G. F., Peirce, M. A.& Ashford, R. W. (1993). Avian Haematozoa, mortality and pathogenicity. *Journal of Natural History* London, Vol. 26, pp. 993-1001

Bensch, S.; Stjernman, M.; Hasselquist, D.; Östman, O.; Hansson, B.; Westerdahl; H. & Pinheiro, R. T. (2000). Host specificity in avian blood parasites: a study of *Plasmodium* and *Haemoproteus* mitochondrial DNA amplified from birds. *Proceedings of the Royal Society of London* B, Vol. 267, pp. 1583- 1589

Bensch, S.; Pérez-Tris, J.; Waldensrtöm, J. & Hellgren, O. (2004). Linkage between nuclear and mitochondrial DNA sequences in avian malaria parasites: Multiple cases of cryptic speciation? *Evolution*, Vol. 58, pp. 1617-1621

Bensch, S.; Hellgren, O. & Pérez-Tris, J. (2009). MalAvi: A public database of malaria parasites and related haemosporidians in avian hosts based on mitochondrial cytochrome b lineages. *Molecular Ecology Resources*, Vol. 9, pp. 1353-1358

Blackburn, T.M.; Lockwood, J.L. & Cassey, P. (2009). *Avian Invasions. The ecology and evolution of exotic birds*. Oxford University Press, ISBN 978- 0199232550, Oxford, UK

Blossey, B. & Nötzold, R. (1995). Evolution of increased competitive ability in invasive nonindigenous plants: a hypothesis. *Journal of Ecology*, Vol. 83, pp. 887-889

Callaway, R. M. & Ridenour, W. M. (2004). Novel weapons: a biochemically based hypothesis for invasive success and the evolution of increased competitive ability. *Frontiers in Ecology and the Environment*, Vol. 2, pp. 436-433

Charleston, M.A. & Perkins, S.L. (2002). Lizards, malaria, and jungles in the Caribbean. In: *Tangled Trees: Phylogeny, Cospeciation, and Coevolution*, R.D.M. Page (Ed.),. Chicago University Press, pp. 65–92, ISBN 978-0226644677, Chicago, USA

Chen, M.; Shi, L. & Sullivan, D. Jr. (2001). *Haemoproteus* and *Schitosoma* synthesize heme polymers similar to *Plasmodium* hemozoin and β- hematin. *Molecular and Biochemical Parasitology*, Vol. 113, pp. 1-8

Colautti, R. I.; Ricciardi, A.; Grigorovich, I. A. & MacIsaac, H. J. (2004). Is invasion success explained by the enemy release hypothesis? *Ecology Letters*, Vol. 7, pp. 733

Danilewsky, V. (1889). Le parasitologie comparie du sang. I. Nouvelles recherches sur les parasites du sang des oiseaux. A. Dame, Kharkoff.

Davidar, P. & Morton, E. S. (2006). Are multiple infections more severe for purple martins (*Progne subis*) than single infections? *Auk*, Vol. 123, pp. 141–147

Dawson, R. D. & Bortolotti, G. R. (2000). Effects of hematozoan parasites on condition and return rates of American kestrels. *Auk*, Vol. 117, pp. 373-380.

Diamond, J. (1997). *Guns, germs, and steel: the fates of human societies*. Random House, ISBN 978-0393317558, New York, USA

Doré, A. B. (1918). Rat trypanosomes in New Zealand. *New Zealand Journal of Science and Technology* Vol. 1, pp.200

Dufva, R. (1996). Blood parasitism, health, reproductive success, and egg volume in female great tits *Parus major*. *Journal of Avian Biology*, Vol. 27, pp. 83-87

Dufva, R. & Allander, K. (1995). Intraespecific variation in plumage coloration reflects inmune response in great tit (*Parus major*) males. *Functional Ecology*, Vol. 9, pp. 785-789

Evans, M. & Otter, A. (1998). Fatal combined infection with *Haemoproteus noctuae* and *Leucocytozoon ziemanni* in juvenile snowy owls (*Nyctea scandiaca*). *Veterinary Records*, Vol. 143, pp. 72–76

Fairley, N. H. (1947). Sidelights of malaria in men obtained by subinoculation experiments. *Transactions of the Royal Society of Tropical Medicine and Hygiene*, Vol. 40, pp. 621-676

Fallis, A. M. & Desser, S. S. (1977). On species of *Leucocytozoon*, *Haemoproteus*, and *Hepatocystis*. In *Parasitic protozoa*, J.P. Kreier (Ed.), pp. 239-266, Academic Press, ISBN 0 04 591021 9, New York, USA

Fallon, S.M.; Ricklefs, R.E.; Latta, S.C. & Bermingham, E. (2004). Temporal stability of insular avian malarial parasite communities. *Proceedings of the Royal Society of London* B, Vol. 271, pp. 493–500

Fallon, S.; Fleischer, R. & Graves, G. (2006). Malarial parasites as geographical markers in migratory birds? *Biology Letters*, Vol. 2, pp.213–216

Fenwick, P. (1980). The effect of *Plasmodium berghei*, *Trypanosoma lewisi*, *Coryrebacterium parvum*, and *Mycobacterium bovis* (BCG) on the growth and survival of *Hymenolepis diminuta* in the rat. *Parasitology*, Vol. 81, pp. 175-183

Freed, L.A.; Cann, R.L.; Goff, M.L.; Kuntz, W.A. & Bodner, G.R. (2005). Increase in avian malaria at upper elevation in Hawai'I. *The Condor*, Vol. 107, pp. 753

Garvin, M. C.; Homer, B. L. & Greiner, E. C. (2003). Pathogenicity of *Haemoproteus danilewskyi*, Kruse, 1890, in blue jays (*Cyanocitta cristata*). *Journal of Wildlife Diseases*, Vol. 39, pp.161–169

Garamszegi, L. Z. (2011). Climate change increases the risk of malaria in birds. *Global Change Biology*, Vol. 17, pp. 1751–1759

Graham, A.L.; Lamb, T.J.; Read, A.F.& Allen, J.E. (2005). Malaria filaria co-infection in mice makes malarial disease more severe unless filarial infection achieves patency. *Journal of Infectious Diseases*, Vol. 191, pp. 410–421

Hellgren, O. (2005). The occurrence of haemosporidian parasites in the Fennoscandian bluethroat (*Luscinia svecica*) population. *Journal of Ornithology*, Vol. 146, pp. 55-60

Hobson, K.A.; McFarland, K.P.; Wassenaar, L.I.; Rimmer, C.C. & Goetz, J.E. (2001) Linking breeding and wintering grounds of Bicknell's thrushes using stable isotope analyses of feathers. *Auk*, Vol. 118, pp. 16–23

Hobson, K.A.; Bowen, G.; Wassenaar, L., Ferrand, Y. & Lormee, H. (2004). Using stable hydrogen and oxygen isotope measurements of feathers to infer geographical origins of migrating European birds. *Oecologia*, Vol. 141, pp. 477-488.

Hobson, K.A. (2005). Stable isotopes and the determination of avian migratory connectivity and seasonal interactions. *Auk*, Vol. 122, pp.1037-1048

Huijben, S.; Schaftenaar, W.; Wijsman, A.; Paaijmans, K. & Takken, W. (2007). Avian malaria in Europe: an emerging infectious disease? In: *Emerging pests and vector-borne diseases in Europe*, W. Takken & B.G.J. Knols (eds), 59 – 74, Wageningen Academic Publishers, ISBN 978-90-8686-053-1, Wageningen, The Netherlands

Ishtiaq, F.; Beadell, J.S.; Baker, A.J.; Rahmani, A.R.; Jhala, Y.V. & Fleischer, R. C. (2006). Prevalence and evolutionary relationships of haematozoan parasites in native versus introduced populations of common myna *Acridotheres tristis*. *Proceedings of the Royal Society of London* B, Vol. 273, pp. 587–594

Jarvi, S.I., Atkinson, C.T. & Fleischer, R.C. (2001). Immunogenetics and resistance to avian malaria in Hawaiian honeycreepers (Drepanidinae). *Studies in Avian Biology*, Vol. 22, pp. 254-263

Jovani, R. (2002). Malaria transmission, sex ratio and erythrocytes with two gametocytes. *Trends in Parasitology*, Vol. 18, pp. 537–539

Juhl, J. & Permin, A. (2002). The effect of *Plasmodium gallinaceum* on a challenge infection with *Ascaridia galli* in chickens. *Veterinary Parasitology*, Vol. 105, pp. 11-19

Keymer, A. E. & Read, A. F. (1991). Behavioural ecology: the impact of parasitism. In: *Parasite-host associations: coexistance or conflict*, C. A. Toft, A. Aeschlimann & L. Boils (Eds.), 37-61, Oxford University Press, ISBN 978-0198548348, Oxford, UK

Knowles, S. C. L., Palinauskas, V. & Sheldon, B. (2010). Chronic malaria infections increase family inequalities and reduce parental fitness: experimental evidence from a wild bird population. *Journal of Evolutionary Biology*, Vol. 23, pp. 557-569

Korpimäki, E., Hakkarainen, H. & Bennett, G. F. (1993). Blood parasites and reproductive success of Tengmalm´s owl: detrimental effects on females but not on males? *Functional Ecology*, Vol. 7, pp. 420-423

Korpimäki, E., Tolonen, P. & Bennett, G. F. (1995). Blood parasites, sexual selection and reproductive seccess of European kestrels. *Ecoscience*, Vol. 2, pp. 335-343

Krettli, A.U.; Andrade-Neto, V.F.; Brandao, M.G.L. & Ferrari, W.M.S. (2001). The search for new antimalarial drugs from plants used to treat fever and malaria or plants ramdomly selected: a review. *Memórias do Instituto Oswaldo Cruz*, Vol. 96, pp. 1033-1042

Krettli, A.U. (2009). Antimalarial drug discovery: screening of Brazilian medicinal plants and purified compounds. *Expert Opinion on Drug Discovery*, Vol. 4, pp. 1-14

Krettli, A.U.; Adebayo, J.O. & Krettli, L.G. (2009). Testing of Natural Products and Synthetic Molecules Aiming at New Antimalarials. *Current Drug Targets*, Vol. 10, pp. 261-270

Laird, M. (1995). Background and findings of the 1993-94 New Zealand mosquito survey. *New Zealand Entomologist*, Vol. 18, pp. 77-90

Levine, N.D. (1988). *The Protozoan Phylum Apicomplexa*. CRC Press, ISBN 978-0849346538, Boca Ratón, Florida, USA

Lima, M.R.; Simpson, L.; Fecchio, A. & Kyaw, C. (2010). Low prevalence of haemosporidian parasites in the introduced house sparrow (*Passer domesticus*) in Brazil. *Acta Parasitologica*, Vol. 55, pp. 297–303

Mac, M.J.; Opler, P.A.; Puckett Haecker, C.E. & Doran, P.D. (1998). *Hawaii and Pacific islands. Status and Trends of the Nation's Biological Resources*. U.S. Department of the Interior, U.S. Geological Survey, ISBN 978-0160532856, Reston, VA, USA

Mack, R.N.; Simberloff, D.; Lonsdale, W.M.; Evans, H., Clout, M. & Bazzaz, F.A. (2000). Biotic invasions: causes, epidemiology, global consequences and control. *Ecological Applications*, Vol. 10, pp. 10-689

MacLeod, C.J.; Duncan, R.P.; Parish, D.M.B.; Wratten, S.D. & Hubbard, S.F. (2005). Can increased niche opportunities and release from enemies explain the success of introduced yellowhammer populations in New Zealand? *Ibis*, Vol. 147, pp. 598– 607

Martínez-De-La-Puente, J.; Merino, S.; Tomás, G.; Moreno, J.; Morales, J.; Lobato, E.; García-Fraile, S. & Belda, E. J. (2010). The blood parasite *Haemoproteus* reduces survival in a wild bird: A medication experiment. *Biology Letters*, Vol. 6, pp. 663-665

Martinsen, E.S.; Perkins, S.L. & Schall, J.J. (2008). A three-genome phylogeny of malaria parasites (*Plasmodium* and closely related genera): Evolution of life-history traits and host switches. *Molecular Phylogenetics and Evolution*, Vol. 47, pp. 261-273

Marzal, A.; de Lope, F.; Navarro, C. & Møller, A. P. (2005). Malarial parasites decrease reproductive success: an experimental study in a passerine bird. *Oecologia*, Vol. 142, pp. 541-545

Marzal, A.; Bensch, S.; Reviriego, M.; Balbontín, J. & De Lope, F. (2008). Effects of malaria double infection in birds: one plus one is not two. *Journal of Evolutionary Biology*, Vol. 21, pp. 979-987

Marzal, A.; Ricklefs, R.E.; Valkiūnas, G.; Albayrak, T.; Arriero, E.; Bonneaud, C.; Czirják, G.A.; Ewen, J.; Hellgren, O.; Hořáková, D.; Iezhova, T.A.; Jensen, H.; Križanauskienė, A.; Lima, M.R.; de Lope, F.; Magnussen, E.; Martin, L.B.; Møller, A.P.; Palinauskas, V.; Pap, P.L.; Pérez-Tris, J.; Sehgal, R.N.; Soler, M.; Szöllősi, E.; Westerdahl, H.; Zetindjiev, P. & Bensch, S. (2011). Diversity, Loss, and Gain of Malaria Parasites in a Globally Invasive Bird. *PLoS ONE* Vol. 6, e21905, doi:10.1371/journal.pone.0021905

Merino, S.; Moreno, J.; Sanz, J. J. & Arriero, E. (2000). Are avian blood parasites pathogenic in the wild? A medication experiment in blue tits (*Parus caeruleus*). *Proceedings of the Royal Society of London*. B, Vol. 267, pp. 2507-2510

Mooney, H.A. & Cleland, E.E. (2001). The evolutionary impact of invasive species. *Proceedings of the National Academy of Sciences of the United States of America*, Vol. 98, pp. 5446-5451

Mu, J.; Joy, D.A.; Duan, J.; Huang, Y.; Carlton, J.; Walker, J.; Barnwell, J.; Beerli, P.; Charleston, M.A.; Pybus, O.G. & Su, X.Z. (2005). Host switch leads to emergence of *Plasmodium vivax* malaria in humans. *Molecular Biology and Evolution*, Vol. 22, pp. 1686–1693

McGhee, R. B.; Singh, S. D. & Weathersby, A. B. (1977). *Plasmodium gallinaceum*: vaccination in chickens. *Experimental Parasitology*, Vol. 43, pp. 231- 238

Pagenkopp, K.M.; Klicka, J.; Durrant, K.L.; Garvin, J.C. & Fleischer, R.C. (2008) Geographic variation in malarial parasite lineages in the common yellowthroat (*Geothlypis trichas*). *Conservation Genetics*, Vol. 9, pp. 1577–1588

Palinauskas, V.; Markovets, M.Yu; Kosarev, V.V.; Efremov, V.D.; Sokolov, L.V. & Valkiunas, G. (2005). Occurrence of avian haematozoa an Ekaterinburg and Ircutsk districts of Russia. *Ekologija* Vol. 4, pp. 8–12

Palinauskas, V.; Valkiūnas, G.; Bolshakov, V. C. & Bensch, S. (2008). Effects of *Plasmodium relictum* (lineage P-SGS1) on experimentally infected passerine birds. *Experimental Parasitology*, Vol. 120, pp. 372-380

Palinauskas, V.; Valkiūnas, G.; Križanauskienė, A.; Bensch, S. & Bolshakov, C. V. (2009). *Plasmodium relictum* (lineage P-SGS1): Further observation of effects on experimentally infected passeriform birds, with remarks on treatment with Malarone™. *Experimental Parasitology*, Vol. 123, pp. 134-139

Palinauskas V.; Valkiūnas G.; Bensch S. & Bolshakov V. C. (2011). *Plasmodium relictum* (lineage SGS1) and *Plasmodium ashfordi* (lineage GRW2): The effects of the co-infection on experimentally infected passerine birds. *Experimental Parasitology*, Vol. 127, pp. 527-533

Paul, R.E.; Nu, V.A.; Krettli, A.U. & Brey, P.T. (2002). Interspecific competition during transmission of two sympatric malaria parasite species to the mosquito vector. *Proceedings of the Royal Society of London.* B, Vol. 269, pp. 2551- 2557

Pérez-Tris, J. & Bensch, S. (2005). Diagnosing genetically diverse avian malaria infections using mixed-sequence analysis and TA-cloning. *Parasitology*, Vol. 131, pp. 1-9

Perez-Tris, J.; Hasselquist, D.; Hellgren, O.; Krizanauskiene, A.; Waldenstrom, J. & Bensch, S. (2005). What are malaria parasites? *Trends in Parasitology*, Vol.. 21, pp. 209–211

Perez-Tris, J.; Hellgren, O.; Krizanauskiene, A.; Waldenstrom, J.; Secondi, J.; Bonneaud, C.; Fjeldsa, J.; Hasselquist, D. & Bensch, S. (2007). Within-host speciation of malaria parasites. *PLoS ONE*, Vol. 2, pp. 1–7

Prenter, J.; MacNeil, C.; Dick, J. T. A. & Dunn, A. M. (2004). Roles of parasites in animal invasions. *Trends in Ecology and Evolution*, Vol. 19, pp. 385-390

Råberg, L; Graham, A. & Read, A.F. (2009). Decomposing health: tolerance and resistance to parasites in animals. *Proceedings of the Royal Society of London.* B, Vol. 364, pp. 37–49.

Rätti, O.; Dufva, R. & Alatalo, R. V. (1993). Blood parasites and male fitness in the pied flycatcher. *Oecologia*, Vol. 96, pp. 410-414

Rintamäki, P.T.; Ojanen, O., Pakkala, H. & Tynjälä, M. (1998). Blood parasites of migrating Willow Warblers (*Phylloscopus trochilus*) at a stopover site. *Canadian Journal of Zoology*, Vol. 76, pp.984–988

Roehl, W. (1926). Die Wirkung des Plasmochins auf die Vogelmalaria. *Naturwissenschaften*, Vol. 14, pp. 1156–1159

Sá, M. R. (2011). Studies of avian malaria and Brazil in the international scientific context (1907-1945). *História, Ciências, Saúde-Manguinhos*, Vol. 18, pp. 499-518

Sanz, J.J.; Arriero, E.; Moreno, J. & Merino, S. (2001). Interactions between hemoparasite status and female age in the primary reproductive output of Pied Flycatchers. *Oecologia*, Vol. 126, pp.339–344

Schall, J.J. (2002). Parasite virulence. In: *The Behavioural Ecology of Parasites*, E.E. Lewis, J.F. Cambell & M.V.K. Sukhdeo (Eds.), 283–313, CABI Publishing, ISBN 978-0851996158, Oxon, UK

Sergent, E. & Sergent E. (1921). Étude expérimentale du Paludisme des oiseaux à *Plasmodium relictum*, transmis par *Culex pipiens*. *Archives des Instituts Pasteur de l'Afrique du Nord*, Vol 1, pp. 1–32

Shwartz, A.; Strubbe, D.; Butler, C.J.; Matthysen, E. & Kark, S. (2009). The effect of enemy-release and climate conditions on invasive birds: a regional test using the Rose-ringed Parakeet (*Psittacula krameri*) as a case study. *Diversity and Distributions*, Vol. 15, pp. 310-318

Shurulinkov, P. & Ilieva, M. (2009). Spatial and temporal differences in the blood parasite fauna of passerine birds during the spring migration in Bulgaria. *Parasitology Research*, Vol. 104, pp. 1453—1458

Sillett, T. S. & Holmes, R.T. (2002). Variation in survivorship of a migratory songbird throughout its annual cycle. *Journal of Animal Ecology*, Vol. 71, pp. 296-308

Slater, L.B. (2009). *War and disease: biomedical research on malaria in the twentieth century*. Rutgers University Press, ISBN 978-0813544380, New Brunswick, NJ, USA

Spencer, K.A.; Buchanan, K.L.; Leitner, S.; Goldsmith, A.R. & Catchpole, C.K. (2005). Parasites affect song complexity and neural development in a songbird. *Proceedings of the Royal Society of London*. B, Vol. 272, pp. 2037–2043

Svennson, E.I. & Råberg, L. (2010). Resistance and tolerance in animal enemy–victim coevolution. *Trends in Ecology & Evolution*, Vol. 25, pp. 267-274

Sweeney, A. W. (2000). Wartime research on malaria chemotherapy. *Parassitologia*, Vol. 42, pp. 33-45

Tang, J.; Inoue, M.; Sunahara, T.; Kanda, M.; Kaneko, O. & Culleton, R. (2010) Intra-host dynamics of mixed species malaria parasite infections in mice and mosquitoes. *Malaria Journal*, Vol. 9, pp. O31

Taylor, L. H.;MacKinnon, M. J. & Read, A. (1998). Virulence of mixed-clone and single-clone infections of the rodent malaria *Plasmodium chabaudi*. *Evolution*, Vol. 52, pp. 583-591

TEEB. (2008). The Economics of Ecosystems and Biodiversity: An Interim Report', European Commission, Brussels. URL: www.teebweb.org/LinkClick.aspx?fileticket=u2fMSQoWJf0%3d&tabid=1278&language=en-US.

Tomás, G.; Merino, S.; Martínez, J.; Moreno, J. & Sanz, J. J. (2005). Stress protein levels and blood parasite infection in blue tits (*Parus caeruleus*): a medication field experiment. Annales Zoologici Fennici, Vol. 42, pp. 45-56

Tompkins, D.M. & Poulin, R. (2006). Parasites and biological invasions. In: *Biological Invasions in New Zealand* , R.B. Allen & W.G. Lee (Eds.),67-84, Springer-Verlag, ISBN 978-3-540-30022-9, Berlin Heidelberg, Germany

Torchin, M. E.; Lafferty, K. D.; Dobson, A. P.; McKenzie, V. J. & Kuris, A. M. (2003). Introduced species and their missing parasites. *Nature*, Vol. 421, pp. 628-630

Trager, W. (1950). Studies on the extracellular cultivation of an intracellular parasite (avian malaria). *The Journal of Experimental Medicine*, Vol. 92, pp. 349- 365

Valkiūnas, G. (2005). *Avian malaria parasites and other haemosporidia*. CRC Press, ISBN 978-0415300971, Boca Raton, Florida, USA

Valkiunas, G.; Anwar, A.M.; Atkinson, C.T.; Greiner, E.C.; Paperna, I. & Peirce, M.A. (2005). What distinguishes malaria parasites from other pigmented haemosporidians? *Trends in Parasitology*, Vol. 21, pp. 357–358

Valkiūnas, G.; Žičkus, T.; Shapoval, A. P. & Iezhova, T. A. (2006a). Effect of *Haemoproteus belopolskyi* (Haemosporida: Haemoproteidae) on body mass of the Blackcap *Sylvia atricapilla*. *Journal of Parasitology*, Vol. 92, pp. 1123–1125

Valkiūnas, G.; Bensch, S.; Iezhova, T. A.; Križanauskienė, A.; Hellgren, O. & Bolshakov, C. (2006b). Nested cytochrome b polymerase chain reaction diagnostics underestimate mixed infections of avian blood haemosporidian parasites: microscopy is still essential. *Journal of Parasitology*, Vol. 92, pp. 418–422

Van Riper III, C.; Van Riper, S. G.; Goff, M. L. & Laird, M. (1986). The epizootiology and ecological significance of malaria in Hawaiian land birds. *Ecological Monographs*, Vol. 56, pp. 327 – 344

von Rönn, J. (2010). *Migration and blood parasites in barn swallows*. PhD thesis, Max-Planck-Institute for Evolutionary Biology, Plön, Germany.

Wakelin, D. (1996). *Immunity to parasites: How parasitic infections are controlled*. Cambridge University Press, ISBN 978-0521436359, Cambridge, UK

Waldenström, J.; Bensch, S.; Kiboi, S.; Hasselquist, D. & Ottosson, U. (2002). Cross-species infection of blood parasites between resident and migratory songbirds in Africa. *Molecular Ecology*, Vol. 11, pp. 1545–1554

Wasielewski, T. K. W. N. (1904). *Studien und Mikrophotogramme zur Kenntnis der Pathogenen Protozoen*. Nabu Press, ISBN 978-1143527210, Leipzig, Germany.

Wassenaar, L.I. & Hobson, K.A. (2000). Stable-carbon and hydrogen isotope ratios reveal breeding origins of red-winged blackbirds. *Ecological Applications*, Vol. 10, pp. 911–916

Weatherhead, P. J. & Bennett, G. F. (1992). Ecology of parasitism of brown-headed cowbirds by haematozoa. *Canadian Journal of Zoology*, Vol. 70, pp. 1-7

Webster, M. S.; Marra, P. P.; Haig, S. M.; Bensch, S. & Holmes, R. T. (2002). Links between worlds: unravelling migratory connectivity. *Trends in Ecology and Evolution*, Vol. 17, pp. 76–83

Wilson, M.L. (2001). Ecology and infectious disease. In: *Ecosystem change and public health*, J. Aron, J.A. Patz (eds), 283-324, The Johns Hopkins University Press, ISBN 978-0801865824, Baltimore, USA

Yohannes, E.; Križanauskienė, A.; Valcu, M.; Bensch, S. & Kempenaers, B. (2008). Prevalence of malaria and related haemosporidian parasites in two shorebird species with different winter habitat distribution. *Journal of Ornithology*, Vol. 150, pp. 287-291

Zehtindjiev, P.; Ilieva, M.; Westerdahl, H.; Hansson, B.; Valkiūnas, G. & Bensch, S. (2008). Dynamics of parasitemia of malaria parasites in a naturally and experimentally infected migratory songbird, the great read warbler *Acrocephalus arundinaceus*. *Experimental Parasitology*, Vol. 119, pp. 99-110

6

Intraerythrocytic *Plasmodium falciparum* Growth in Serum-Free Medium with an Emphasis on Growth-Promoting Factors

Hiroko Asahi
Department of Parasitology,
National Institute of Infectious Diseases,
Japan

1. Introduction

Malaria remains a devastating disease, particularly in the tropics. The annual incidence of malaria worldwide is estimated to be between 294 and 500 million clinical cases, while estimates of annual mortality from malaria, caused largely by the protozoan *Plasmodium falciparum*, range from 0.97 to 2.7 million worldwide (World Malaria Report 2010[1], World Health Organization; Snow et al., 2005). The emergence of resistance to conventional antimalarial drugs and insecticides means that new chemotherapeutic approaches with alternative targets are needed (Ridley, 2002). Better understandings of antimalarial drugs and the biology of the parasites are needed to allow the development of new medications.

A review of the impact of continuous cultures of *P. falciparum* underscores their significant contributions to malaria research (Trager & Jensen, 1997). The mechanisms responsible for the growth of the parasite, however, remain largely unknown. Culture media for *P. falciparum* require human serum, a growth-promoting fraction derived from adult bovine plasma (GFS), or lipid-enriched bovine albumin (Asahi & Kanazawa, 1994; Asahi et al., 1996; Cranmer et al. 1997; Jensen, 1979). Elucidation of the factors able to induce the growth of *P. falciparum* could be of help, not only for successful culture of the parasite, but also for providing critical clues to understanding the biology of parasite proliferation during the erythrocytic phase.

In order to identify the factors controlling parasite development, and the effects of growth-promoting factors on the parasite, we initially investigated growth-promoting substances to formulate a chemically defined culture medium (CDM) suitable for sustaining the complete development and intraerythrocytic growth of *P. falciparum*. We also developed a simple and sensitive flow-cytometry-based assay for following each developmental stage of the parasite's erythrocytic growth. The distinct roles of the growth-promoting factors in the growth of *P. falciparum* were then investigated.

---

[1]http://www.who.int/malaria/world_malaria_report_2010/en/index.htm

2. Parasites and culture

Cultures of the FCR3/FMG (ATCC Catalogue No. 30932, Gambia) strain of *P. falciparum* were used in all experiments. The parasites were routinely maintained using *in vitro* culture techniques. The culture medium was devoid of whole serum, and consisted of basal medium supplemented with 10% GFS (Daigo's GF21; Wako Pure Chemical Industries, Japan), as previously reported (Asahi, 2009; Asahi & Kanazawa, 1994; Asahi et al., 1996; Asahi et al., 2005; Asahi et al., 2011). This complete medium is referred to as GFSRPMI. The basal medium consisted of RPMI-1640 containing 2 mM glutamine, 25 mM 4-(2-hydroxylethyl)-piperazine ethanesulfonic acid, 24 mM $NaHCO_3$ (Invitrogen Ltd., USA), 25 µg/ml gentamycin (Sigma-Aldrich Corp., USA) and 150 µM hypoxanthine (Sigma-Aldrich). Briefly, erythrocytes (RBC) were preserved in Alsever's solution (Sigma-Aldrich; Asahi et al., 1996) for 3–30 days. They were then washed, dispensed into 24-well culture plates at a hematocrit (% of packed RBC in medium) of 2% (1 ml of suspension/well), and cultured in a humidified atmosphere of 5% CO_2, 5% O_2, and 90% N_2 at 37°C. For subculture, 3-4 days after inoculation, infected RBC and uninfected RBC were washed. Parasitemia (% of infected RBC in total RBC) was adjusted to 0.1% (for subculture) or 0.4% (for growth tests), by adding uninfected RBC, and the hematocrit was adjusted to 2% by adding the appropriate volume of either GFSRPMI or the test medium. The cultures were synchronized at the ring stage by three successive exposures to 5% (w/v) D-sorbitol (Sigma-Aldrich) at 41- and 46-h intervals. After the third sorbitol treatment, residual schizonts and cell debris were removed by isopycnic density centrifugation on 63% Percoll PLUS (GE Healthcare Bio-Science Corp., USA). The current cultivation method remains essentially the same as initially described (Jensen, 2002), with a few refinements, particularly in terms of the culture medium. The growth experiments were performed by replacing GFSRPMI with test samples. Growth rate was estimated by dividing the parasitemia of the test sample after incubation by the initial parasitemia.

3. CDM for continuous intraerythrocytic growth of *P. falciparum* using lipids

The *P. falciparum* parasite develops through three distinct stages within RBC during its cycle of approximately 48 h: ring, trophozoite, and schizont (Bannister et al., 2000). However, the development of *P. falciparum* requires the presence of currently unknown factors present in human serum (Jensen, 1979). Although numerous studies have attempted to identify the factors and substances able to sustain parasite growth (Asahi & Kanazawa, 1994; Asahi et al., 1996, 2005; Cranmer et al., 1997; Divo and Jensen. 1982; Lingnau et al., 1994; Mi-Ichi et al., 2006; Nivet et al., 1983; Ofulla et al., 1993; Willet and Canfield, 1984), the establishment of a fully-defined culture medium for the parasite has represented a major challenge. We previously reported that GFS supported intraerythrocytic growth of *P. falciparum* (Asahi and Kanazawa, 1994; Asahi et. al., 1996; Asahi et al., 2005). GFS contains lipid-rich albumin as a major component. Similarly, Cranmer et al. (1997) described a commercially available lipid-enriched bovine albumin (Albumax II; Invitrogen) that could replace human serum for the *in vitro* cultivation of *P. falciparum*. These serum substitutes are currently widely employed to maintain parasite cultures. However, there is still insufficient information on these indispensable additives to allow direct identification of the functional components required for the growth of *P. falciparum*. The replacement of human serum or GFS in culture medium with chemically- or functionally-defined substances could not only be advantageous for parasite culture, but could also provide critical clues about the parasite's biology and its requirements for proliferation at the erythrocyte stage. To establish a CDM for continuous, intraerythrocytic growth of *P. falciparum*, we initially characterized the ability of the various components of GFS to sustain parasite growth (Asahi et al., 2005). Based on these results, we subsequently determined the ability of structurally defined chemicals to sustain parasite growth, and formulated a CDM for *P. falciparum* growth (Asahi, 2009).

3.1 The ability of GFS components to sustain parasite growth

We investigated the components of GFS and related substances that have shown an ability to sustain parasite growth (Asahi et al., 2005). A simple total lipid fraction of GFS obtained by lipid extraction has been shown to sustain complete parasite development. However, specific proteins such as bovine and human albumin, as well as the simple total lipid fraction of GFS, have also been shown to be important (Figure 1a). The simple total lipid fraction of GFS contained phospholipids, diacylglycerides (DAG), cholesterol, monoglycerides, nonesterified fatty acids (NEFA) and cholesteryl esters. The components of the NEFA fraction were mainly *cis*-9-octadecenoic acid (C18:1-*cis*-9, 43%), hexadecanoic acid

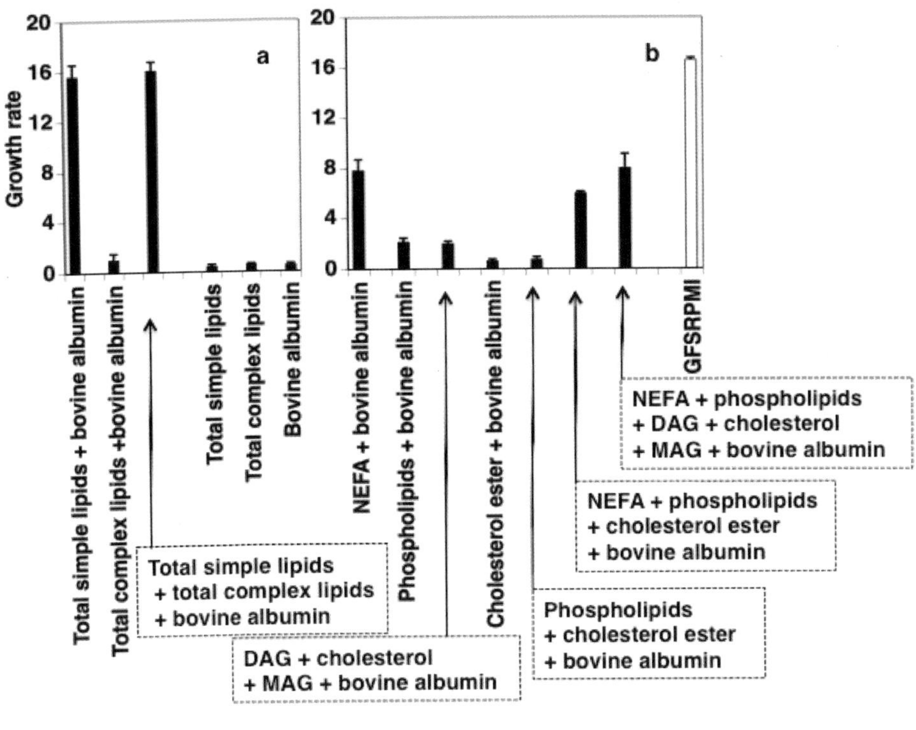

Fig. 1. Abilities of fractions derived from GFS (a) and a total simple lipid fraction of GFS (b) to sustain growth of *P. falciparum*. Growth rate was estimated 4 days after inoculation.

(C16:0, 21%), octadecanoic acid (C18:0, 14%), *cis,cis*-9,12-octadecadienoic acid (C18:2), *cis*-9-hexadecenoic acid (C16:1), *cis*-5,8,11,14-eicosatetraenoic acid (C20:4), *cis*-5,8,11,14,17-eicosapentaenoic acid (C20:5), and *cis*-4,7,10,13,16,19-docosahexaenoic acid (C22:6). Each NEFA enriched with bovine albumin (fatty-acid free) was tested for its ability to promote parasite growth. Mixtures of NEFA, but not individual NEFA, sustained parasite growth to a low extent (Figure 1b), but parasite growth in the presence of various combinations of NEFA was still lower than that achieved with a simple total lipid fraction of GFS, or with GFS- or human serum-containing medium. These results implied that, although the NEFA components of the simple total lipid fraction are functional factors in promoting parasite growth, other factor (s) must also contribute to the high growth-promoting activity of GFS.

3.2 CDM for intraerythrocytic growth of *P. falciparum*

Initial experiments designed to determine the factor (s) responsible for the high growth-promoting activity of GFS involved culture of *P. falciparum* with the lipid classes found in the simple total lipid fraction of GFS, and different concentrations of a mixture of the two most abundant NEFA, C18:1-*cis*-9 (0–60 μg/ml [212.4 μM]) and C16:0 (0–30 μg/ml [117.0 μM]) at a ratio of 2:1. The growth rate was dependent on the concentrations of the NEFA in the mixture: the maximum effect was obtained with 30 μg/ml C18:1-*cis*-9 plus 15 μg/ml C16:0, with declines at lower and higher concentrations. However, the growth rates were much lower than that obtained with a simple total lipid fraction of GFS or with GFSRPMI.

A mixture of all the constituents detected in a simple total lipid fraction of GFS sustained complete parasite growth. In an attempt to identify the factor (s) responsible for this growth-promoting effect, each lipid was omitted from the medium in turn. Parasite growth in the absence of phosphatidylcholine (PC) decreased to a level similar to that seen with the NEFA mixture (Figure 2a). Phospholipids were also tested for their possible efficacies in augmenting the ability of NEFA to promote parasite growth, by adding each phospholipid to cultures with NEFA. Phospholipids, even PC alone, markedly amplified the growth-promoting ability of the NEFA mixture (Figure 2b). These results indicate the critical importance of PC for amplifying the parasite-growth-promoting ability of NEFA mixtures. Phospholipids other than PC, such as phosphatidylethanolamine (PE), phosphatidylserine (PS), and phosphatidic acid (PA), were also beneficial for parasite growth, while the growth rates in the absence of phosphatidylinositol (PI), cholesterol, and cholesterol ester were significantly higher (Figure 2a), indicating these phospholipids were detrimental. DAG had no effect on the growth rate of the parasite at the concentrations tested.

The effects of various types of NEFA mixtures enriched with phospholipids were tested for their abilities to promote parasite growth. The growth rate was dependent on the ratios of the two NEFA; the highest growth rate occurred at 2:1 (C18:1-*cis*-9 to C16:0) at a total concentration of 45 μg/ml. The growth rates with the best mixtures of NEFA in the presence of phospholipids were significantly higher than those with the same NEFA in the absence of phospholipids (Figure 3). The culture media were also reconstituted by mixing phospholipids with two types of NEFA (either C18:1-*cis*-9 plus a saturated NEFA or C16:0 plus an unsaturated NEFA). The best combination of NEFA was C18:1-*cis*-9 plus C16:0, followed by *cis*-11-octadecenoic acid (C18:1-*cis*-11) plus C16:0, C18:1-*cis*-9 plus pentadecanoic acid (C15:0), C18:1-*cis*-9 plus C18:0, and C18:1-*cis*-9 plus tetradecanoic acid (C14:0). The combinations of C16:1 plus C16:0, *cis*-6-octadecenoic acid (C18:1-*cis*-6) plus

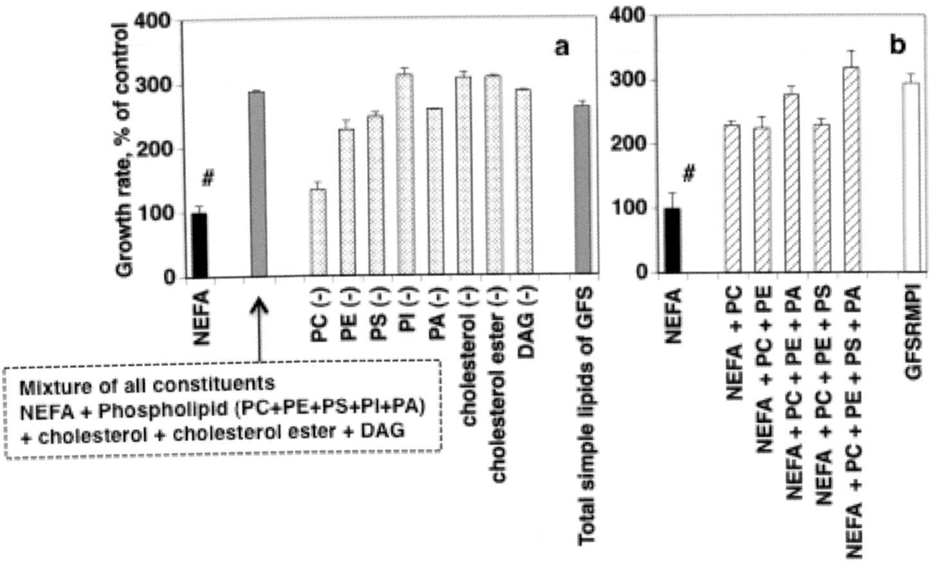

Fig. 2. Effects of various classes of lipids and combinations of phospholipids on abilities of NEFA to sustain growth of *P. falciparum.* The combination of 30 µg/ml C18:1-*cis*-9 and 15 µg/ml C16:0 served as a control. Growth rate was estimated 4 days after inoculation.

C16:0, *cis*-13-octadecenoic acid (C18:1-*cis*-13) plus C16:0, and C18:2 plus C16:0 showed similar growth-promoting effects to that seen with C18:1-cis-9 plus C16:0 in the absence of phospholipids. Combinations of C18:1-*cis*-9 plus dodecanoic acid (C12:0), C18:1-*cis*-9 plus docosanoic acid (C22:0), *cis,cis,cis*-6,9,12-octadecatrienoic acid (C18:3) plus C16:0, C20:4 plus C16:0, C20:5 plus C16:0, and C22:6 plus C16:0 were detrimental to parasite growth. The combination of *trans*-9-octadecenoic acid (C18:1-*trans*-9) plus C16:0 also deterred parasite growth (Figure 4). The efficacies of NEFA in sustaining the growth of *P. falciparum* thus varied markedly, depending on the type, total amount, and combinations used; saturated or unsaturated NEFA with longer or shorter carbon-chain lengths than the optimal combination (C18:1-*cis*-9 plus C16:0) promoted growth to lesser extents, or were detrimental to the growth of *P. falciparum*. Higher degrees of unsaturation were also detrimental to parasite growth. The growth-promoting effects of NEFA with 18 carbons and one double bond are specific to the *cis*-form, and the position of the double bond in these NEFA influences their growth-promoting effects.

Various PC containing different fatty acid moieties, such as two of hexanoic acid, C12:0, C14:0, C16:0, C18:1, C18:1 in racemic form, C18:2, and C20:4, two different fatty acids of C18:1 and C16:0, and C20:4 and C16:0, and PC derived from soy beans and egg yolk, were tested at graded concentrations ranging from 20–320 µM, for their abilities to augment the effects of the NEFA mixture on parasite growth. Among the 12 tested PC, 1,2-dioleoyl-sn-glycero-3-phosphocholine (PC-di18:1) markedly amplified the growth-promoting ability of the NEFA mixture in a dose-dependent manner and over a wide range of concentrations, to a level similar to that seen with GFSRPMI (Figure 5). This was followed by 1,2-dipalmitoyl-sn-glycero-3-phosphocholine (PC-di16:0) and 2-oleoyl-1-palmitoyl-sn-glycero-3-phosphocholine (PC-18:1/16:0). The addition of PC other than PC-di18:1 at certain concentrations also augmented the growth-promoting ability of the NEFA mixture to various extents, ranging from 0–270%.

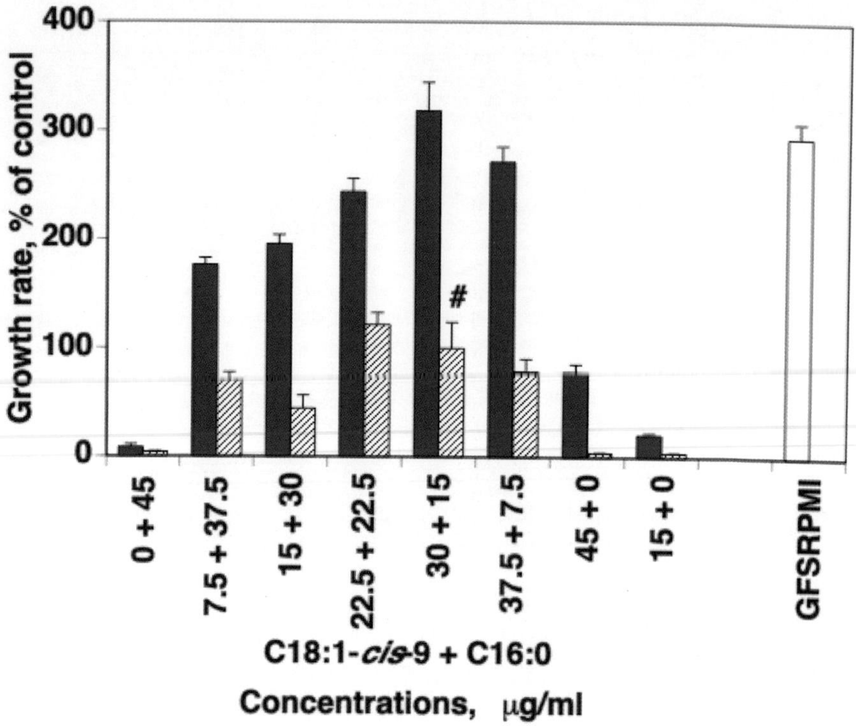

Fig. 3. Growth of *P. falciparum* with NEFA (C18:1-*cis*-9 plus C16:0) in the presence (■) or absence (▨) of phospholipids. Growth rate was estimated 4 days after inoculation. #, A paired NEFA of C18:1-*cis*-9 and C16:0 served as a control.

Specific proteins such as bovine and human albumin were shown to be required for *P. falciparum* growth in serum-free culture with lipids, as stated above. Recombinant human albumin could replace serum albumin for sustaining parasite growth in the presence of lipids (Figure 6).

All stages of *P. falciparum* cultured in the formulated CDM containing the best combination of two NEFA, phospholipids, and human, bovine, or recombinant albumin were morphologically indistinguishable from growth in complete medium (Figure 7).

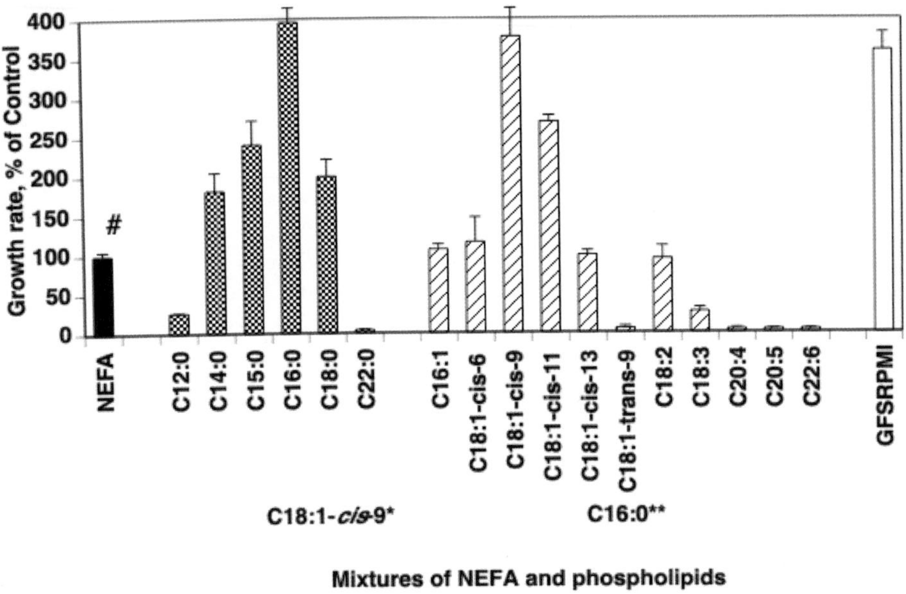

Fig. 4. Growth of *P. falciparum* in the presence of various combinations of paired NEFA. Each saturated NEFA was added at 15 μg/ml in the presence of 30 μg/ml C18:1-*cis*-9 (*) and each unsaturated NEFA at 30 μg/ml in the presence of 15 μg/ml C16:0 (**). These culture media contained phospholipids. #, NEFA (C18:1-*cis*-9 + C16:0) in the absence of phospholipids served as a control. Growth rate was estimated 4 days after inoculation.

4. Development of a measure of intraerythrocytic growth of *P. falciparum* using flow cytometry and SYBR Green I

Growth-promoting and antimalarial effects on plasmodia can be assessed both quantitatively and qualitatively by directly examining RBC smears from blood or cultures under a microscope; however, this method is tedious and subjective. Numerous novel *in vitro* assays have been introduced that are more objective, faster, more sensitive, and designed to be easier to handle. The most common of these include isotopic, enzymatic, and enzyme-linked immunosorbent assays (ELISA) (Noedl et al., 2003). Isotopic assays rely on the incorporation of radioactive ^{3}H-hypoxanthine into the parasite DNA (Noedl et al., 2003; Webster et al., 1985; Yayon et al., 1983). These methods are relatively reliable and objective, but not sufficiently sensitive, and require the use of hazardous radioactive material. The assays are well suited for screening large numbers of compounds. Parasite lactate dehydrogenase levels have also been used to assess the growth of malarial parasites (Asahi, et al., 2005; Makler and Hinrichs, 1993; Noedl et al., 2003). ELISA-based assays can provide measures of parasite growth by quantifying biomolecules produced during parasite development, such as histidine-rich protein 2 or parasite lactate dehydrogenase, by double-site sandwich ELISA (Druihe, et al., 2001; Noedl et al., 2002; Noedl et al., 2003). ELISA-based tests are rapid and easy to perform, and are also well suited for the screening of large number of drugs. These methods have been widely employed to detect and analyze the growth of parasites, although they are poorly suited for discriminating the developmental stages of the parasite in parasitized RBC. Flow cytometry using nucleic acid staining offers the possibility of studying the cell cycle and developmental stages of intraerythrocytic growth of malaria parasites. Flow cytometric analysis using intercalating dyes, such as acridine orange, thiazole orange, hydroethidine, propidium iodine, YOYO-1, and SYTO-16, has already been used successfully to test human and murine samples (Barkan et al., 2000; Janse and Van Vianen, 1994; Jimenez-Diaz et al., 2009; Jouin et al., 1995; Li et al., 2007; Nyakeriga, 2004; Persson et al., 2006). However, the use of flow cytometry has been limited by its lack of specificity and the complicated preparation required. We modified the flow cytometry system and introduced SYBR Green I as an intercalating dye, allowing the growth and development of *P. falciparum* to be analyzed with a high degree of accuracy (Izumiyama et al., 2009).

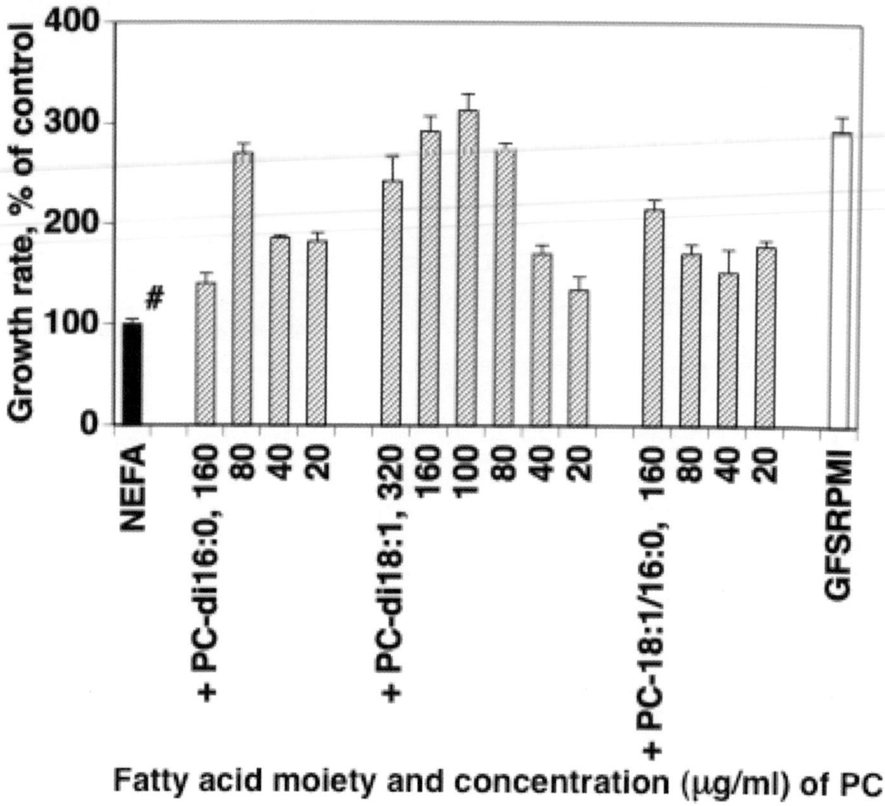

Fig. 5. Effects of various types of PC containing different fatty acid moieties on the abilities of NEFA to sustain growth of *P. falciparum*. Growth rate was estimated 4 days after inoculation. #, A paired NEFA of C18:1-*cis*-9 and C16:0 served as a control.

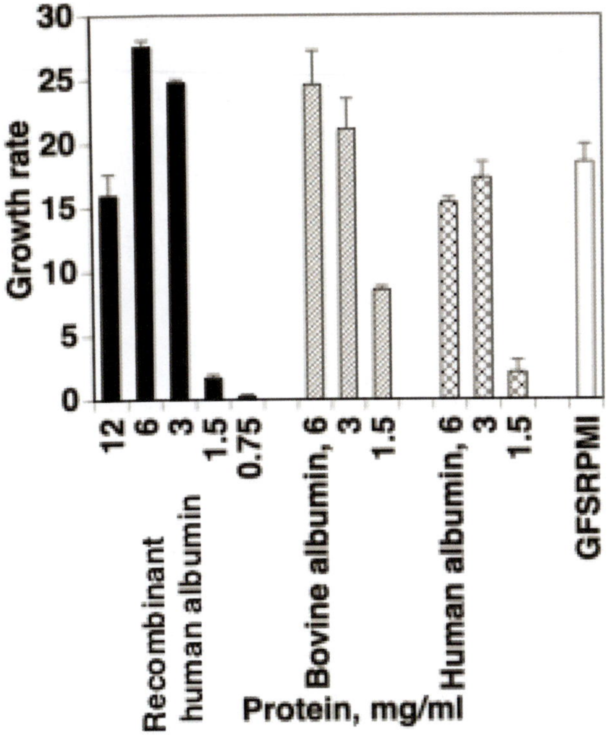

Fig. 6. Effects of various proteins on the ability of a mixture of NEFA and phospholipids to sustain growth of *P. falciparum*. Growth rate was estimated by dividing the parasitemia of the test sample 4 days after inoculation by the initial parasitemia.

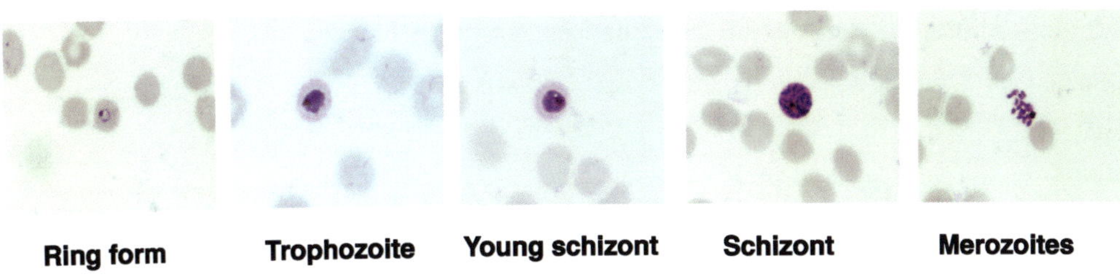

Fig. 7. Different stages of the parasite cultured in the formulated CDM, stained with Giemsa.

4.1 Optimization of flow cytometric measurement of infected RBC with SYBR Green I

The cytometer was equipped with a single argon-ion laser tuned to a fluorescence excitation of 488 nm for 15 mW output (PAS flow cytometer, Partec Co. Ltd., Germany). A FACSCalibur (Becton Dickinson Immunocytometry Systems, USA) was also used with a single fluorescence measurement (530 nm). Analysis was performed using FCS express software (De Novo Software Inc., Canada).

In order to distinguish infected RBC or merozoites from platelets, leukocytes, and RBC debris by flow cytometry, it is essential for them to retain their normal morphological characteristics and membrane integrity, without disruption. We evaluated the effects of (1) fixatives, (2) dilution buffer and concentration range of SYBR Green I, and (3) staining period on the intensity of fluorescence of infected RBC. (1) Infected RBC in culture were fixed using fixatives such as 1% paraformaldehyde or 1% glutaraldehyde in Tris-saline solution (20 mM Tris (hydroxymethyl) aminomethane hydrochloride at pH 7.2 and 138 mM NaCl), phosphate-buffered saline (PBS) (10 mM phosphate buffer at pH 7.2 and 138 mM NaCl), or Alsever's solution. Paraformaldehyde combined with Alsever's solution proved the most useful fixative, with no noticeable lysis or deformity of infected/uninfected RBC, such as often occurs when Tris-saline or PBS is used to dilute fixatives. (2) Concentration ranges and dilution buffers for SYBR Green I were tested to determine the optimal solution for producing clearly resolved peaks of fluorescence. Individual peaks in histograms corresponding to the development stages of infected RBC showed most clearly with SYBR Green I diluted at concentrations ranging from 0.00625–2× in Tris-saline at pH 8.8 (SYBR Green I-basic). Both fixed and unfixed infected RBC gave the best results at 1× dilution of SYBR Green I. (3) The dependence of fluorescence with time for fixed or unfixed infected RBC in SYBR Green I-basic at 1× dilution was evaluated over 30 min by time-curve analysis of *P. falciparum* cultures. The frequency distribution of fluorescence was similar after staining for 5 min or longer with SYBR Green I-basic, although fluorescence could be detected within seconds after addition of the fluorescent stain to fixed or unfixed infected RBC. SYBR Green I in Tris-saline at pH 6.8 and PBS resulted in inadequate signals for infected RBC stained for less than 30 min, and in deformation and hemolysis of infected RBC. Accordingly, the optimized protocol was fixation of infected/uninfected RBC by the addition of 1% paraformaldehyde combined with Alsever's solution, and staining the fixed RBC, at measure by flow cytometry, by adding into SYBR Green I-basic solution containing SYBR Green I at x1 dilution for 5 min.

4.2 Visualization of infected RBC populations with SYBR Green I-basic

Infected RBC populations were stained as described above. All developmental stages were clearly stained with SYBR Green I with no autofluorescence of RBC (Figure 8).

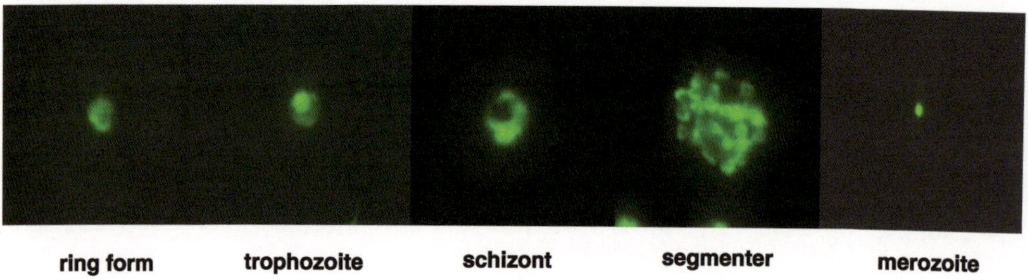

Fig. 8. Developmental stages of *P. falciparum* stained with SYBR Green I-basic.

Infected RBC were stained with SYBR Green I-basic by adding 8 x 10^5 cells into 1 ml staining solution, followed by analysis with flow cytometry. SYBR Green I-basic provided brilliant resolution of infected versus uninfected RBC and permitted visualization of infected RBC populations with high accuracy. Infected RBC were located as three clusters in two-parameter dot-plot presentations of infected/uninfected RBC from *P. falciparum* cultures: (1) cluster 1 (C1) contained predominantly ring forms with low DNA content (low fluorescence intensity); (2) cluster 2 (C2) contained predominantly late trophozoites and young schizonts with moderate DNA content (moderate fluorescence intensity); and (3) cluster 3 (C3) contained late schizonts and segmenters with high DNA content (high fluorescence intensity) (Figures 9a, b).

In regular cultures, schizonts burst spontaneously to release free merozoites, which then enter new RBC and increase the number of infected RBC. While the majority of released free merozoites remain in culture for a while, the merozoites after culture indicate the completion of schizogony. Parasites were synchronized at the ring form stage and cultured over 45 h under the pressure of various concentrations of the anti-schizogony drug chloroquine, to confirm the accuracy of counting the number of merozoites by flow cytometry. Merozoites released from mature schizonts were counted clearly and sensitively by flow cytometry (Figures 10a,b).

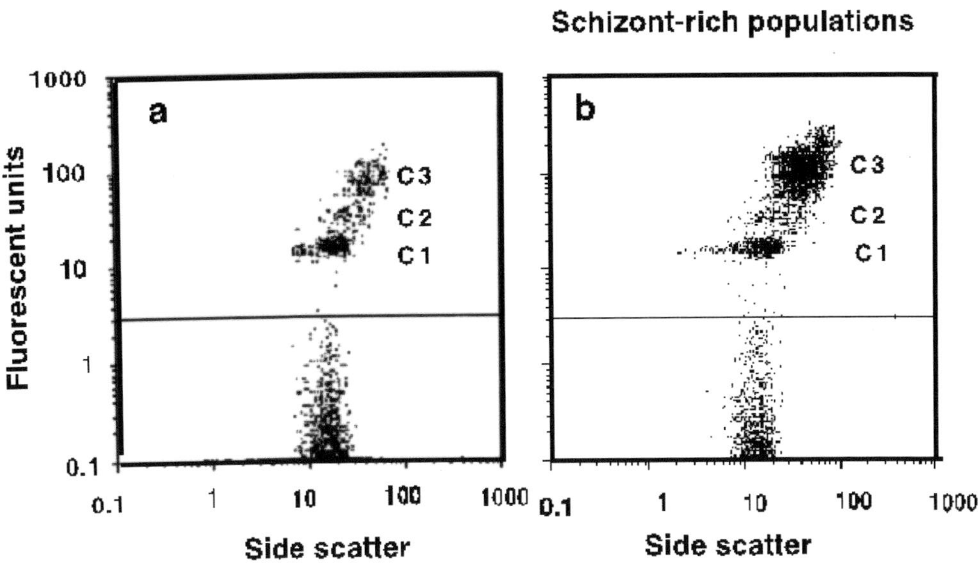

Fig. 9. Two-parameter dot-plot representation of fluorescent units and side scatter from asynchronous culture (a) of *P. falciparum* and schizont-rich populations (b) separated by Percoll sedimentation.

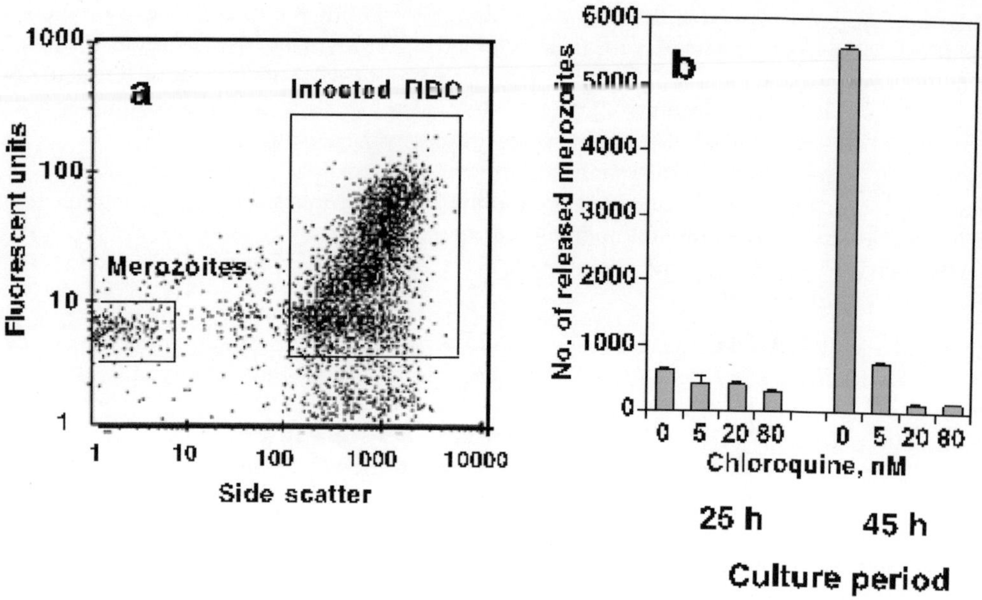

Fig. 10. Merozoites released into surrounding medium were counted (a) and the number of merozoites decreased under the pressure of graded concentrations of chloroquine (b). The numbers of merozoites are shown per 5,000 infected RBC (b).

5. Differing effects of NEFA and phospholipids on intraerythrocytic growth of *P. falciparum* in serum-free medium

The efficacies of NEFA in sustaining general growth of *P. falciparum* varied markedly, depending on the type, total amount, and combinations. Certain structural characteristics of NEFA, such as carbon-chain length, degree and position of unsaturation, and isomerism were important. However, the mechanisms responsible for the different abilities of the various NEFA in the presence or absence of phospholipids, and of specific proteins such as bovine and human albumin for promoting parasite growth are unknown. Subsequent experiments therefore investigated the distinct effects of various NEFA on each developmental stage of *P. falciparum*, including schizogony, merozoite formation, and reinvasion of RBC, to provide clues to the mechanisms underlying the growth-promoting properties of NEFA.

5.1 Four typical growth patterns

To assess the effects of NEFA on each developmental stage of the parasite (schizogony, merozoite formation, and reinvasion of RBC), synchronized *P. falciparum* were cultured in the presence of phospholipids and bovine albumin, further supplemented with one or two NEFA. The distribution of the parasites among the different developmental stages was determined using flow cytometry with SYBR Green I-basic at 25 and 45 h during the first cycle of growth (Izumiyama et al., 2009). Late schizonts at 25 h (schizont-25h), released merozoites at 45 h (released merozoite-45h), new ring forms at 45 h (ring form-45h), and parasitemia at 45 h (parasitemia-45h) were compared between parasites grown under test conditions and those grown in complete medium GFSRPMI. Different types and combinations of NEFA exerted markedly distinct effects on parasite growth in the presence/absence of phospholipids. Four typical growth patterns were defined: no inhibition (comparable to growth in complete medium); and three rate-determining steps in growth including suppressed schizogony (SS); suppressed formation of merozoites (SMF); and inhibited invasion of merozoites into new RBC (IMI)/formation of incomplete merozoites (Figure 11).

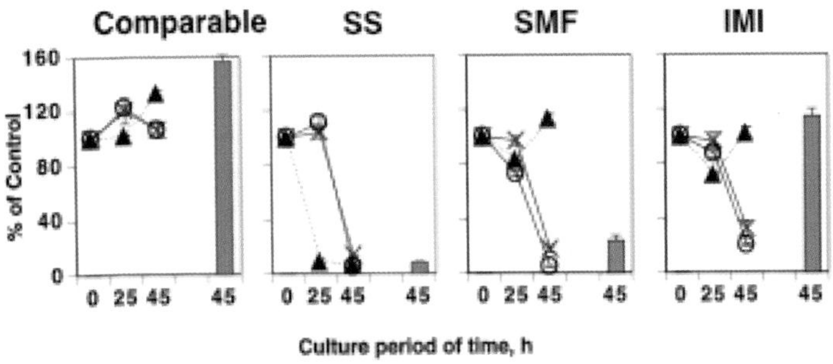

Schizont-25h	High	Low	High	Moderate~High
Released merozoite-45h	High	Low	Low	High
Ring form-45h	High	Low	Low	Low
Parasitemia-45h	High	Low	Low	Low

Fig. 11. Representative modification of growth of *P. falciparum* cultured synchronously in the presence of various growth promoters, indicating comparable growth, SS, SMF, and IMI. Each developmental stage was compared with complete growth in GFSRPMI (control): ring forms (—○—), late schizonts (...▲...), parasitemia (—X—), and released merozoites (closed bars). Parasites at the ring stage (adjusted to 5.0% parasitemia) were maintained in different culture media.

5.2 Growth-rate-determining steps in development of *P. falciparum* cultured in various growth factors

All stages of the parasite cultured in medium supplemented with NEFA (C18:1-*cis*-9 plus C16:0) in the presence of phospholipids were comparable to those grown in GFSRPMI. Medium containing C18:1-*cis*-9 and C12:0 caused parasites to accumulate in clusters of ring forms, by an SS effect. SS was also observed in the presence of C16:0 alone, C18:2 plus C16:0, C20:4 plus C16:0, or C18:1-*trans*-9 plus C16:0. Partial SS (less suppressed) was detected when the mixture of C18:1-*cis*-13 plus C16:0 was added. C18:1-*cis*-9 alone and C18:1-*cis*-9 plus C22:0 suppressed the progression of parasites to merozoites following schizont formation, by an SMF effect. SMF was also observed in parasites cultured in C18:1-*cis*-9 plus C16:0 in the absence of phospholipids, indicating that exogenous phospholipids were crucial for the development of complete merozoites. Adding C18:1-*cis*-13 plus C16:0 or C16:1 plus C16:0 to the media caused accumulation of the merozoites released from mature schizonts, but the merozoites did not invade new RBC, by the IMI effect. Partial IMI (less inhibited) was detected when C18:1-*cis*-9 plus C14:0, C18:1-*cis*-6 plus C16:0, C18:1-*cis*-11 plus C16:0, or C18:1-*cis*-9 plus C18:0 were added. Any effects on steps that governed parasite growth rate disrupted the cyclic behavior of the parasite, and reduced parasitemia at 45 h culture. These results indicate that different NEFA exert distinct roles in parasite development by arresting development at different stages (Figure 12).

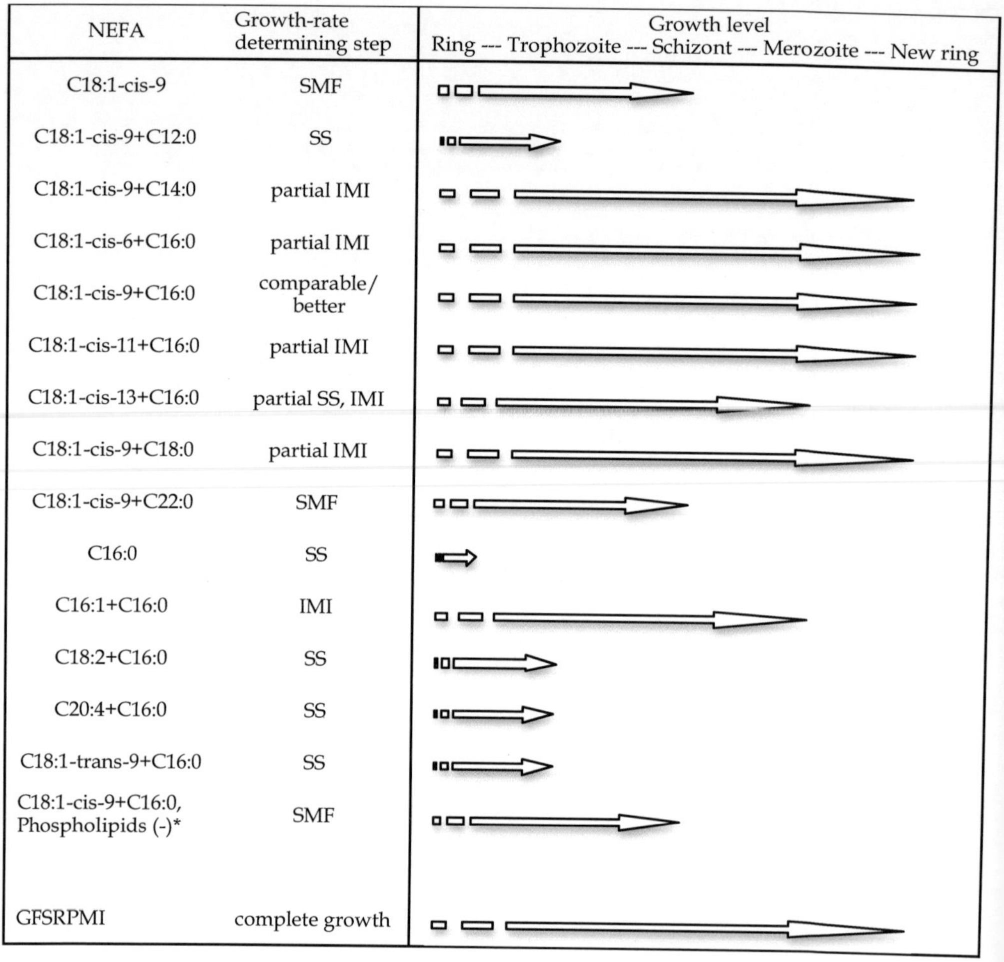

Fig. 12. Growth-rate-determining step and growth level in development of *P. falciparum* cultured in the presence of NEFA alone or in combination. Growth of the parasite was examined in the presence of optimal phospholipids, except for C18:1-*cis*-9 plus C16:0 in the absence of phospholipids (*) and GFSRPMI. Bovine albumin was added to the medium, except for GFSRPMI.

5.3 Microscopic examination of *P. falciparum* cultured with NEFA exerting IMI and SMF effects

Microscopic examination revealed that parasites cultured in medium containing NEFA (C18:1-*cis*-9 plus C16:0), phospholipids and bovine albumin closely resembled parasites grown in GFSRPMI. In contrast, the majority of ring forms cultured in media containing C16:1 plus C16:0 or C18:1-*cis*-13 plus C16:0 (IMI effect) for 45 h were devoid of normal structures. The majority of schizonts cultured in media containing C18:1-*cis*-9 alone, C18:1-*cis*-9 plus C22:0, C18:1-*cis*-9 plus C16:0 in the absence of phospholipids (SMF effect) for 45 h were found to be degenerate (Figure 13).

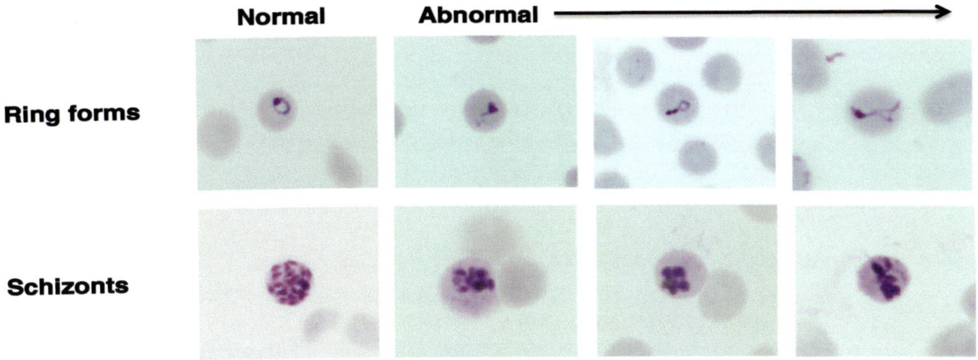

Fig. 13. Abnormal parasites (ring forms and schizonts) grown in non-optimal culture media.

6. Conclusions and future perspectives

In an attempt to elucidate the mechanisms responsible for growth of *P. falciparum*, growth-promoting factors were identified and a CDM suitable for complete growth of the parasite was established. The CDM consists of paired NEFA, phospholipids with specific fatty acid moieties, and specific proteins dissolved in basal medium RPMI1640 supplemented with hypoxanthine. The most effective combination of NEFA was C18:1-*cis*-9 and C16:0. The best phospholipid crucial for serum-free culture medium supplemented with NEFA was PC-di18:1 at concentrations of 80–320 μg/ml. A simple protocol for flow cytometry with SYBR Green I was developed and used to analyze the various developmental stages of *P. falciparum*. Different stages of the parasite in RBC and released merozoites were quantified using this flow cytometry protocol. These techniques were applied to investigate the distinct roles of the identified growth-promoting factors in the development of the parasite, demonstrating that different combinations of NEFA and phospholipids exerted distinct roles in the growth of *P. falciparum* by sustaining development at different stages.

These findings can be usefully applied in diverse aspects malaria research, including drug resistance, vaccine development, genetics, parasite biochemistry, and studies of the relationship between the parasites and the host RBC. Culture in CDM produces similar results to those using the original culture method with human serum (Trager & Jensen, 1997), with the added advantage of avoiding the adverse effects caused by human serum. In particular, the methods reported here will allow the components crucial to each developmental stage of the parasite to be established. We have already performed a large-scale analysis of the genome-wide gene expression in *P. falciparum* cultured in the various CDM established here, to investigate the relationship between gene expression regulation and parasite development at different stages. This comprehensive analysis identified a number of genes possibly involved in arresting parasite development. These results will be reported elsewhere. Interactions between growth-promoting factors and parasite components can provide critical clues to the understanding of the general biology of *P. falciparum,* and will provide the foundations for future drug and vaccine development efforts aimed at eradicating this disease.

7. Acknowledgment

I thank Dr. S. Izumiyama of the National Institute of Infectious Diseases, Tokyo, Japan, for performing flow cytometry.

8. References

Asahi, H. & Kanazawa, T. (1994). Continuous cultivation of intraerythrocytic *Plasmodium falciparum* in a serum-free medium with the use of a growth-promoting factor, *Parasitology,* Vol. 109, pp. 397-401,

Asahi, H., Kanazawa, T., Kajihara, Y., Takahashi, K. & Takahashi, T. (1996). Hypoxanthine: a low molecular weight factor essential for growth of erythrocytic *Plasmodium falciparum* in a serum-free medium. *Parasitology,* Vol. 113, pp. 19-23,

Asahi, H., Kanazawa, T., Hirayama, N. & Kajihara, Y. (2005). Investigating serum factors promoting erythrocytic growth of *Plasmodium falciparum. Exp. Parasitol.,* Vol. 109, pp. 7-15,

Asahi, H. (2009). *Plasmodium falciparum*: Chemically defined medium for continuous intraerythrocytic growth using lipids and recombinant albumin. *Exp. Parasitol.,* Vol. 121, pp. 22-28.

Asahi, H., Izumiyama, S., Tolba, M.E. & Kwansa-Bentum, B. (2011). *Plasmodium falciparum*: Differing effects of non-esterified fatty acids and phospholipids on intraerythrocytic growth in serum-free medium. *Exp. Parasitol.,* Vol. 127, pp. 708-713,

Bannister, L.H., Hopkins, J.M., Fowler, R.E., Krishna, S. & Mitchell, G.H. (2000). A brief illustrated guide to the ultrastructure of *Plasmodium falciparum* asexual blood stages. *Parasitol. Today,* Vol. 16, pp. 427-433,

Barkan, D., Ginsburg, H. & Golenser, J. (2000). Optimisation of flow cytometric measurement of parasitemia in *Plasmodium*-infected mice. *Int. J. Parasitol.,* Vol. 30, pp. 649-635,

Cranmer, S.L., Magowan, C., Liang, J., Coppel, R.L. & Cooke, B.M. (1997). An alternative to serum for cultivation of *Plasmodium falciparum* in vitro. *Trans. Roy. Soc. Trop. Med. Hyg.,* Vol. 91, pp. 363-365,

Divo, A.A. & Jensen, J.B. (1982). Studies on serum requirements for the cultivation of *Plasmodium falciparum.* 2. Medium enrichment. *Bull. World Health Organ.,* Vol. 60, pp. 571-575,

Druilhe, P., Moreno, A., Blanc, C., Brasseur, P.H. & Jacquier, P. (2001). A colorimetric in vitro drug sensitivity assay for *Plasmodium falciparum* based on a highly sensitive double-site lactate dehydrogenase antigen-capture enzyme-linked immunosorbent assay. *Am. J. Trop. Med. Hyg.,* Vol. 64, pp. 233-241,

Izumiyama, S., Omura, M., Takasaki, T., Ohmae, H. & Asahi, H. (2009). *Plasmodium falciparum*: Development and validation of a measure of intraerythrocytic growth using SYBR Green I in a flow cytometer. *Exp. Parasitol.*, Vol. 121, pp. 144-150,

Janse, C.J. & Van Vianen, P.H. (1994). Flow cytometry in malaria detection. *Meth. Cell Biol.*, Vol. 42 Part B, pp. 295-318,

Jensen, J.B. (1979). Some aspects of serum requirements for continuous cultivation of *Plasmodium falciparum. Bull. World Health Org.*, Vol. 57 Suppl. 1, pp. 27-31,

Jensen, J.B. (2002). In vitro culture of *Plasmodium* Parasites. In: *Methods in Molecular Medicine, Vol.72: Malaria Methods and Protocols,* Denise L. Doolan (Ed.), pp. 477-488. Humana Press Inc., ISBN 0-89603-823-8, New Jersey, USA

Jimenez-Diaz, M.B., Mulet, T., Gomez, V., Viera, S., Alvarez, A., Garuti, H., Vazquez, Y., Fernandez, A., Ibanez, J., Jimenez, M., Gargallo-Viola, D. & Angulo-Barturen, I. (2009). Quantitative measurement of *Plasmodium*-infected erythrocytes in murine models of malaria by flow cytometry using bidimensional assessment of SYTO-16 fluorescence. *Cytometry A*, Vol. 75, pp. 225-235,

Jouin, H., Goguet de la Salmoniere, Y.O., Behr, C., Huyin Qan Dat, M., Michel, J.C., Sarthou, J.L., Pereira da Silva, L. & Dubois, P., 1995. Flow cytometry detection of surface antigens on fresh, unfixed red blood cells infected by *Plasmodium falciparum. J. Immunol. Meth.*, Vol. 179, pp. 1-12,

Li, Q., Gerena, L., Xie, L., Zhang, J., Kyle, D. & Milhous, W. (2007). Development and validation of flow cytometric measurement for parasitemia in cultures of *P. falciparum* vitally stained with YOYO-1. *Cytometry A*, Vol. 71, pp. 297-307,

Lingnau, A., Margos, G., Maier, W.A. & Seitz, H.M. (1994). Serum-free cultivation of several *Plasmodium falciparum* strains. *Parasitol. Res.*, Vol. 80, pp. 84-86,

Makler, M.T. & Hinrichs, D.J. (1993). Measurement of the lactate dehydrogenase activity of *Plasmodium falciparum* as an assessment of parasitemia. Am. J. Trop. Med. Hyg., Vol. 48, pp. 205-210,

Mi-Ichi, F., Kita, K. & Mitamura, T. (2006). Intraerythrocytic *Plasmodium falciparum* utilize a broad range of serum-derived fatty acids with limited modification for their growth. *Parasitology, Vol.* 133, pp. 399-410,

Nivet, C., Guillotte, M. & Pereira da Silva, L. (1983). *Plasmodium falciparum*: one-step growth in a semi-defined medium and the stimulatory effect of human seric lipoproteins and liposomes. *Exp. Parasitol.*, Vol. 55, pp. 147-151,

Noedl, H., Wernsdorfer, W.H., Miller, R.S. & Wongsrichanalai, C. (2002). Histidine-rich protein II: a novel approach to malaria drug sensitivity testing. *Antimicrobial Agents and Chemotherapy, Vol.* 46, pp. 1658-1664,

Noedl, H., Wongsrichanalai, C. & Wernsdorfer, W.H. (2003). Malaria drug-sensitivity testing: new assays, new perspectives. Trends Parasitol. 19, 175-181,

Nyakeriga, A. (2004). In vitro reinvasion and growth inhibition assay by flow cytometric measurement of parasitemia using propidium iodide (PI) staining. In: *Method in Malaria Research*, Ljungstrom, I., Perlmann, H., Schlichtherle, M., Scherf, A., & Wahlgren, M. (Eds.), pp. 85-86, MR4/ATCC, Virginia, USA

Ofulla, A.V., Okoye, V.C., Khan, B., Githure, J.I., Roberts, C.R., Johnson, A.J. & Martin, S.K. (1993). Cultivation of *Plasmodium falciparum* parasites in a serum-free medium. *Am. J. Trop. Med. Hyg.*, Vol. 49, pp. 335-340,

Persson, K.E., Lee, C.T., Marsh, K. & Beeson, J.G. (2006). Development and optimization of high-throughput methods to measure *Plasmodium falciparum*-specific growth inhibitory antibodies. *J. Clin. Microbiol.*, Vol. 44, pp. 1665-1673,

Ridley, R.G. (2002). Medical need, scientific opportunity and the drive for antimalarial drugs. *Nature*, Vol. 415, pp. 686-693,

Snow, R.W., Guerra, C.A., Noor, A.M., Myint, H.Y. & Hay, S.I. (2005). The global distribution of clinical episodes of *Plasmodium falciparum* malaria. *Nature*, Vol. 434, pp. 214-217,

Trager, W. & Jensen, J.B. (1997). Continuous culture of *Plasmodium falciparum*: its impact on malaria research. *Int. J. Parasitol.*, Vol. 27, pp. 989-1006,

Webster, H.K., Boudreau, E.F., Pavanand, K., Yongvanitchit, K. & Pang, L.W. (1985). Antimalarial drug susceptibility testing of *Plasmodium falciparum* in Thailand using a microdilution radioisotope method. *Am. J. Trop. Med. Hyg.*, Vol. 34, pp. 228-235,

Willet, G.P. & Canfield, C.J. (1984). *Plasmodium falciparum*: continuous cultivation of erythrocyte stages in plasma-free culture medium. *Exp. Parasitol.*, Vol. 57, pp. 76-80,

Yayon, A., Vande Waa, J.A., Yayon, M., Geary, T.G. & Jensen, J.B. (1983). Stage-dependent effects of chloroquine on *Plasmodium falciparum* in vitro. *J. Protozool.*, Vol. 30, pp. 642-647,

7

Development of Humanized Mice to Study Asexual Blood Stage *Plasmodium falciparum* Infection

R.K. Tyagi[1,2*], N.K. Garg[3], T. Sahu[4] and P. Prabha[5]

[1]Department of Global Health, College of Public Health, University of South Florida, Tampa, Florida,
[2]Malaria Vaccine Development Laboratory, Institute Pasteur Paris,
[3]Shantha Biotechnics Ltd., (A Part of Sanofi Aventis Group), Hyderabad, AP,
[4]National Institute of Allergy and Infectious Diseases, National Institutes of Health, Rockville, MD,
[5]Gene Regulation Laboratory, School Of Biotechnology, Jawaharlal Nehru University, New Delhi,
[1,4]USA
[2]France
[3,5]India

1. Introduction

Infectious diseases continue to heavily burden our global society. Endemic and epidemic malaria results in severe disease in an estimated half-a-billion people each year, and causes over 1.5 million deaths annually. Although progress has been made in the prevention and treatment of *falciparum* malaria infections, more effective, tolerable and affordable therapies are urgently needed. This deadly parasite displays unique human tropism, and the development of novel intervention strategies have been hampered by the lack of robust, cost effective, and predictive animal models that accurately reproduce the hallmark of human infections. While rodents and non-human primates have been employed in biomedical research and drug/vaccine development, they often do not yield reliable preclinical results that translate into effective human treatments. "Humanized" mice have recently emerged as powerful tools in the investigation of human diseases (Legrand et al., 2006; Manz, 2007; Shultz et al., 2007). These are amenable animal models transplanted with various kinds of human cells and tissues (and/or equipped with human transgenes) that may be ideally suited for direct investigation of human infectious agents such as malaria. Despite the challenges, humanized mouse technology has made rapid progress over the last few years, and it is now possible to achieve significant levels of human chimerism in various hosts, organ/tissues, particularly the immune systems, liver and muscles. Such humanized mice provide a new opportunity to perform preclinical studies of intractable human malaria

*Corresponding Author

parasite. However, the relevance of *Plasmodium falciparum*-infected humanized mice for malaria studies has been questioned because of the low percentage of mice in which the parasite develops. Malaria caused by *Plasmodium falciparum* is difficult to model in the laboratory because of the specificity of this parasite for its human host, the complexity of its life cycle and the substantial diversity of parasite strains. Consequently, most experimental in vivo studies on malaria have heavily relied on different combinations of various murine strains and Plasmodium spp. of rodent (Carlton et al., 2001; Hernandez-Valladares et al., 2005) but biological differences between parasite species remain a major limitation. For example, there are many indications that in human cerebral malaria, the preferential sequestration of parasitized erythrocytes in the brain capillaries is the central precipitating step (Medana and Turner, 2006), whereas this phenomenon is much less evident in rodent models (Lou et al., 2001).

Limitations of experimental models have also hampered the evaluation of the impact of new drugs or vaccines prior to clinical trials. During the preclinical screening of a new drug, its activity has to be evaluated first against the development of *P. falciparum* in vitro, then against the infection of a rodent Plasmodium in a mouse model and, finally, against *P. falciparum* infection in a monkey model (Fidock et al., 2004) or in a humanized mouse model.

1.1 Perspectives

The stability, reproducibility and long-standing tendency of parasitaemia in the developed humanized model based on NOD/SCID/IL2Rγ-null mouse (NSG), a mouse strain with profoundly deficient adaptive and innate immunity (NSG-IV model) might be validated by selecting artesunate resistant mutants of *P. falciparum* through prolonged exposure of the parasite to increasing levels of the drug.

2. The development of humanized mice

Advances in the ability to generate humanized mice have depended on a systematic progression of genetic modifications to develop immunodeficient host mice. Three main breakthroughs have occurred in this field (TIMELINE). First, the discovery of the *Prkdcscid* (protein kinase, DNA activated, catalytic polypeptide; severe combined immunodeficiency, abbreviated *scid*) mutation in CB17 mice (Bosma et al., 1983) was soon followed by the observation that human PBMCs (Mosier et al., 1988), fetal haematopoietic tissues (McCune et al., 1988) and HSCs (Lapidot et al., 1992) could engraft in these mice. However, engraftment occurred at only a very low level, and the engrafted human cells failed to generate a functional human immune system. The limitations impeding human-cell engraftment in CB17-*scid* mice include the spontaneous generation of mouse T and B cells during aging (known as leakiness) and high levels of host natural killer (NK)-cell and other innate immune activity, which limit the engraftment of the human hematopoietic compartment (Greiner et al., 1998). The *scid* mutation also results in defective DNA repair and, consequently, an increase in radio sensitivity. Targeted mutations at the recombination-activating gene 1 (*Rag1*) and *Rag2* loci prevent mature T- and B-cell development in the mice but do not cause leakiness or radio sensitivity. However, these mice retained high levels of NK-cell activity and had limited engraftment of human HSCs (Greiner et al., 1998; Mombaerts et al., 1992; Shinkai et al., 1992).

The second breakthrough was the development of immunodeficient non-obese diabetic (NOD)-*scid* mice (Shultz et al., 1995). Crossing the *scid* mutation onto different strain backgrounds led to the observation that NOD-*scid* mice supported higher levels of engraftment with human PBMCs than did any of the other strains that were tested, including C3H/HeJ-*scid* and C57BL/6-*scid* mice (Hesselton et al., 1995). Furthermore, it was observed that NK-cell activity, which is one of the main impediments to the engraftment of human haematopoietic cells (Christianson et al., 1996), was lower in NOD-*scid* mice than in CB17-*scid* mice (Shultz et al., 1995). NOD-*scid* mice also have additional defects in innate immunity that allow higher levels of human PBMC (Hesselton et al., 1995) and HSC (Lowry et al., 1996; Pflumio et al., 1996) engraftment. Incremental improvements in the extent of human-cell engraftment as a result of the development of new genetic variations of NOD-*scid* mice occurred over the following 10 years (TIMELINE), but the use of humanized NOD-*scid* mice as a model for human immunity remains limited by their relatively short life span, and the residual activity of NK cells and other components of innate immunity, which impedes the engraftment of the human lymphoid compartment.

The third breakthrough was the humanization of immunodeficient mice homozygous for targeted mutations at the interleukin-2 receptor (IL-2R) γ-chain locus (*Il2rg*; also known as the common cytokine-receptor γ-chain, γc) (Ishikawa et al., 2005; Ito et al., 2002; Shultz et al., 2005;Traggiai et al., 2004). These mice support greatly increased engraftment of human tissues, HSCs and PBMCs compared with all previously developed immunodeficient humanized mouse models. The IL-2R γ-chain is a crucial component of the high-affinity receptors for IL-2, IL-4, IL-7, IL-9, IL-15 and IL-21, and it is required for signaling through these receptors (Sugamura et al., 1996). The absence of the IL-2R γ-chain leads to severe impairments in T- and B-cell development and function, and completely prevents NK-cell development (Cao et al., 1995; DiSanto et al., 1995; Ohbo et al., 1996).

3. Optimization of immunosuppression protocols: Engraftment of *P. falciparum* in humanized mice

After an obtainment of proliferation of *Theileria sergenti* in scid mouse grafted with bovine-RBC (Tsuji et al., 1992), several studies raised the possibility of obtaining *P. falciparum* in immune deficient mice grafted with huRBCs (Badell et al., 2000; Moore et al., 1995; Tsuji et al., 1995). The researchers used different strategies to improve parasite survival considering the fast clearance of the parasite in few hours after being inoculated. Moore *et al* tried to adapt parasite *in vitro* partially in the serum of scid mice in place of human serum before being inoculated into the mouse (Moore et al., 1995). A concentration of mouse serum higher than 5% was found toxic for the parasite in culture. In this study, the NOD/scid mice were intraperitoneally infected with 1% adapted parasite followed by 1 ml huRBCs injection everyday. The parasite survival lasting up to 10 days was achieved with this protocol. Although splenectomized mice had shown an improvement of parasite growth (>15 days), variations in the parasitaemia from one mouse to another was detected. Another research group (Badell et al., 1995) developed another strategy of *P. falciparum* survival in the immunodeficient mice. They also noted that parasite inoculated through i.p. route into the scid mouse was eliminated in few hours from the circulation. Moreover, mouse serum added in *in vitro* cultures did not show any toxicity to parasite growth and parasite survival was observed even at 10% serum. This experiment further confirmed the important role of residual innate immune effectors of mice in the clearance of parasite. The efforts have been made to control innate immune effectors by various means such as irradiation and cyclophosphamide treatment however with limited success. This group was able to establish an immunomodulatory protocol for BXN mouse to deplete innate immune regulatory cells and could achieve an average of 0.1% parasitaemia. This immunomodulatory protocol comprised of an i.p. injection of 0.2 ml of dichloro-methylene-diphosphonate (CL_2MDP) loaded liposome once per week to destroy the murine macrophages in conjunction with an administration of an anti-PMN monoclonal antibody at every 5th day to block the polymorphonuclear cells and also the injection of 1 ml of huRBCs & AB+ human serum in 1 ml of 10%-RPMI every day. Tsuji *et al*, used splenectomized scid mice and administered huRBCs by intravenous route from day 1 to 5. As from day 1 to 4 mice received an intraperitoneal injection of 500µl of human serum as well as a subcutaneous injection of an anti-mouse RBC antibody to replace murine RBC by huRBCs. Afterwards, the mouse was reconstituted with the huRBCs followed by the irradiation, and was also injected with 1.6-4% parasitized huRBCs through an intravenous route. By employing this protocol almost complete substitution of murine RBC by huRBCs was achieved (Tsuji et al., 1995). Until recently, immunomodulatory protocol (destroying macrophages with CL2MDP-lip and blocking PMN with an anti-PMN monoclonal antibody) was applied to the NOD/scid mice (Moreno Sabater et al., 2005). Moreover, a comparative study was carried out to show differences in the capabilities of *P. falciparum* survival in BXN and NOD/scid mice using the protocol with two intraperitoneal infections (i.e. primary infection on 3rd day and secondary infection on 18th day) and with the injection of immunosuppressors along with fresh huRBCs at every three days interval. In brief NOD/scid mouse allowed a better development of the parasite for 35 days with 75% infectivity compared to only 8% with BXN mice. In the BXN mouse strain the parasite could grow until day 7 post second infections followed by a gradual decrease in parasitaemia. On the contrary NOD/scid mice showed 0.25% average parasitaemia until day 17 post second infection. Therefore this protocol with NOD/scid mice showed an improvement of parasite survival (Moore et al., 1995). Interestingly, this protocol does not imply either the need of splenectomy or *in vitro* adaptation of the parasite prior to infection. Recently Inigo *et al* (Angulo-Barturen et al., 2008), developed a murine model (NOD/scidβ2m-/-) to study *falciparum*-malaria in non-myelodepleted mice grafted with human erythrocytes with considerable success in terms of parasitaemia and with 100% infectivity. They claimed to generate *in vivo* strains of *P. falciparum* able to grow reproducibly in peripheral blood of humanized mouse with out using immunosuppressors to deplete murine phagocytes. Despite the significant success with this model cumbersome administration of 1ml RBC pellet i.p. everyday and *in vitro* adaptation of *falciparum* strains prior to infection raise questions over its ideal nature. The same group (Jimenez-Diaz et al., 2009) came up with the same protocol applied to NOD/SCIDIL-2Rγ-/- strain with slight modifications for the survival of the parasite.

Therefore to complement the descriptive analysis in humans by an experimental approach in a model, we decided to perform in *P. falciparum* NOD/SCID model a systematic and stepwise analysis of innate cell responses and inflammation mediators produced in response to the grafting of HuRBC, of *P. falciparum*, as well as to agents employed to control innate defences. The results brought new insights about the role and potency of innate defences against human xenografts, such as HuRBC, and human pathogens, such as *P. falciparum* (Arnold et al.).

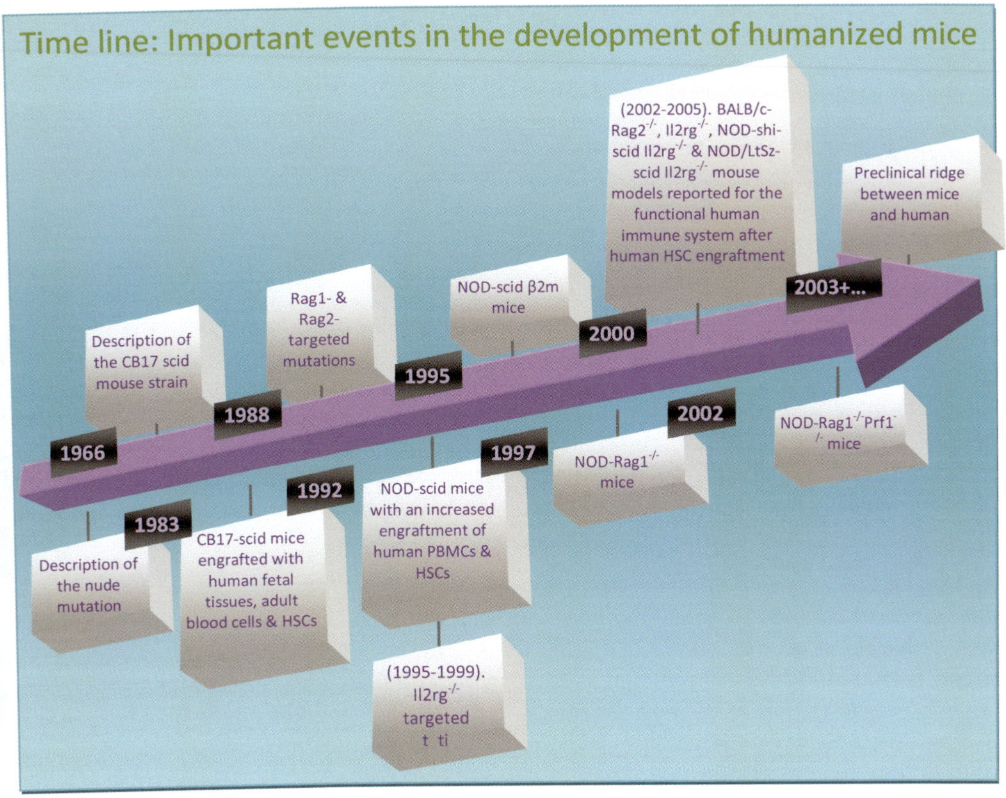

Fig. 1. Chronological events in the development of humanized mouse model

A main barrier to achieving an improved, workable *P. falciparum* mouse model is the strong pro-inflammatory effect of the parasite itself. In humans the asexual erythrocytic stages of *P. falciparum* are known to result in a systemic inflammatory process that is responsible for many of the symptoms of the disease. A second significant practical problem with all existing models developed to date is that huRBC are injected by the intra-peritoneal (IP) route, which relies on the successful migration of huRBC into the blood stream across the peritoneum. This is a process that is not properly understood, and, therefore, prevents any rational analysis and further improvement of the model. With these limitations of current models in mind, we thought to improve the *P. falciparum* humanized mouse model, particularly in terms of control of inflammatory reactions, and reproducibility of parasitemia. We decided to address these issues by using the IV route for huRBC and parasite administration, and by investigating other means to increase control over the mouse innate immune response. The use of this IV model led us to identify, among several factors investigated, the effect of aging and that of inosine as significant in reducing inflammatory reactions, and therefore improving *P. falciparum* growth. Moreover, after using various strains of immunodeficient mice, we investigated, as others [14], the value of the NOD/SCID/IL-2Rc-null mouse (NSG mouse) which, due to the knock out of the γ-chain of the IL-2 receptor, has been shown to better tolerate a variety of transplanted human cells (Ito et al., 2002; King et al., 2007; Watanabe et al., 2007). The resulting now IV model based on NSG mice presents several advantages over previously available models. It offers greater reproducibility, with 100% of mice successfully grafted without the need for mouse-adapted parasites, consistent curves of parasitemia, and high levels of infection with up to 40–50% of total erythrocytes infected (Arnold et al., 2010).

4. Strategic planning for the development of humanized mouse model

4.1 Materials and methods

4.1.1 Mice

BALB/c, NOD/SCID and NSG mice are purchased from Charles River. Immunodeficient mice were kept in sterile isolators. They are housed in sterilized cages equipped with filter tops during the experimentation, and are provided with autoclaved tap water and a γ-irradiated pelleted diet ad libitum. They are manipulated under pathogen free conditions using laminar flux hoods.

4.1.2 Human red blood cells

Human whole blood is provided by the blood bank. Blood donors had no history of malaria and all the blood groups are used without observing any difference on parasite survival. Whole blood is washed three times by centrifugation at 900 ×g, 5 minutes at room temperature and buffy coat was separated in order to eliminate white blood cells and platelets. Packed huRBCs are suspended in SAGM (Adenine, Glucose and mannitol solution) and kept at 4°C for a maximum of 2 weeks. Before use huRBCs are washed three times in RPMI-1640 medium (Gibco/BRL, Grand Island, N.Y.) supplemented with 1 mg hypoxanthine per liter (Sigma, St Louis, MO) and warmed 10 minutes at 37°C.

4.1.3 Parasites

P. falciparum lines 3D7, UPA, and K1 are employed in the study, along with clinical isolates taken from a patient at Bichat Hospital, Paris (which was used the day after being sampled). The Uganda Palo Alto (UPA) strain employed is the Palo Alto Marburg line, used for all the experiments conducted. Parasite cultures are not synchronized and therefore a mix of various developmental stages was injected to infect mice. Parasites are maintained under *in vitro* conditions at 5% hematocrit at 37°C in a candle jar in complete culture medium (RPMI-1640 medium (Gibco/BRL), 35mM HEPES (Sigma), 24mM $NaHCO_3$, 10% albumax (Gibco/BRL) and 1mg of hypoxanthine (Sigma) per liter. Parasite samples are cryopreserved using the glycerol/sorbitol method (Rowe et al., 1968). The cultures are controlled for mycoplasma contamination by using polymerase chain reaction (PCR) technique. A non-lethal rodent parasite strain *Plasmodium yoelii* XNL1.1 is preserved in 500µl aliquot of cryo-preserving buffer at -80°C at 22% parasitaemia. The strain is thawed at room temperature, diluted twice in RPMI-1640 medium followed by the injection of 50×10^6 parasite directly into the mice.

5. Protocols to control residual innate immunity

5.1 (I.P. Protocol)

5.1.1 Immunomodulatory agents to suppress innate immunity

Numerous attempts have been made to increase the success rate of the grafting of infected RBC. Un-sized dichloromethylene diphosphonate (Cl_2-MDP) encapsulated in liposome (clo-lip) (provided by N. Van Rooijen, Amsterdam, The Netherlands) is injected through intraperitoneal (i.p.) route in order to reduce the number of tissue MP, as described previously (van Rooijen and van Kesteren-Hendrikx, 2003). The anti-PMN monoclonal antibody NIMP-R14 (Lopez et al., 1984) is purified from a hybridoma. Its activity is compared to that of two other anti-PMN monoclonal antibodies: RB6-8C5 (purified from the hybridoma) and 1A8 (BioXcell, Lebanon). The NIMP-R14 monoclonal antibody is used in all the studies, unless specified. Various agents (from Sigma) (Table 1) are used to further reduce innate immunity such as dexamethasone (1-5 mg/kg/day), TGF-β (100 ng - 1 µg/day) (PeproTech, Rocky Hill, NJ), cyclophosphamide (75 mg/kg/day), cisplatinium (1-10 mg/kg/day), and TMβ-1 monoclonal antibody that targets NK cells (1 mg/kg/day).

Experiments Performed Using I.P. Protocol With Vaious Immunomodulatory Reagent					
Protocol tested	**Dose**	**Nb of mouse**	**% of sucrose(more than 2 days**	**Paracitemia length average (days)**	**Best parasitemia (days)**
DSMO	5 %	18	88.8	7.18	12
TGFβ	100 ng/day	17	23.5	7.25	8
	100 µg/day	3	66.6	10	13
Splenctomy		5	60	7	10
Cyclophopshamide	75 mg/Kg	7	100	7.6	9
	50 mg/Kg	12	41.6	6.8	9
Coinfection *P.Chabaudi* P.Falciparum		7	71.42	11	24
Coinfection *P.Yoellii* *P.Falciparum*		52	90.24	11.09	34
NAC	100 mg/Kg	25	56	11.07	19
Vitamine E	200 mg/kg	13	77	8.25	34
Trolox	4 mg/Kg	5	60	3.85	6
Anti-NK(TMBβ-1)	1 mg	15	53.3	4.12	8
Futhan	200 µg/day	4	50	2.75	4
Bleeding		20	35	7.42	14
P.Falciparum with various amount	0.3	2	100	2	2
	1%	2	100	4	4
	5%	2	100	5.5	6
	7%	2	100	4	4
	10%	2	100	5.5	6
pABA	400 mg/Kg	4	100	4.5	5
Folinic acid	mg/Kg	4	100	4.5	5
Coinfection *P.Chabaudi* and *P.Yoellii*, NAC and Vitamine E seem to have a beneficial effect in *P.Falciparum* survival; however results are very heterogeneous form one mouse to other and from one experiment to other one					

Table 1. Various immune suppressants to control innate immunity

The effect of splenectomy and of irradiation (100 - 300 cGy) is also tested. Other experiments that evaluates the addition of metabolic agents such as pABA (400 mg/kg/day), and folinic acid (400 mg/kg/day), or of antioxidants, such as vitamin E (20 mg/kg/day, Nepalm, Cenexl, Fontenay-sous, France), N-acetyl cysteine (100 mg/kg/day), trolox (4-100 mg/kg /day), 8-aminoguanidine (100 mg/kg/day).

5.1.2 Chemical immunomodulation protocol and mouse infection

A previously described immunomodulation protocol (Badell et al., 2000), modified as described in (Moreno et al., 2006) is employed. On day -13, each mouse receives a dose of 10 mg/kg of mAb NIMP-R14 by i.p. injection. On day -12, each mouse receives 0.2 ml of the suspension of clo-lip by the same route. On days -9, -6, -3 each mouse receives 0.5 ml of huRBCs i.p. mixed with a dose of 10 mg/kg of mAb NIMP-R14 and 0.2 ml of clo-lip. On day 0 mice are infected with 50µl huRBCs parasitized by *P. falciparum* at a parasitaemia of 1% (all the developmental forms, i.e. trophozoite, schizont and rings, were present) mixed with a dose of 10 mg/kg of NIMP-R14 antibody. Afterwards, a dose of 10 mg/kg of antibody NIMP-R14, 0.2 ml of clo-lip and 0.5 ml of huRBCs is injected i.p. at 3 day intervals, until the end of the study. The infection is followed-up by daily Giemsa stained thin blood films drawn from the tail vein.

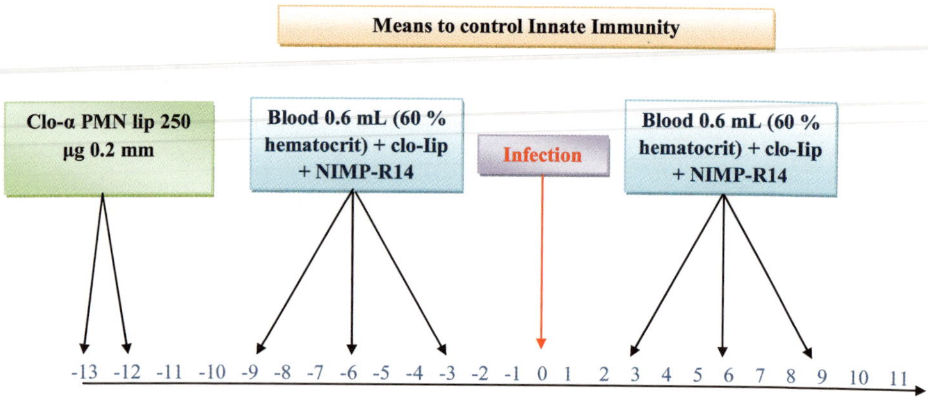

Fig. 2. Schematics of intraperitoneal immunomodulation protocol

5.2 Protocol for intravenous injection

5.2.1 Mouse infection and immunomodulation protocol

NOD/SCID mice are retro-orbitally injected with 400 µl huRBCs every 3 days to ensure a satisfactory proportion of huRBCs (i.e. chimerism), at the time of infection (≈ 60%). Simultaneously, 0.1 ml of un-sized dichloromethylene diphosphonate (Cl_2MDP) encapsulated in liposome (clo-lip) (provided by Nico Van Rooijen) diluted in 0.4 ml RPMI is intraperitoneally injected. Four injections at 2-3 day intervals are given before parasite infection. At the time of the fifth injection, mice are retro-orbitally injected with 300 µl of a *P. falciparum* infected huRBCs suspension in RPMI at a parasitaemia of 1% (all the developmental forms, i.e. rings, trophozoites and schizonts were present). After infection huRBCs and clo-lip are supplied every 3 days as described for the pre-infection step. In some experiments, 250 mg/kg of inosine (Sigma) is injected intraperitoneally every day as the half-life of inosine is very short (Mabley et al., 2009). In experiments using NSG mice the protocol has been adopted in order to achieve varying levels of adequate huRBCs chimerism and to avoid overloading the mice. As such, different amounts of blood are employed, and either 200, 400, 550 or 750 μl huRBCs are injected 3 times per week (i.e. Monday, Wednesday and Friday) mixed with 250 μl human AB serum, as it has previously been described that human serum improves huRBCs survival in immunocompromised mice (Angulo-Barturen et al., 2008); 4 injections are done prior to infection, and clo-lip is injected as described above. The infection is followed-up by daily Giemsa stained thin blood films drawn from the tail vein.

5.2.2 Haematological parameters and grafting of *P. falciparum*-huRBCs

The study blood samples are collected from mice retro-orbital sinus on heparin. Various haematological parameters such as haematocrit, leukocyte number and phenotype (Ly-6C APC, Ly-6G APC (Miltenyi Biotec, Germany), CD115 PE, CD43 FITC, CD62L FITC, CD11b FITC, DX5 FITC, CD122 PE (BD Biosciences, UK) in peripheral blood samples were monitored, as well as the phenotype characterization of monocytes (CD11b+,CD115+), inflammatory monocytes (CD43-, CD62L+, Ly-6C+), PMN (CD11b+, ly6G+), and natural killer cells (DX5+, CD122+). Total leukocyte number (leukocytes/μl blood) is evaluated by lysing 20μl of total blood with BD FACS™ Lysing solution, and counting on Malassez haematocytometer. Since successfully grafted mice have a significant, but variable, percentage of huRBCs in their peripheral blood, parasitaemia in mice is expressed as the overall percentage of *P. falciparum* infected RBCs among total RBCs, i.e. both human and mouse RBCs observed on thin blood smears. In addition, the peritoneal blood parasitaemia is measured on the smears drawn from the peritoneum.

Blood samples drawn from mice are used to determine the percentage of huRBCs in mouse peripheral blood at regular intervals by flow cytometry on a FACScalibur (BD biosciences) using FITC labeled anti-human glycophorin monoclonal antibody (Dako, Denmark).

5.2.3 Mouse cell isolation

In NOD/SCID mice inflammation is induced by IP injection of 1ml 3% thioglycolate (Sigma) diluted in sterile PBS. 4-5 days after, the peritoneal cavity is washed with HBSS without Ca^{++} and Mg^{++}. The collected cells are washed twice in RPMI supplemented with L-glutamine, Penicillin (100U/ml), Streptomycin (100ug/ml), and 10% Fetal Calf Serum (FCS) and seeded at $3x10^5$ per well in a 96-well culture plate. Cell suspensions of splenocytes are prepared in cold RPMI 1640 medium supplemented with 10% FCS and filtered on a 100 μm cell strainer to remove debris. Erythrocytes are lysed with ACK lysis buffer, and the splenocytes are washed 2 times with RPMI supplemented with 10% FCS and seeded at $3x10^5$ per well of a 96 well culture plate.

5.2.4 Cytokines/chemokine/chemiluminesence assay

100 μl blood samples are collected from the retro-orbital plexus with a Pasteur pipette, and sera are stored at -80°C. Conditioned media obtained after 16h stimulation of peritoneal cells and splenocytes with lipopolysaccharide (LPS, 1 μg/ml) (Sigma) are stored at -80°C. Cytokines and chemokines (IL-6, MCP-1, IFNγ, TNFα, IL-12p70 and IL-10) are quantified

using the BD™ Cytometric Bead Array mouse inflammatory kit (BD biosciences) following the manufacturer's recommendations on a FACScalibur (BD biosciences).

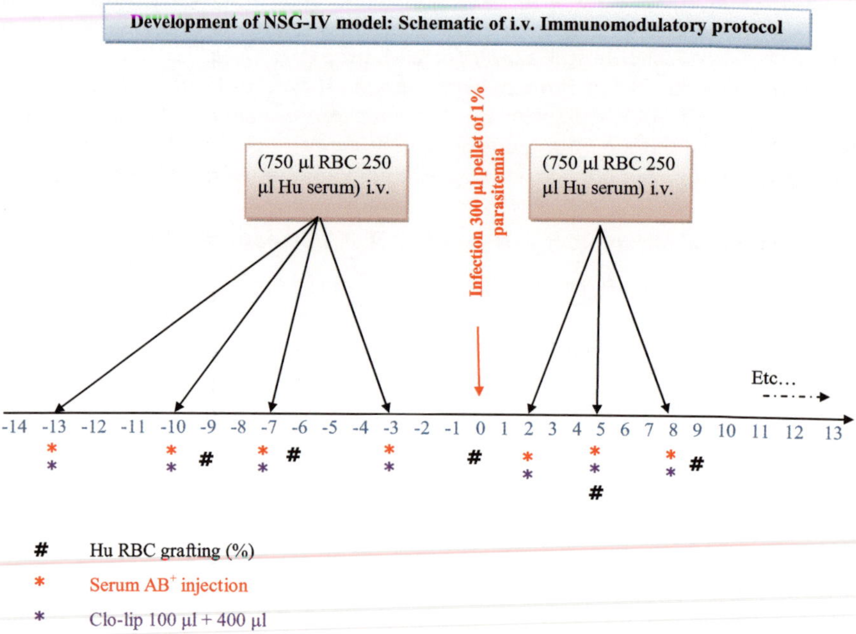

Fig. 3. Development of NSG-IV (NOD/SCIDIL2Rγ-/-) model: schematic of immunomodulatory protocol

Since production of reactive oxygen intermediates (ROI) closely mirrors the state of activation of macrophages and polymorphonuclear cells, luminol dependent photometric assay is used to measure Reactive Oxygen Intermediates (ROI). Blood samples are collected from NOD/SCID mice, washed with HBSS with freshly added Ca^{++} and Mg^{++}. Washed blood is diluted 1/10 in HBSS and 90 µl blood were added to each well in a 96 well plate (Nunc, Denmark) and incubated for 30 minutes at 37°C after adding 10 µl PMA (final concentration 1 µg/ml) to stimulate the cells. 50µl of luminol (final concentration 200 µg/ml) solution are added immediately before measuring emissions.

5.2.5 Analysis of deep-seated organs for parasite differential count

NSG mice are used for the comparison of parasite differential counts in the peripheral blood, with that in deep-seated organs. Four mice are infected with UPA strain, and when a parasitaemia of >10% is reached a thin smear from peripheral blood is drawn before killing the mouse, and harvesting its organs. Kidney, Liver, Spleen, Lung, and Brain are removed from each mouse. Parasite content is assessed from blots made by repeatedly spotting sections from each organ. These slides are then stained with Giemsa. The last blots taken, are considered to be the most representative of the parasite content in the organ's vascular bed, and are examined at 1000x magnification to perform differential counts of each stage (> 200 parasites from each organ counted).

6. Anticipated results

The present protocols illustrate an improvement of the mice with genetic deficiencies in adaptive immunity for successful grafting of human cells or pathogens to study human biological processes *in vivo*. Since non-adaptive immunity received little attention, we have deployed our efforts to study innate defences, responsible for the substantial control of *P. falciparum* and highlighted some of the remaining limitations on the development of the optimal humanized mouse. In addition, numerous attempts were made to enhance the success rate of infected huRBC by employing various immunomodulatory agents intraperitoneally to further suppress the residual innate immunity. This study came up with some conclusions such as, 1) stable parasitaemia with only a subset of mice 2) parasite clearance and *P. falciparum* induced inflammation are correlated 3) *P. yoelii* induces less inflammation than *P. falciparum* 4) huRBC, and the anti-inflammatory agents, induce low grade inflammation. 5) repeated administrations of huRBC, clo-lip and anti-PMN reduce inflammation and improve HuRBC grafting 6) MO/MPs are critical in controlling *P. falciparum* and huRBC grafting in NOD/SCID. A strong pro-inflammatory effect of the parasite itself and poor understanding of migration of infected and uninfected huRBC into blood stream across the peritoneum and subsequently, uneven distribution of huRBC are two barriers to achieving an improved, workable humanized mouse model. The results obtained by the IP protocols indicate that the SCID mice to study human biological processes *in vivo* need to be carefully explored and that further attempts are required to address the remaining limitations such as residual innate immunity and route of delivery of huRBC to create an optimized humanized mouse model.

The complex biological processes often require *in vivo* analysis of human cells: humanized mice or mouse-human chimeras have been developed to meet this requirement, however, with low percentage of infectivity and reproducibility supporting a long standing parasitaemia only in a proportion of animals. We have obtained improved parasitaemias based on intravenous delivery of huRBC and *P. falciparum* instead of the intraperitoneal route (IP) by testing various immunosuppressive drugs.

In essence the genetic background has also played an important role to optimize the humanized mouse model. The intravenous mouse model (NSG-IV) shows the role of ageing and inosine in controlling *P. falciparum* induced inflammation. The success of humanized mouse (NSG mice) model, with IV delivery of huRBC and *P. falciparum* in clo-lip treated (immunosuppression of macrophages) mice, was 100% in terms of infectivity and reproducibility. Synchronization, partial sequestration and receptivity to various strains of *P. falciparum* without preliminary adaptation are some of the lucrative features of the developed mouse model which is reliable and more relevant, and better meet the needs of biomedical translational research.

7. Conclusion

In conclusion, the chapter demonstrates that the careful selection of mice with combined deficiencies of adaptive and innate immunity, and the better control of innate immune defenses by improving immunomodulatory protocols and using anti-inflammatory substances, could provide a reproducible, long lasting and straightforward mouse model of

P. falciparum infection. This model may be further used to obtain malaria parasites that present a high level of resistance to different anti-malarial drugs such as artemisinin *in vivo* and *in vitro*. Interestingly, the same model could be also used to test the efficacy of new drugs, and in particular could be used to screen novel drugs for their effectiveness against ART resistant *P. falciparum* parasites

8. Abbreviations

NOD- Non-Obese Diabetic; SCID-Severe Combined Immunodeficiency; IL2Rγ- Interleukin-2 Receptor γ-chain; NK- Natural Killer; PBMCs: Peripheral Blood Monocytes; HSCs: Hematopoietic stem cells; *Rag*-Recombination-Activating Gene; IL-Interleukin; huRBCs—Human Red Blood Cells; PMN-Polymorphonuclear; SAGM- Adenine, Glucose and Mannitol solution; CL_2MDP- Dichloro-Methylene-Diphosphonate; NSG-NOD scid gamma; TGF-Tumor Growth Factor; APC-Antigen Presenting Cell; FACS- Fluorescence Activated Cell sorting; FCS- Fetal Calf Serum; FITC- Fluorescein isothiocyanate, phorbol-12-myristate-13-acetate (PMA)

9. References

Angulo-Barturen, I.; Jimenez-Diaz, M.B.; Mulet, T.; Rullas, J.; Herreros, E.; Ferrer, S.; Jimenez, E.; Mendoza, A.; Regadera, J.; Rosenthal, P.J. et al. (2008). A murine model of falciparum-malaria by in vivo selection of competent strains in non myelodepleted mice engrafted with human erythrocytes. *PLoS ONE*, e2252.

Arnold, L.; Tyagi, R.K.; Meija, P.; Swetman, C.; Gleeson, J.; Perignon, J.L., & Druilhe, P.(2011). Further improvements of the P. falciparum humanized mouse model. *PloS ONE*, e18045.

Arnold, L.; Tyagi, R.K.; Mejia, P.; Van Rooijen, N.; Perignon, J.L. & Druilhe, P. (2010).Analysis of innate defences against Plasmodium falciparum in immunodeficient mice. *Malaria Journal*, pp 197..

Badell, E.; Oeuvray, C.; Moreno, A.; Soe, S.; van Rooijen, N.; Bouzidi, A. & Druilhe, P. (2000). Human malaria in immunocompromised mice: an in vivo model to study defense mechanisms against Plasmodium falciparum. *The Journal of Experimental Medicine*,pp 1653-1660.

Badell, E., Pasquetto, V., Eling, W., Thomas, A., & Druilhe, P. (1995). Human Plasmodium liver stages in SCID mice: a feasible model? *Parasitology today*,pp 169-171.

Bosma, G.C.; Custer, R.P. & Bosma, M.J. (1983). A severe combined immunodeficiency mutation in the mouse. *Nature*, pp 527-530.

Cao, X.; Shores, E.W.; Hu-Li, J.; Anver, M.R.; Kelsall, B.L.; Russell, S.M.; Drago, J.; Noguchi, M.; Grinberg, A.; Bloom, E.T. et al. (1995). Defective lymphoid development in mice lacking expression of the common cytokine receptor gamma chain. *Immunity*, 223-238.

Carlton, J.M.; Hayton, K.; Cravo, P.V. & Walliker, D. (2001). Of mice and malaria mutants: unravelling the genetics of drug resistance using rodent malaria models. *Trends in Parasitology*, pp 236-242.

Christianson, S.W.; Greiner, D.L.; Schweitzer, I.B.; Gott, B.; Beamer, G.L.; Schweitzer, P.A. Hesselton, R.M. & Shultz, L.D. (1996). Role of natural killer cells on engraftment of human lymphoid cells and on metastasis of human T-lymphoblastoid leukemia cells in C57BL/6J-scid mice and in C57BL/6J-scid bg mice. *Cellular immunology,* pp 186-199.

DiSanto, J.P.; Muller, W.; Guy-Grand, D.; Fischer, A. & Rajewsky, K. (1995). Lymphoid development in mice with a targeted deletion of the interleukin 2 receptor gamma chain. *Proceedings of the National Academy of Sciences of the United States of America,* pp 377-381.

Fidock, D.A.; Rosenthal, P.J.; Croft, S.L.; Brun, R. & Nwaka, S. (2004). Antimalarial drug discovery: efficacy models for compound screening. *Nature Reviews Drug Discovery,* pp 509-520.

Greiner, D.L.; Hesselton, R.A. & Shultz, L.D. (1998). SCID mouse models of human stem cell engraftment. *Stem Cells (Dayton, Ohio),* pp 166-177.

Hernandez-Valladares, M.; Naessens, J. & Iraqi, F.A. (2005). Genetic resistance to malaria in mouse models. *Trends in Parasitology,* pp 352-355.

Hesselton, R.M.; Greiner, D.L.; Mordes, J.P.; Rajan, T.V.; Sullivan, J.L. & Shultz, L.D. (1995). High levels of human peripheral blood mononuclear cell engraftment and enhanced susceptibility to human immunodeficiency virus type 1 infection in NOD/LtSz-scid/scid mice. *The Journal of Infectious Diseases,*pp 974-982.

Ishikawa, F.; Yasukawa, M.; Lyons, B.; Yoshida, S.; Miyamoto, T.; Yoshimoto, G.; Watanabe, T.; Akashi, K.; Shultz, L.D. & Harada, M. (2005). Development of functional human blood and immune systems in NOD/SCID/IL2 receptor {gamma} chain(null) mice. *Blood,* pp 1565-1573..

Ito, M.; Hiramatsu, H.; Kobayashi, K.; Suzue, K.; Kawahata, M.; Hioki, K.; Ueyama, Y.; Koyanagi, Y.; Sugamura, K.; Tsuji, K. et al. (2002). NOD/SCID/gamma(c)(null) mouse: an excellent recipient mouse model for engraftment of human cells. *Blood,* pp 3175-3182.

Jimenez-Diaz, M.B.; Mulet, T.; Viera, S.; Gomez, V.; Garuti, H.; Ibanez, J.; Alvarez-Doval, A.; Shultz, L.D.; Martinez, A.; Gargallo-Viola, D. & Angulo-Barturen, I. (2009). Improved murine model of malaria using Plasmodium falciparum competent strains and non-myelodepleted NOD-scid IL2Rgammanull mice engrafted with human erythrocytes. *Antimicrobial Agents and Chemotherapy,* pp 4533-4536.

King, M.; Pearson, T.; Shultz, L.D.; Leif, J., Bottino, R.; Trucco, M.; Atkinson, M.; Wasserfall, C.; Herold, K.; Mordes, J.P. et al. (2007). Development of new-generation HU-PBMC-NOD/SCID mice to study human islet alloreactivity. *Annals of the New York Academy of Sciences,* pp 90-93.

Lambros, C. & Vanderberg, J.P. (1979). Synchronization of Plasmodium falciparum erythrocytic stages in culture. *The Journal of Parasitology,* pp 418-420.

Lapidot, T.; Pflumio, F.; Doedens, M.; Murdoch, B.; Williams, D.E. & Dick, J.E. (1992). Cytokine stimulation of multilineage hematopoiesis from immature human cells engrafted in SCID mice. *Science (New York, N.Y,* pp 1137-1141.

Legrand, N.; Weijer, K., & Spits, H. (2006). Experimental models to study development and function of the human immune system in vivo. *Journal of Immunology*, pp 2053-2058.

Lopez, A.F.; Strath, M. & Sanderson, C.J. (1984). Differentiation antigens on mouse eosinophils & neutrophils identified by monoclonal antibodies. *British Jornal Haematology*, pp 489-494.

Lou, J.; Lucas, R., Grau, G.E. (2001). Pathogenesis of cerebral malaria: recent experimental data and possible applications for humans. *Clinical Microbiology Reviews*, Vol 14, pp 810-820. table of contents.

Lowry, P.A.; Shultz, L.D.; Greiner, D.L.; Hesselton, R.M.; Kittler, E.L.; Tiarks, C.Y.; Rao, S.S.; Reilly, J.; Leif, J.H.; Ramshaw, H. et al. (1996). Improved engraftment of human cord blood stem cells in NOD/LtSz-scid/scid mice after irradiation or multiple-day injections into unirradiated recipients. *Biology of Blood and Marrow Transplantationt*, pp 15-23.

Mabley, J.G.; Pacher, P.; Murthy, K.G.; Williams, W.; Southan, G.J.; Salzman, A.L. & Szabo, C. (2009). The novel inosine analogue, INO-2002, exerts an anti-inflammatory effect in a murine model of acute lung injury. *Shock*, pp 258–262.

Manz, M.G. (2007). Human-hemato-lymphoid-system mice: opportunities and challenges. *Immunity*, pp 537-541.

McCune, J.M.; Namikawa, R.; Kaneshima, H.; Shultz, L.D.; Lieberman, M. & Weissman, I.L. (1988). The SCID-hu mouse: murine model for the analysis of human hematolymphoid differentiation and function. *Science (New York, N.Y*, pp 1632-1639.

Medana, I.M. & Turner, G.D. (2006). Human cerebral malaria and the blood-brain barrier. *International journal for parasitology*, pp 555-568.

Mombaerts, P., Iacomini, J., Johnson, R.S., Herrup, K., Tonegawa, S., & Papaioannou, V.E. (1992). RAG-1-deficient mice have no mature B and T lymphocytes. *Cell*, pp 869-877.

Moore, J.M.; Kumar, N.; Shultz, L.D. & Rajan, T.V. (1995). Maintenance of the human malarial parasite, Plasmodium falciparum, in scid mice and transmission of gametocytes to mosquitoes. *The Journal of Experimental Medicine*, pp 2265-2270.

Moreno, A.; Ferrer, E.; Arahuetes, S.; Eguiluz, C.; Van Rooijen, N. & Benito, A. (2006). The course of infections and pathology in immunomodulated NOD/LtSz-SCID mice inoculated with Plasmodium falciparum laboratory lines & clinical isolates. *International Journal of Parasitology*, pp 361-369.

Moreno Sabater, A.; Moreno, M.; Moreno, F.J.; Eguiluz, C.; van Rooijen, N. & Benito, A. (2005). Experimental infection of immunomodulated NOD/LtSz-SCID mice as a new model for Plasmodium falciparum erythrocytic stages. *Parasitology Research*, pp 97-105.

Mosier, D.E.; Gulizia, R.J.; Baird, S.M. & Wilson, D.B. (1988). Transfer of a functional human immune system to mice with severe combined immunodeficiency. *Nature*, pp 256-259.

Ohbo, K.; Suda, T.; Hashiyama, M.; Mantani, A.; Ikebe, M.; Miyakawa, K.; Moriyama, M.; Nakamura, M.; Katsuki, M.; Takahashi, K. et al. (1996). Modulation of hematopoiesis in mice with a truncated mutant of the interleukin-2 receptor gamma chain. *Blood,* pp 956-967.

Pflumio, F.; Izac, B.; Katz, A.; Shultz, L.D.; Vainchenker, W. & Coulombel, L. (1996). Phenotype and function of human hematopoietic cells engrafting immune-deficient CB17-severe combined immunodeficiency mice and nonobese diabetic-severe combined immunodeficiency mice after transplantation of human cord blood mononuclear cells. *Blood,* pp 3731-3740.

Reese, R.T.; Langreth, S.G. & Trager, W. (1979). Isolation of stages of the human parasite Plasmodium falciparum from culture and from animal blood. *Bulletin World Health Organization* Suppl 1, 53-61.

Rowe, A.W.; Eyster, E. & Kellner, A. (1968). Liquid nitrogen preservation of red blood cells for transfusion; a low glycerol-rapid freeze procedure. *Cryobiology,* pp 119-128.

Shinkai, Y.; Rathbun, G.; Lam, K.P.; Oltz, E.M.; Stewart, V.; Mendelsohn, M.; Charron, J., Datta M.; Young, F.; Stall, A.M. & et al. (1992). RAG-2-deficient mice lack mature lymphocytes owing to inability to initiate V(D)J rearrangement. *Cell,* pp 855-867.

Shultz, L.D.; Ishikawa, F. & Greiner, D.L. (2007). Humanized mice in translational biomedical research. *Nature Reviews,* pp 118-130.

Shultz, L.D.; Lyons, B.L.; Burzenski, L.M.; Gott, B.; Chen, X.; Chaleff, S.; Kotb, M.; Gillies, S.D.; King, M.; Mangada, J. et al. (2005). Human lymphoid and myeloid cell development in NOD/LtSz-scid IL2R gamma null mice engrafted with mobilized human hemopoietic stem cells. *Journal of Immunology,* pp 6477-6489.

Shultz, L.D.; Schweitzer, P.A.; Christianson, S.W.; Gott, B.; Schweitzer, I.B.; Tennent, B.; McKenna, S.; Mobraaten, L.; Rajan, T.V.; Greiner, D.L. et al. (1995). Multiple defects in innate and adaptive immunologic function in NOD/LtSz-scid mice. *Journal of Immunology,* pp 180-191.

Sugamura, K.; Asao, H.; Kondo, M.; Tanaka, N.; Ishii, N.; Ohbo, K.; Nakamura, M. & Takeshita, T. (1996). The interleukin-2 receptor gamma chain: its role in the multiple cytokine receptor complexes and T cell development in XSCID. *Annual Review of Immunology,* pp 179-205.

Traggiai, E.; Chicha, L.; Mazzucchelli, L.; Bronz, L.; Piffaretti, J.C.; Lanzavecchia, A. & Manz, M.G. (2004). Development of a human adaptive immune system in cord blood cell-transplanted mice. *Science* (New York, N.Y. pp 104-107.

Tsuji, M.; Hagiwara, K.; Takahashi, K.; Ishihara, C.; Azuma, I. & Siddiqui, W.A. (1992). Theileria sergenti proliferates in SCID mice with bovine erythrocyte transfusion. *The Journal of Parasitology,*pp 750-752.

Tsuji, M.; Ishihara, C.; Arai, S.; Hiratai, R. & Azuma, I. (1995). Establishment of a SCID mouse model having circulating human red blood cells and a possible growth of Plasmodium falciparum in the mouse. *Vaccine,* pp 1389-1392.

van Rooijen, N. & van Kesteren-Hendrikx, E. (2003). "In vivo" depletion of macrophages by liposome-mediated "suicide". *Methods Enzymology,* pp 3-16.

Watanabe, S.; Terashima, K.; Ohta, S., Horibata, S.; Yajima, M.; Shiozawa, Y.; Dewan, M.Z.; Yu, Z.; Ito, M.; Morio, T. et al. (2007). Hematopoietic stem cell-engrafted NOD/SCID/IL2Rgamma null mice develop human lymphoid systems and induce long-lasting HIV-1 infection with specific humoral immune responses. *Blood,* pp 212-218.

8

Human Erythrocyte Remodelling by *Plasmodium falciparum*

Xue Yan Yam[1,2], Alassane Mbengue[1] and Catherine Braun-Breton[1]
[1]*University Montpellier II, CNRS UMR5235, University Montpellier I, Dynamique des Interactions Membranaires Normales et Pathologiques,*
[2]*School of Biological Sciences, Nanyang Technological University, Singapore,*
[1]*France*
[2]*Singapore*

1. Introduction

Making the erythrocyte its home for 48 hours has important consequences for the human malaria parasite *Plasmodium falciparum*. Indeed, erythrocytes are terminally differentiated cells that lack a nucleus as well as intracellular organelles, are thus unable to endocytose or exocytose macromolecules, and have lost several membrane transport activities upon differentiation. Consequently, the parasite has to deeply remodel its host cell, from the very beginning to ensure its entry into the red blood cell, throughout its growth and multiplication to fulfil its needs for extracellular nutrients, and to the very end of its intra-erythrocytic development with the parasite-induced opening and curling of the red cell membrane leading to the dispersion of newly formed merozoites into the blood flow. The most spectacular, and first reported, modifications of the red blood cell membrane induced by *P. falciparum* are electron dense protrusions named knobs and consisting of parasite proteins exported to the red cell membrane and sub-membrane skeleton where they eventually interact with host cell proteins. Knobs are directly related to the severity of *falciparum* malaria because they mediate adherence of infected erythrocytes to the microvasculature endothelium. More recent studies have revealed that the parasite might export several hundreds of proteins, as well as membrane compartments, to the red cell and divert enzymatic and structural host proteins to make the erythrocyte a suitable environment for its growth. In the last decade, remodelling of its host cell by *Plasmodium falciparum* has become an important and growing field of research. In this review, we will describe the current stage of knowledge concerning red blood cell remodelling by *Plasmodium falciparum* and the role of these parasite-induced modifications for its growth and survival.

2. Early modifications of the red blood cell

Apicomplexan parasites share a conserved mode of invasion by actively entering their host cell with the formation of a specialised junction with the host cell membrane and the establishment of the parasite inside a self-induced parasitophorous vacuole (Aikawa *et al.*, 1978). Initial attachment of the parasite to the host cell surface results from low-affinity reversible interactions (Dvorak *et al.*, 1975) and induces the sequential discharge of two types of apical secretory organelles: 1/ the micronemes, small secretory organelles underlying the parasite's apical pole and providing a variety of adhesive proteins and 2/ the pear-shaped rhoptries providing rhoptry neck proteins that, in collaboration with microneme proteins establish a junction between the invading parasite and its host cell membrane named the "moving junction" (Aikawa *et al.*, 1978). For malaria parasites, initial attachment triggers waves of deformation of the red cell membrane (Figure 1) (Gilson & Crabb, 2009), that cover the merozoite and might facilitate the formation of the junction between the merozoite's apical pole and the host cell membrane. Noteworthy, to form this junction, the parasite exports to the host cell membrane its own receptor, Ron2, for the parasite surface ligand AMA1 (Besteiro *et al.*, 2009). Additional rhoptry neck proteins, Ron4, Ron5 and Ron8, are secreted to the cytosolic face of the host cell plasma membrane and participate in the junction formation that provides the parasite an anchoring to the host cell membrane supporting forward motion of the parasite with the apical pole leading the way (Besteiro *et al.*, 2011). This active penetration promotes invagination of the host cell plasma membrane with the moving junction acting as a sieve excluding host cell integral membrane proteins from the nascent parasitophorous vacuole membrane (PVM) while some glycosyl-phosphatidylinositol (GPI)-anchored and lipid raft-associated proteins enter the vacuole (Aikawa *et al.*, 1981; Atkinson *et al.*, 1988; Dluzewski *et al.*, 1989; Dluzewski *et al.*, 1988). Noteworthy, the malarial parasite seems to exploit glyco-sphingolipids and cholesterol enriched microdomains of the erythrocyte membrane known as lipid rafts for invasion: this is supported by the evidence that the merozoite infection is halted following disruption of raft-cholesterol using the cholesterol depleting agent, methyl-β-cyclodextrin (MBCD) (Samuel *et al.*, 2001). In addition, *P. falciparum* entry is blocked by lidocaine hydrochloride, a local anaesthetic agent reversibly disrupting the lipid rafts without altering the cholesterol content of the erythrocyte membrane (Koshino & Takakuwa, 2009). A proposed mechanism for this is that the disruption of rafts alters an erythrocyte raft hetero-trimeric guanine nucleotide-binding protein-mediated signal transduction pathway that induces the phosphorylation of sub-membrane skeletal proteins (Kamata *et al.*, 2008). These phosphorylations can modify the mechanical properties of the erythrocyte membrane [reviewed in (Zuccala & Baum, 2011)] and favour membrane invagination. The major and raft-associated erythrocyte membrane protein Band 3 appears to be phosphorylated on tyrosine residues upon invasion (Pantaleo *et al.*, 2010). This phosphorylation should result in the clustering of Band 3 and thus be important for parasite entry by de-connecting Band 3 from the erythrocyte sub-membrane skeleton (Ferru *et al.*, 2011). In addition, G-protein coupled signalling through the β2-adrenergic receptor, has also been shown to regulate the parasite invasion efficiency (Harrison *et al.*, 2003) and growth (Murphy *et al.*, 2006a). All these studies strongly imply that erythrocyte rafts are functionally exploited for parasite invasion and also serve as a platform for signalling events to take place.

The biogenesis of the PVM is dynamic and has not been completely resolved. Immuoelectron microscopy studies have provided evidences that apical organelles of the merozoite contain and release into the erythrocyte lipidic lamellar materials which could participate in the PVM expansion (Bannister & Mitchell, 1989; Bannister *et al.*, 1986; Mikkelsen *et al.*, 1988). Additionally, as described in (Dluzewski *et al.*, 1995) the PVM does not contain lipids solely from the host cell membrane as the surface area of newly infected erythrocytes had not evidently decreased in size, suggesting the contribution of lipids from the parasite itself. On the other hand, exchange of lipids between the parasite and erythrocyte membrane have also been reported (Hsiao *et al.*, 1991) and studies using fluorescent lipophilic probes revealed that the PVM does contain lipids from the host cell membrane (Haldar *et al.*, 1989; Ward *et al.*, 1993). All these data illustrate that the biogenesis of the PVM appears to have relative contributions from both parasite- and host cell erythrocyte-derived lipids. In addition, a lipid raft based biogenesis of the PVM has been proposed (Hiller *et al.*, 2003).

Although there is no formal proof for a role of rhoptry bulb proteins in the formation of the parasitophorous vacuole, their association to the parasitophorous vacuole membrane suggests that they participate in early stages of its biogenesis. However, direct evidences have been obtained in *T. gondii*, showing that rhoptry proteins, particularly protein kinases and phosphatase, secreted to the parasitophorous vacuole membrane or host cell nucleus serve as effectors, and constitute major virulence factors that counteract the immune response of the host (Behnke *et al.*, 2011; El Hajj *et al.*, 2007; Gilbert *et al.*, 2007; Saeij *et al.*, 2006). The Band 3 phosphorylation on tyrosine residues mentioned above might be induced by a, yet unidentified, secreted parasite protein kinase or by the activation of an erythrocyte tyrosine-kinase.

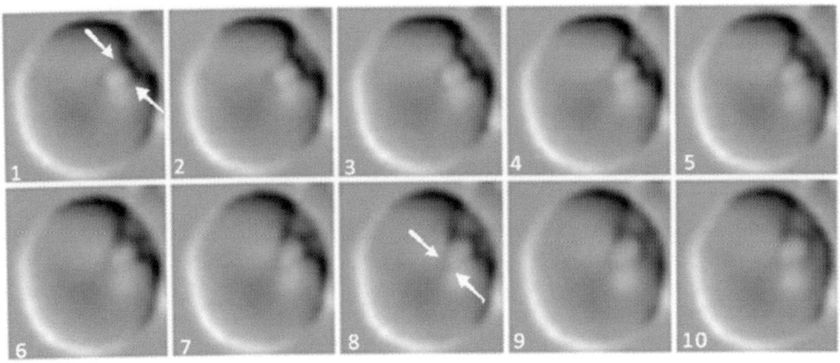

Fig. 1. Erythrocyte membrane deformations generated by a *P. falciparum* merozoite. The merozoite glides on the surface of a red blood cell membrane prior to entrance (Time lapse of 0.5 s between each frame). The membrane is deformed by the strength of adhesion. The adhesion site is transferred from the back of the merozoite (frame 1, white arrows) to its apical pole (frame 8, white arrows). High speed live imaging with the participation of Magali Roques and Manouk Abkarian.

Host proteins also participate in the development of the parasitophorous vacuole since the selective vacuolar uptake of several DRM-associated erythrocyte membrane proteins has been reported, including both transmembrane and GPI-anchored proteins (Lauer *et al.*, 2000; Murphy *et al.*, 2004; Bietz *et al.*, 2009). However, not all proteins derived from the erythrocyte DRMs are recruited to the PVM, suggesting that the recruitment does not depend only on their DRMs association. The moving junction is likely playing a central role in this selection process that might participate in changing the physical properties of the erythrocyte for efficient parasite entry (Mordue *et al.*, 1999; Murphy *et al.*, 2004). Interestingly, dematin, an erythrocyte sub-membrane skeleton binding protein, was also recently found to be internalized by the parasite (Lalle *et al.*, 2011). The biological functions of these internalized proteins remain enigmatic and further studies are necessary to determine whether internalization of these proteins is essential for the parasite survival and in maintaining the stability of the vacuolar environment. However, both Band 3 tyrosine-phosphorylation and dematin internalisation participate in a parasite-induced fragility of the red cell membrane likely required for efficient merozoite entry (Ferru *et al.*, 2011; Khanna *et al.*, 2002) while the Ring-infected Erythrocyte Surface Antigen (RESA) released by the merozoite into the red blood cell upon invasion stabilizes spectrin tetramers and confers the infected erythrocyte enhanced resistance to mechanical and thermal degradation (Pei *et al.*, 2007). Noteworthy, the binding of RESA to spectrin tetramers also confers the newly infected erythrocyte resistance to further invasion (Pei *et al.*, 2007).

Moreover, using *Plasmodium knowlesi* parasites, Torii and collaborators have observed the release of the dense granule contents into the lumen of the parasitophorous vacuole and the concomitant invagination of the PVM adjacent to the released contents (Torii *et al.*, 1989). These results suggested that the dense granules, another type of apical secretory organelles of the merozoite, play a role in forming finger-like channels extending into the surrounding erythrocyte cytoplasm. Numerous studies using primarily *Toxoplasma gondii* parasites but also *Plasmodium falciparum* showed that the released dense granule contents transform the parasitophorous vacuole into a metabolically active compartment [reviewed in (Mercier *et al.*, 2005)].

3. Living within the parasitophorous vacuole

The intracellular parasite living in the vacuole acquires nutrients by uptake from the host cell cytosol and extracellular milieu, hence the PVM has dual roles: (i) protect the parasite from extracellular harmful substances and (ii) facilitate nutrients access to parasite needs (Lingelbach & Joiner, 1998). Upon parasite growth and parasitophorous vacuole enlargement, extensions from the PVM form membranous whorls and loops and tubular elements projecting to the host cell periphery without fusing with the red blood cell membrane. These PVM extensions form an interconnected network of tubular and vesicular membranes known as the tubovesicular network (TVN) (Atkinson & Aikawa, 1990; Elmendorf & Haldar, 1994; Grellier *et al.*, 1991). Inhibition of the parasite sphingomyelin synthase activity, localised to the TVN (Elmendorf & Haldar, 1994), by dl-threo-1-phenyl-2-palmitoylamino-3-morpholino-1-propanol (PPMP) arrested the assembly of the interconnected TVN network and resulted in the blockage of the delivery of extracellular nutrients to the parasite (Lauer *et al.*, 1997), indicating the importance of TVN in nutrients import for the intracellular parasite. In addition, using a comparative transcriptomic analysis of PPMP-treated *P. falciparum* infected erythrocytes, Tamez and colleagues have identified erythrocyte vesicle protein 1 (EVP1), a parasite protein implicated in the maintenance of the TVN for nutrients import (Tamez *et al.*, 2008). Furthermore, van Ooij *et al.* have shown that the exported protein PfC435 localises at vesicles proposed to connect the PVM and TVN and to be involved in the TVN formation (van Ooij *et al.*, 2008). There are most probably more proteins involved in the formation of this network, which call for further investigations.

3.1 Nutrient uptake and induction of new permeability pathways

The trophozoite growth is accompanied by extensive digestion of the red blood cell cytoplasm. However, it is not sufficient to provide the parasite all the nutrients it needs to sustain its growth: for example, haemoglobin does not contain isoleucine, and several other amino acids such as glutamate, methionine, cysteine and proline are under represented; in addition, the red blood cell has lost many membrane transporter activities upon differentiation from reticulocytes, thus limiting the parasite's access to extracellular nutrients. Consequently, the intra-erythrocytic growth of the parasite depends on its ability to efficiently uptake a range of essential nutrients from the extracellular milieu through the host cell membrane to the TVN (Lauer *et al.*, 1997). This is achieved by both the use of constitutively active host cell transporters and by the creation of new permeability pathways (NPPs) in the host cell membrane [reviewed in (Kirk, 2001)].

The permeability to a wide range of physiologically relevant solutes is newly detected in the infected erythrocyte membrane at the trophozoite stage of the parasite (Ginsburg *et al.*, 1985; Homewood & Neame, 1974; Staines *et al.*, 2001). They might originate both from parasite-encoded transporters that are delivered to the host cell membrane, and from the modulation of endogenous transporters of the erythrocyte by parasite-encoded proteins. Indeed, the NPPs depend on parasite proteins either as components of the NPPs or as modulators of endogenous erythrocytic transporters as first demonstrated by their re-appearance in intact infected erythrocytes following inactivation by chymotrypsin treatment and further suspension in a chymotrypsin-free medium (Baumeister *et al.*, 2006). NPPs re-appearance depends on the parasite viability and ability for protein secretion. Nguitragool and collaborators have recently determined that the parasite Clag3 proteins, exported to the red blood cell membrane, contribute to a novel ion channel with unusual selectivity and conductance properties (Nguitragool *et al.*, 2011). Moreover, several parasite protein-kinases are exported to the erythrocyte cytosol (Nunes *et al.*, 2007) that might modulate the activity and specificity of pre-existing inactive membrane transporters. A specific and high affinity interaction of serum albumin with the surface of infected erythrocytes has also been shown to stimulate anion conductance in the host erythrocyte membrane, thus clearly illustrating the participation of both parasite and host factors in the activation of NPPs (Duranton *et al.*, 2008).

3.2 Protrusions at the cell surface mediate sequestration of *P. falciparum*-infected erythrocytes

The parasite-induced changes at the red blood cell membrane described above, would end up in a very efficient splenic removal of infected erythrocytes from the blood circulation if the parasite had not been able to confer adhesive properties to its host cell. Indeed, cytoadherence of *P. falciparum*-infected erythrocytes to the microvasculature endothelium has been observed which results in their sequestration at the mature trophozoite and schizont stages of the parasite. This cytoadherence is mediated by the parasite adhesin, PfEMP1, exposed at electron-dense protrusions of the erythrocyte surface, referred to as knobs (Baruch *et al.*, 1995; Fairhurst & Wellems, 2006; Fremount & Miller, 1975). The key player in knobs formation is the knob-associated histidine-rich protein (KAHRP or HRP-1) as absence of this protein results in knobless infected erythrocytes (Crabb *et al.*, 1997; Kilejian, 1979). In addition, the C-terminal region of this protein has been shown to be essential for the formation of functional knobs (Rug *et al.*, 2006). The knobs-mediated cytoadherence of *P. falciparum*-infected erythrocytes and its implication in the pathogenesis of severe malaria [reviewed in (Rowe *et al.*, 2009) have been the subject of numerous studies and reviews and will only be shortly described here with special focus on the molecular organization of knobs.

As the parasite matures from trophozoite to schizont, the knobs increase in density (from 10-35 to 45-75 knobs/μm^2) and eventually cover the entire red blood cell surface while their size varies inversely from 160-110 nm to 70-100 nm in diameter (Gruenberg *et al.*, 1983). Their formation implies dynamic changes to the erythrocyte membrane and sub-membrane skeleton, which involve redistribution and organization of constituents from both parasite and host cell origin. The knob-associated histidine-rich protein (KAHRP) self-aggregates (Kilejian *et al.*, 1991) and anchors the carboxy-terminal domain of PfEMP1 to the erythrocyte sub-membrane skeleton at the actin-protein 4.1-spectrin junction (Waller *et al.*, 1999; Waller *et al.*, 2002). In addition, extractability data strongly suggest that other red blood cell membrane-associated proteins are implicated because the insertion of PfEMP1 in the red blood cell membrane seems to rely more on protein-protein interactions than protein-lipid interactions (Papakrivos *et al.*, 2005). Indeed, beside KAHRP, other parasite and erythrocyte proteins affect the amount and distribution of PfEMP1 at the red blood cell surface (Allred *et al.*, 1986; Fairhurst & Wellems, 2006). Many studies have contributed to provide an integrated model of the knob structure [reviewed in (Maier *et al.*, 2009)], implicating erythrocyte cytoskeletal components such as spectrin, ankyrin and actin and thus altering the physical properties of the erythrocyte by increasing its rigidity and adhesiveness (Pei *et al.*, 2005). However, while the 5' repeat region of KAHRP is required for the knob protrusion (Rug *et al.*, 2006), the precise interactions at the red blood cell membrane and sub-membrane skeleton causing protrusion of the red blood cell plasma membrane still need further investigations.

Besides the TVN and knobs, many other parasite-induced changes in the red blood cell and different populations of vesicular-like membrane compartments have been observed in the infected erythrocyte which might be implicated in the trafficking of nutrients, lipids and parasite-encoded proteins within the host cell (Grellier *et al.*, 1991; Hanssen *et al.*, 2010; Külzer *et al.*, 2010; Tamez *et al.*, 2008).

4. The Maurer's clefts, a novel secretory compartment transposed in the host cell cytosol

Within tens of seconds after merozoites entry and sealing of the parasitophorous vacuole, the erythrocyte membrane deforms from its biconcave disc shape to an echinocyte shape and returns to its normal state after several minutes (Gilson & Crabb, 2009) (Figure 2). This echinocytosis might be the result of the invagination of the red cell membrane and changes to the host cell cytoskeleton (Pantaleo *et al.*, 2010) or induced by an efflux of potassium and chloride ions (Gilson & Crabb, 2009). In addition, these fluctuations of the red cell membrane might correlate with 1) the insertion of lipids in the external leaflet of the host cell membrane likely secreted with the rhoptry content upon invasion that would result in increasing the area of the red cell membrane external leaflet and explain the formation of spicules; 2) modifications of the erythrocyte membrane / sub-membrane skeleton interactions upon parasite entry. Two modifications of the erythrocyte Band 3 necessary for efficient parasite entry have been observed: cleavage by the rhoptry protease Pfgp76 resulting in increased uptake of phospholipids by the red cell membrane (Braun-Breton *et al.*, 1992; Roggwiller *et al.*, 1996) and hyper-phosphorylation resulting in the dissociation of Band 3 interactions with the cytoskeleton (Ferru *et al.*, 2011; Pantaleo *et al.*, 2010). Such a detachment is concordant with the spectacular echinocytic and transient shape transformation of the erythrocyte after invasion. At approximately the time of resumption of the erythrocyte to its normal shape, parasite-induced membranous compartments termed Maurer's clefts are present and observed to be scattered within the host cell cytoplasm (Gruring *et al.*, 2011) before predominantly residing in close vicinity of the erythrocyte periphery.

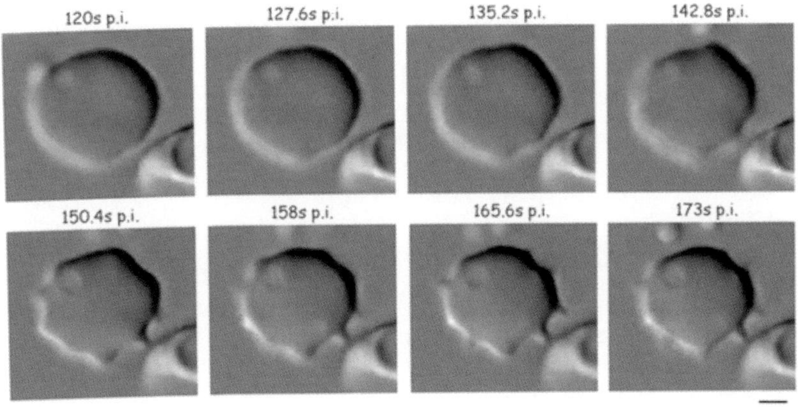

Fig. 2. Red blood cell deformations following the entry of a *P. falciparum* merozoite. Change of the erythrocyte shape started about 2 min following entry of a *P. falciparum* merozoite, with the formation of membrane spicules and generating an echinocyte morphology. The time scale post-invasion is indicated on each snap-shot. High speed live imaging with the participation of Magali Roques and Manouk Abkarian

In 1902, the German physician Georg Maurer has described a peculiar dotted staining pattern in the cytoplasm of *P. falciparum*-infected erythrocytes stained with Giemsa. Georg Maurer has provided a complete and in-depth description of these structures that were then named Maurer's clefts in his honour (Lanzer *et al.*, 2006). The significance of the discovery of Maurer's clefts remained unrecognized for almost a century till presently it has become one of the focuses of intense malaria research concerning their morphology, biogenesis and functional roles.

4.1 Morphology of Maurer's clefts

Trager and co-worker were among the first researchers to resolve the dotted pattern as long, narrow, slender single membrane surrounded clefts (Trager *et al.*, 1966). Ultra-structural studies showed that Maurer's clefts have a distinct morphology as stacks of flattened lamellae of long slender membrane of about 0.2-0.5 µm in length with translucent lumen and electron dense coat of variable thickness (60-100 nm) located predominantly at the erythrocyte membrane periphery as the parasite matures (Etzion & Perkins, 1989; Wickert &

Krohne, 2007). 3D reconstructions have added another level of complexity to the organization and structure of Maurer's clefts. The simplest form of Maurer's clefts is a single, disc-shaped cistern localized beneath the erythrocyte membrane with height and width of at least 500 nm. Maurer's clefts with more complex morphology are formed by small stacks of parallel cisternae with height of 650-800 nm and width of 300 nm (Wickert *et al.*, 2004; Wickert & Krohne, 2007). In addition, electron tomography, a technique collecting a series of images titled at different angles and tomography reconstruction of the aligned electron micrographs to generate a 3D model, has been recently applied to obtain a spatial image of Maurer's clefts (Hanssen *et al.*, 2010; Hanssen *et al.*, 2008b; Henrich *et al.*, 2009; Tilley & Hanssen, 2008). Hanssen and colleagues have revealed the 3D complexity of Maurer's clefts with convoluted flotillas of flattened disc-shape structures with translucent lumen and a more electron dense coat; some regions are decorated with surface nodules each of ~25 nm in diameter (Hanssen *et al.*, 2008b; Tilley & Hanssen, 2008). Differences were also observed in the complexity of the clefts between different *P. falciparum* strains. In D10 strain, more than 60% of Maurer's clefts have more than two cisternae, while in 3D7, only 10% show such complex organization (Frischknecht & Lanzer, 2008; Hanssen *et al.*, 2008b), suggesting that additional studies with a range of field and laboratory strains are needed to have a complete overview of the Maurer's clefts morphology (Hanssen *et al.*, 2008b).

4.2 Biogenesis of the Maurer's clefts

The biogenesis of Maurer's clefts still remains an open area of research. Wickert and colleagues proposed that Maurer's clefts form a continuous network from the PVM/ TVN with Maurer's clefts arising at one or more sites from the PVM/ TVN membrane and extending across the host cell cytoplasm to the inner leaflet of the erythrocyte plasma membrane (Wickert *et al.*, 2004; Wickert *et al.*, 2003). Consistently, using a fluorescent lipid and 3D reconstructions of sequential confocal images, Haldar and colleagues observed a continuous, membranous tubular network and vesicular structures within the cytoplasm of infected erythrocytes with dots, presumably Maurer's clefts, connected by fine threads originating from the PVM (Haldar *et al.*, 2001). Additionally, electron tomography studies showed stalk-like structures connecting one end of Maurer's clefts body to the PVM (Hanssen *et al.*, 2008b). These findings are consistent with the Maurer's clefts originating from the PVM.

However, FRAP-fluorescence recovery after photobleaching using a fluorescent lipid probe and GFP chimeras of Maurer's clefts proteins such as MAHRP1 and REX1 (Ring Exported Protein 1) (Hanssen *et al.*, 2008a; Spielmann *et al.*, 2006b; Spycher *et al.*, 2006) showed that although nascent Maurer's clefts seem to bud from the PVM, they further diffuse in the host cell cytoplasm as distinct, independent entities. Moreover, proteomic and immunofluorescence studies have revealed different sets of proteins residing in the parasitophorous vacuole and Maurer's clefts (Nyalwidhe & Lingelbach, 2006; Vincensini *et al.*, 2005).

4.3 Connectivity of the Maurer's clefts with the host cell membrane

A recent study by Gruring *et al* shows that Maurer's clefts are highly mobile structures in the ring stage parasites and with transition to trophozoite stage, the position of clefts become fixed and with smaller rearrangement in the later stage as clefts predominantly move to host cell periphery before merozoite formation and egress (Gruring *et al.*, 2011). Consistently, using limited osmotic lysis of infected erythrocytes, Blisnick and colleagues showed that Maurer's clefts are attached to the erythrocyte membrane and sub-membrane skeleton (Blisnick *et al.*, 2000). The binding of Maurer's clefts to the erythrocyte membrane in the late stage parasite partly depends on the interaction of a Maurer's clefts resident protein, PfSBP1 (*P. falciparum* skeleton binding protein1) (Blisnick *et al.*, 2000) with an erythrocyte host peripheral membrane protein, LANCL1 (lantibiotic synthetase component C-like protein) through its carboxy-terminal domain (Blisnick *et al.*, 2005). This interaction is dependent on the phosphorylation status of PfSBP1 which is regulated by a Maurer's cleft protein phosphatase, PfPP1, in the late stage parasite (Blisnick *et al.*, 2006). However, Maurer's clefts are attached to the erythrocyte membrane throughout the intra-erythrocytic development of the parasite (Blisnick *et al.*, 2005). Hence, it is believed that there must be other forms of interaction between Maurer's clefts and the erythrocyte membrane probably involving binding of Maurer's clefts proteins to erythrocyte skeleton proteins such as actin (Etzion & Perkins, 1989) or ankyrin (Atkinson *et al.*, 1988).

Indeed, electron tomography studies revealed that some Maurer's clefts are tethered to the erythrocyte membrane with stalk-like profiles (Hanssen *et al.*, 2008b). High resolution at the tethered region reveals a membrane bilayer tube of a diameter of ~30 nm, with a striated appearance and a more electron dense luminal compartment as compared to the Maurer's clefts lumen (Tilley & Hanssen, 2008). The contact between the tether-like structure and the erythrocyte membrane appears to involve an interaction with the cytoplasmic face of the erythrocyte membrane. In addition, a parasite membrane-associated histidine-rich protein 2 (MAHRP2) has also been identified residing specifically at these stalk extensions (Pachlatko *et al.*, 2010). Importantly, all attempts to date to genetically knock out *mahrp2* have failed, indicating its importance, and that of Maurer's clefts, for the parasite survival. Very new and important data have been recently published, showing that the flattened morphology of Maurer's clefts is likely due to the force generated by actin filaments that polymerize from the Maurer's clefts to domains of the red blood cell sub-membrane skeleton underneath the knobs (Cyrklaff *et al.*, 2011). Vesicle-like structures of ~25 nm in diameter were also observed in the erythrocyte cytoplasm which may be involved in the transport of cargoes between the Maurer's clefts and red cell membrane compartments (Hanssen *et al.*, 2008b). Moreover, the actin filaments attaching Maurer's clefts to the knobs seem to provide support and guidance for the transport of such vesicles from the clefts to the host cell plasma membrane (Cyrklaff *et al.*, 2011).

In conclusion, nascent Maurer's clefts are thought to originate from the parasitophorous vacuole membrane and then mature to form functionally independent compartments tethered to the erythrocyte membrane. These membranous compartments are not physically connected, as there is no bilayer continuum between the compartments at either the protein or lipid level but are connected by vesicles, likely transporting parasite proteins from the Maurer's clefts to the host cell surface (Gruring *et al.*, 2011; Hanssen *et al.*, 2008b; Tilley & Hanssen, 2008).

4.4 Biological roles of Maurer's clefts

Maurer's clefts are described as an extracellular secretory organelle which functions as an intermediate compartment or 'pre-assembly' platform for the sorting and delivery of parasite-encoded proteins to their final destinations in the host cell (Przyborski, 2008). In addition to permanent resident proteins (Vincensini *et al.*, 2005), Maurer's clefts appeared to house some transient parasite-encoded proteins such as STEVOR (subtelomeric variable open reading frame) (Przyborski *et al.*, 2005), KAHRP (knob-associated histidine rich protein) (Wickham *et al.*, 2001), PfEMP3 (Knuepfer *et al.*, 2005a) and the virulence factor, PfEMP1 (Knuepfer *et al.*, 2005b) en route to their final destinations at the host cell periphery.

Generation of PfSBP1 knock-out parasites showed that this Maurer's clefts resident protein is essential for the export of the PfEMP1 adhesin to the erythrocyte surface; in addition, in these knock-out parasites, the Maurer's clefts morphology was altered and Maurer's clefts were no longer found close to the periphery of the infected erythrocytes (Cooke *et al.*, 2006). Furthermore, over expression, mutagenesis or deletion of other resident or associated Maurer's clefts proteins such as MAHRP1 (Spycher *et al.*, 2008), REX1 (that associates with the edges of Maurer's clefts) (Hanssen *et al.*, 2008a) and PfEMP3 (Waterkeyn *et al.*, 2000) not only alter the morphology, formation and architecture of Maurer's clefts, but also affect the delivery and presentation of the virulence factor PfEMP1 to the erythrocyte surface (Dixon *et al.*, 2011; Maier *et al.*, 2009). All these data demonstrate that the correct architecture and assembly of Maurer's clefts and their connectivity to the host cell membrane are essential for the delivery of PfEMP1 to knobs and the cytoadhesive properties of *P. falciparum*-infected erythrocytes.

Besides playing a role in protein exporting, Maurer's clefts also potentially house chaperones (HSP), metabolic enzymes and proteins involved in signalling pathways (Vincensini *et al.*, 2005). This indicates that Maurer's clefts could be a multifunctional organelle serving as a platform for metabolic pathways and signalling processes such as phospholipids biosynthesis, protein modulation by phosphorylation and dephosphorylation eventually affecting merozoite egress or other biological processes as reviewed in (Lanzer *et al.*, 2006). Hence, it is crucial to have a deeper insight of the organization and compositions of this membrane compartment.

5. Export of parasite proteins to the host cell

Upon merozoites invasion and trophozoite growth, huge erythrocyte remodelling has been made as discussed before for the parasite growth, nutrients acquisition, pathogenesis and immune evasion, by exporting parasite-encoded proteins to the host cell (Figure 3). In doing so, the parasite has to establish its own novel secretory and trafficking system in the host cell that lacks secretory pathways. In higher eukaryotes, the secretion or trafficking of proteins requires a chain of sequential and highly regulated steps that involve budding and fusion of small vesicles. Most proteins destined to be secreted or exported have a stretch of amino-terminal hydrophobic signal sequence for translocation into the endoplasmic reticulum (ER) (von Heijne, 1985) then transit through the Golgi apparatus before exiting from the cell by exocytosis. These series of events are termed as the constitutive secretory pathway. In *P. falciparum*, like in other eukaryotes, secreted proteins undergoing a constitutive secretory pathway have a signal sequence composed of a stretch of about 15 to 20 hydrophobic amino acids from the N-terminal or a recessed N-terminal signal sequence up to 80 amino acids from the N-terminus addressing the protein to the ER (Lingelbach, 1993). Proteins either with the classical or recessed signal sequences are able to follow the "constitutive" or "default" secretory pathway into the parasitophorous vacuole (soluble proteins) or the

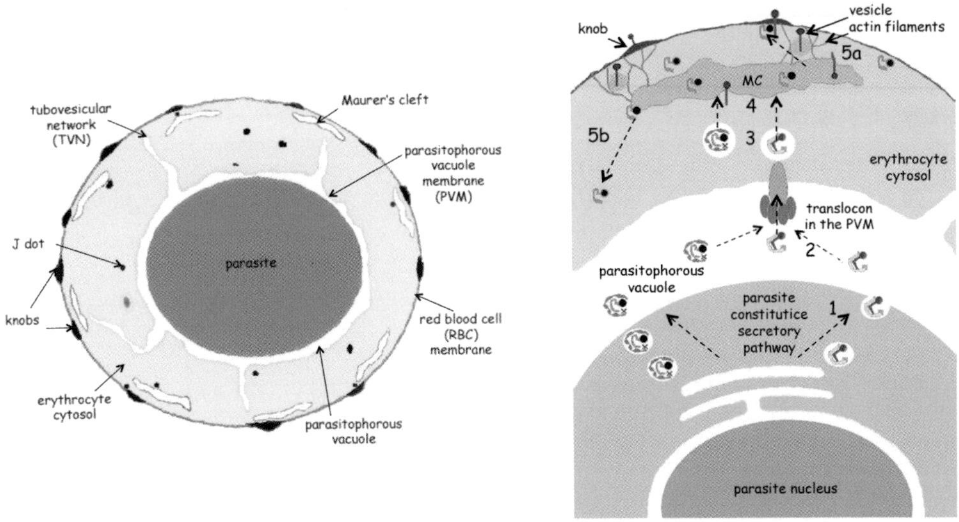

Fig. 3. Scheme of a *P. falciparum*-infected erythrocyte focusing on the host cell major changes (left panel) and a proposed model for export of parasite proteins beyond the confines of the parasite (right panel). The parasite is growing inside the parasitophorous vacuole, the membrane of which constitutes the interface between the parasite and its external environment. Extensions of the parasitophorous vacuole membrane (PVM) form the tubuvesicular network (TVN) extending into the host cell cytosol. Various parasite structures are transposed into the red cell cytosol: the Maurer's clefts are flat and elongated membrane vesicles at the host cell periphery and linked to the host cell membrane and sub-membrane skeleton; J dots are likely membrane structures that might traffic some parasite proteins through the erythrocyte cytosol. Complexes of exported parasite proteins interacting with the erythrocyte membrane and sub-membrane skeleton forms protrusions of the red cell membrane, referred to as knobs, that mediate adhesion of the infected erythrocyte to host cells.Parasite proteins exported to the host cell traffic through the parasite constitutive secretory pathway as soluble proteins (1) (membrane proteins are likely interacting with chaperones to maintain them as unfolded and soluble) and are released in the lumen of the parasitophorous vacuole (2). Interacting with chaperones in the parasitophorous vacuole, they are addressed to a translocon in the parasitophorous vacuole membrane (PVM) (2) and released in the host cell cytosol (3). The proteins are further addressed to the Maurer's clefts, as soluble complexes and also possibly associated with J-dots (4). Finally, soluble proteins are sorted from the Maurer's clefts to the red cell cytosol and sub-membrane skeleton (5b) and membrane proteins are trafficked to the red cell plasma membrane (5a), likely by vesicles that fuse with the host cell membrane.

parasite plasma membrane (integral membrane proteins) (Adisa *et al.*, 2003; Tonkin *et al.*, 2006; Wickham *et al.*, 2001). An example is the integral membrane *P. falciparum* exported protein-1 (PfEXP1), which possesses a classical N-terminal signal sequence and is exported beyond the parasite to the PVM (Günther *et al.*, 1991). Another exported protein KHARP, involved in the cytoadherence complex, has a recessed N-terminal signal that contains information both necessary and sufficient for entry into the ER and trafficking to the parasitophorous vacuole (Wickham *et al.*, 2001). These data indicate that the parasite's translocation machinery is able to recognize both the classical and recessed signal peptides, and in the absence of any additional sorting information, proteins are transported into the parasitophorous vacuole. However, a 34 amino acid sequence in the C-terminal region of eight studied PVM proteins was proposed to be the parasitophorous targeting motif (Eksi & Williamson, 2011). On the other hand, additional information is required for most proteins, which are exported beyond the confines of the parasite across the parasitophorous vacuole to the erythrocyte cytosol and surface.

The unusual nature of export process of *Plasmodium* is further signified by the discovery of a novel pentameric amino acid sequence motif that directs the export of parasite encoded proteins beyond the parasitophorous vacuole. This conserved motif (R/KxI/LxE/Q/D) is referred to as *Plasmodium* Export Element (PEXEL) (Marti *et al.*, 2004) or alternatively as Vacuolar Targeting Signal (VTS) (Hiller *et al.*, 2004), which are identified by different algorithms with slightly different specificities but recognizing the same core sequence (van Ooij *et al.*, 2008). Interestingly, a similar Host Cell Targeting motif (HCTM) is also detected in the Irish potato famine pathogen *Phytophthora infestans* for delivering virulence gene products into plant cells (Bhattacharjee *et al.*, 2006). This has provided the first evidence that eukaryotic microbes share equivalent targeting signals and thus possible conserved mechanisms to access host cells (Haldar *et al.*, 2006). The PEXEL motif is located about 20-40 amino acids downstream from the signal sequence and is typically encoded in close proximity to the start of exon 2 in a two-exon gene (Charpian & Przyborski, 2008). The discovery of this motif, allowed the *in silico* prediction of the exported proteins of *P. falciparum* and other *Plasmodium* species. Using different algorithms, the *P. falciparum* exportome was predicted to contain more than 300 proteins (Hiller *et al.*, 2004; Marti *et al.*, 2004; Sargeant *et al.*, 2006). Many of these proteins have one or two predicted trans-membrane domains (Sargeant *et al.*, 2006; van Ooij *et al.*, 2008) indicating that the parasite transport machinery can export both soluble and trans-membrane proteins. In addition, the amino acids surrounding the motif are important for the correct targeting or trafficking to the host cell as demonstrated by (Przyborski *et al.*, 2005) for the efficient trafficking process of STEVOR.

Further dissecting this PEXEL motif, recent studies provided evidence of N-terminal processing of this motif as shown for PfEMP2, PfHRPII (Chang *et al.*, 2008), PfKAHRP and GBP130 (Glycophorin Binding Protein) (Boddey *et al.*, 2009), where this motif is recognized by a novel ER peptidase which cleaves on the C-terminal side of the Leucine residue in the PEXEL motif. Plasmepsin V is proved to be the ER-resident peptidase responsible for this cleavage (Boddey *et al.*, 2010; Russo *et al.*, 2010). The new N-terminus is then further acetylated in the parasite ER in a PEXEL independent process (Boddey *et al.*, 2009; Chang *et al.*, 2008). The processed protein should then present a motif that is recognized by a specific transporter in the parasitophorous vacuole membrane that helps translocating the protein across the PVM to the host cytosol. Indeed, a *Plasmodium* translocon of exported proteins (PTEX) located in the PVM has been identified in *P. falciparum* (de Koning-Ward *et al.*, 2009). This translocon is ATP-powered and comprises heat shock protein 101, which belongs to a super family commonly associated with protein translocons, a novel protein termed PTEX150 (PF14_0344) and a known parasite protein, exported protein 2 (EXP2), which is suggested to be a potential channel since it is the membrane–associated component of the core PTEX complex (de Koning-Ward *et al.*, 2009). PfEXP2 lacks a typical hydrophobic trans-membrane domain but was proved to be membrane-associated via an amphipathic helix located at the N-terminal part of the protein (Fischer *et al.*, 1998). It has been proposed that, like bacterial pore forming proteins to which it shows some structural similarities, PfEXP2 might insert into the PVM by oligomerization (Haase & de Koning-Ward, 2010). N-acetylation may help the PVM translocon to differentiate between proteins to be exported beyond the PVM and those that should reside in the parasitophorous vacuole. In addition, protein unfolding maintained with the help of chaperones is an essential requirement for transport across the PVM (Gehde *et al.*, 2009). Chaperones and proteases are the most abundant proteins in the vacuole, suggesting an important role of the vacuole both in protein folding and processing (Nyalwidhe & Lingelbach, 2006).

Chimeric proteins with (Wickham *et al.*, 2001) or without (Spycher *et al.*, 2006) PEXEL motif located near the parasite periphery have been reported to localize to structures with the appearance of a necklace of beads that are resistant to recovery after photobleaching. These data suggest the presence of sub-compartments within the PVM. In addition, PfEXP1 and ETRAMP locating at the PVM define separate arrays demonstrating that the protein distribution in the PVM is non-random, hence reinforcing the idea of the presence of sub-compartments within the PVM (Adisa *et al.*, 2003; Spielmann *et al.*, 2006a). Such sub-compartments are proposed to house the PTEX translocon (Boddey *et al.*, 2009; de Koning-Ward *et al.*, 2009).

Exceptionally, the PEXEL motif is not sufficient to export a parasite protein into the host cell as illustrated by RIFIN proteins: members of the B-type subfamily of RIFINs are exported to the Maurer's clefts while subfamily A-type RIFINs are retained within the parasite despite having the PEXEL motif (Petter *et al.*, 2007). This observation highlights the role of additional motifs or protein-protein interactions for efficient export that might be even more important than the PEXEL motif since an increasing number of parasite proteins that lack such an export motif are reported. These proteins are termed as PEXEL negative proteins or PNEPs [(Spielmann *et al.*, 2006b) and reviewed in (Spielmann & Gilberger, 2010)]. Some of the PNEPs including PfSBP1 (Saridaki *et al.*, 2009), PfMAHRP1 (Spycher *et al.*, 2008) and PfREX-1 (Spielmann *et al.*, 2006b) are known to be exported to the Maurer's clefts. The trans-membrane domain of PfSBP1 was demonstrated to address the protein to the parasite ER and constitutive secretory pathway. One of the two characterized N-terminal domains of PfSBP1 with high negative net charge and acting independently is necessary for the protein export beyond the parasite to Maurer's clefts (Saridaki *et al.*, 2009). For PfMAHRP1, the second half of the N-terminal part of the protein and the trans-membrane domain contain the essential signal for trafficking to Maurer's clefts (Spycher *et al.*, 2006). As for PfREX-1, a hydrophobic stretch and additional 10 amino acid towards the C-terminal are important for the protein export (Dixon *et al.*, 2008). The $PfSURFIN_{4.2}$ protein was shown to localize at the Maurer's clefts and the infected erythrocyte plasma membrane using immuno-electron microscopy (Winter *et al.*, 2005), and found to be trafficked to the host cell as a PNEP. $PfSURFIN_{4.2}$ protein export to the host cell does not depend on any of its two non consensus PEXEL-like motifs nor on its extracellular domain but requires its predicted trans-membrane domain (Alexandre *et al.*, 2011). Interestingly, $PfSURFIN_{4.2}$ was reported to accumulate in the parasitophorous vacuole in late schizonts, thus suggesting stage-dependent differential localization (Winter *et al.*, 2005). Taken together, these studies showed that no obvious export motif is found among and shared by PNEPs but proved the importance of an hydrophobic trans-membrane domain, likely addressing PNEPs to the parasite ER, and that of protein-protein interactions for their delivery beyond the confines of the parasite. Whether PNEPs indirectly use the PTEX translocon or an alternative export pathway calls for more investigations.

To date, there are many proposed models of protein trafficking pathways across the PVM to the erythrocyte cytosol and surface, based on the studies of different parasite proteins which has broaden our knowledge of the presence of multiple exporting routes. The most popular model of protein export across the PVM is that unfolded proteins are secreted into the parasitophorous vacuole, and translocate through a channel or translocon (PTEX) into the host cytosol as discussed above. Ultrastructural studies showing strings of vesicles budding off from the PVM have provided evidence of vesicle trafficking in the infected erythrocyte cytosol (Trelka *et al.*, 2000). PfEMP1 and PfEMP3 were found to be associated with these vesicles, and proposed to be delivered to the erythrocyte surface in the mode of vesicles (Trelka *et al.*, 2000). In addition, homologues of two components of the classical vesicle-mediated trafficking machinery COPII, PfSar1p and PfSec31p, were reported to be exported to the erythrocyte cytosol, suggesting a vesicle-mediated trafficking pathway for proteins across the erythrocyte cytoplasm (Adisa *et al.*, 2001; Adisa *et al.*, 2002). However, this model has been recently challenged because, even in the presence of slowly hydrolysable GTP analogues blocking vesicular trafficking, PfEMP1 was still properly trafficked to the erythrocyte membrane (Frankland *et al.*, 2006). Moreover, the localization of the COPII proteins has been later redefined inside the parasite cytoplasm (Adisa *et al.*, 2007). Furthermore, PfEMP1 is transported as a soluble chaperoned complex in the erythrocyte cytosol, transiently inserts into the Maurer's clefts membrane and finally inserts into the erythrocyte membrane (Papakrivos *et al.*, 2005). This has revealed another model of non-vesicular mode of protein export where proteins may transport as soluble complexes in the erythrocyte cytosol and then interact transiently with Maurer's clefts before reaching the erythrocyte membrane skeleton (Knuepfer *et al.*, 2005a). Similarly, PfREX1 is exported across the PVM to the host cell cytosol as a soluble form and inserts to Maurer's clefts *via* a putative coiled-coil motif (Dixon *et al.*, 2008). Differently, PfMAHRP1 is trafficked to the Maurer's clefts in a membrane-associated manner budding from the PVM (Spycher *et al.*, 2006), adding to the evidence that nascent Maurer's clefts might be connected to or bud from the PVM as previously discussed.

To further elucidate the mechanisms of protein trafficking, Hanssen and collaborators have applied immunoelectron tomography combined with serial sectioning and immunogold labelling to explore the topography of infected erythrocytes (Hanssen *et al.*, 2010). They proposed that the exported secretory system of *P. falciparum* comprises a series of modular units: TVN, Maurer's clefts, and two different populations of vesicles of 25 and 80 nm in diameter in the erythrocyte cytosol, suggesting the presence of a vesicular-mediated trafficking pathway for the delivery of cargo between compartments to different destinations in the host cell (Hanssen *et al.*, 2010). Recently, other extra-parasitic structures named 'J-dots' and containing the exported parasite Hsp40 co-chaperone, were identified in the infected erythrocyte cytosol and proposed to traffic parasite proteins to the host cell (Külzer *et al.*, 2010). However, all parasite proteins identified so far as exported to the host cell are transiently associated with the Maurer's clefts. Since Maurer's clefts are physically tethered to the erythrocyte membrane, Hanssen and collaborators have proposed that proteins traffic from the Maurer's clefts to the erythrocyte membrane *via* the membranous tubular structure tethering the clefts to the host cell membrane (Hanssen *et al.*, 2010). Alternatively, transport vesicles have been shown to be attached to the actin filaments that connect the Maurer's clefts to the host cell membrane and might sustain the transport of proteins between these two compartments (Cyrklaff *et al.*, 2011).

6. Lipids remodelling: Implications of lipid rafts (DRMs) in human malaria

Despite identifying the roles and biogenesis of specific extracellular compartments of the parasite and the discovery of the protein exporting PEXEL motif with different models of trafficking pathways proposed, the contribution of lipids in these cellular processes is poorly understood even though the exported proteins have to bypass several membrane barriers to reach their final destination. Upon merozoite invasion, there is a change in the lipid and protein compositions of the infected erythrocyte membrane indicating that the parasite also remodels micro-domains of its host cell membrane known as lipid rafts and a lipid raft-based biogenesis of the parasitophorous vacuole membrane has been proposed. In addition, lipid raft-based processes and interactions of both host and parasite origin might be crucial to maintain the stability of the vacuolar environment for the parasite growth and pathogenesis [reviewed in (Murphy *et al.*, 2006)].

Lipid rafts also serve as a stage for protein assemblies, sorting and trafficking through endocytic and secretory pathways in other cell types [reviewed in (Hanzal-Bayer & Hancock, 2007)]. Do DRMs have any contributions to *P. falciparum* protein trafficking pathways in infected erythrocytes? Tamez and colleagues have described a vesicle-like membrane compartment in the infected erythrocyte cytosol, which might be implicated in the import of lipids from the erythrocyte membrane to the TVN (Tamez *et al.*, 2008). Moreover, the binding of the parasite Hsp40 co-chaperone to "J-dots", proposed to be involved in protein trafficking through the erythrocyte cytosol, was shown to be cholesterol dependent (Külzer *et al.*, 2010). Furthermore, the presentation of the parasite virulence protein PfEMP1 on the erythrocyte surface involves the final insertion of the protein into cholesterol-rich domains of the erythrocyte plasma membrane (Frankland *et al.*, 2006) and with more delivery in the presence of serum lipoproteins (Frankland *et al.*, 2007). Whether all parasite proteins exported to the host cell surface are delivered to lipid rafts needs to be further investigated.

In conclusion, elucidating and characterizing the functional roles of cholesterol rich DRMs during the intra-erythrocytic development of the *P. falciparum* parasite might shed new light on protein trafficking or host cell remodelling processes.

7. Merozoite egress from the red cell: A split second event likely depending on very early changes to the red blood cell membrane

The release of infectious merozoites from the host cell requires the opening of the parasitophorous and red cell membranes. Dvorak and collaborators have first observed that the swelling of the infected erythrocyte precedes the egress of *Plasmodium falciparum* merozoites by a few minutes (Dvorak *et al.*, 1975). In addition, the use of amphiphiles, osmotic stress and protease inhibitors strongly suggested that merozoite release is pressure driven (Glushakova *et al.*, 2009; Glushakova *et al.*, 2005). Shortly before merozoite egress, the intracellular parasites seem to move more freely while the red cell membrane is still intact

(Abkarian *et al.*, 2011), comforting previous studies providing evidence that, when the merozoites are close to egress, the PVM enlarges and ruptures before the erythrocyte membrane (Wickham *et al.*, 2003). What drives a sudden increase in the osmotic pressure? A premature release of immature merozoites has been recently described which results from the inhibition of RNA degradation and is preceded by swelling of the infected erythrocyte (Balu *et al.*, 2011). In addition, parasite proteases specifically active just prior to merozoite release could also participate in the increased osmolarity (Koussis *et al.*, 2009). Noteworthy, proteases of both parasite and host origin have likely numerous roles in merozoite egress and might also participate in both the rupture of the PVM and the subsequent opening of the erythrocyte membrane (Arastu-Kapur *et al.*, 2008; Chandramohanadas *et al.*, 2009; Yeoh *et al.*, 2007).

Indeed, although first considered as an explosive event, merozoite egress from the red blood cell has been shown recently to occur through the opening and stabilization of an osmotic pore in the host cell membrane allowing the release of a limited number of merozoites (Abkarian *et al.*, 2011). The pore opening is followed by the curling and buckling of the erythrocyte membrane, and this results in the wide-angular dispersion of the remaining merozoites. These events happen when a critical radius of the osmotic pore is reached. Abkarian *et al* 2011 hypothesized that this instability is biologically relevant as it disperses the merozoites and contributes to separate them efficiently from the infected cell membrane. Indeed, abortive egress events have been observed with a stop of curling and no buckling, resulting in the merozoites remaining stuck together inside the open erythrocyte and thus unable to further invade new red blood cells (Abkarian *et al.*, 2011). Noteworthy, these data have been obtained with infected erythrocytes in suspension and it is important to determine whether merozoites release proceeds through similar steps *in vivo*, when red cells with mature parasites are sequestered in the microvasculature, adhering to endothelial cells. Observations of infected erythrocytes adhered to a glass substrate shed some light on this process: over 5 merozoites were sequentially released through a pore of similar radius (1 μm) and with higher velocity as compared to non adhering cells, before curling occurred. The membrane was then projected backwards, thereby releasing merozoites but without actually pushing them forward. In brief, while similar steps are involved, the resulting dispersion of the merozoites looks different. These results suggest that adhesion maintains a membrane tension high enough to produce the overpressure driving more merozoites out of the host cell. Considering that *P. falciparum* infected erythrocytes are also able to adhere to non-infected erythrocytes, the merozoites would be released appropriately to re-invade *in vivo* efficiently.

The curling and buckling of the infected erythrocyte membrane can originate from an additional elastic energy due to an asymmetry between the membrane leaflets (Abkarian *et al.*, 2011). A nice illustration of this effect is the curling of a gift ribbon after one slides it between the thumb and a scissor blade, thus creating an excess area of the outer leaflet (Klales *et al.*, 2007). In *P. falciparum*- infected erythrocytes, this asymmetry between the two membrane leaflets could originate from a lipid excess in the inner leaflet caused by a lipid release of parasite origin, a modification of the mechanical properties of the red cell membrane through changes of the cytoskeleton/membrane interactions [reviewed in (An & Mohandas, 2010)] and/or interactions of the erythrocyte membrane with the Maurer's clefts.

As described before, parasite-induced changes at the red blood cell membrane affecting its stability occur as early as parasite entry and very early intra-erythrocytic growth. Moreover, phosphorylation of host peripheral proteins increases upon parasite growth and might modulate the bio-physical properties of the red cell membrane throughout the parasite development (Pantaleo *et al.*, 2010). One might thus consider that on one hand the parasite weakens its host cell membrane and on the other hand it stabilizes it by exporting proteins to the red cell sub-membrane skeleton and recruiting host proteins to or from the sub-membrane skeleton.

However, the ability to curl and buckle has also been proposed to be an intrinsic property of the erythrocyte membrane when the cell is exposed to certain osmotic stress (Lew, 2011) although with marked kinetic differences as compared to the infected erythrocyte. Whether the parasite explores a property of its host cell and at what extent the changes of the red cell membrane and sub-membrane skeleton induced by the parasite are essential for efficient merozoite release need further investigations.

8. Concluding remarks

As described in this chapter, Apicomplexan parasites widely transform the parasitophorous vacuole in which they grow and multiply and which constitutes the interface between the parasite and its extracellular environment. Changes of its closed environment, the red blood cell cytoplasm and plasma membrane, induced by the life-threatening human malaria parasite *Plasmodium falciparum* have been extensively studied because these changes are crucial for the parasite development and some, referred to as knobs, are specific for this species and central to the pathogenesis of severe malaria. In the last decade, the set up of *P. falciparum* genetic engineering and the spectacular advances of imaging technologies, have considerably highlighted our knowledge of the red cell remodelling by the parasite, the processes involved and their importance for the parasite survival.

Upon intra-erythrocytic parasite growth, new permeation pathways in the red cell membrane and extensions of the parasitophorous vacuole membrane in the host cell cytosol, named the tubovesicular network, participate in the import of nutrients from the extracellular milieu. Other membrane structures transposed by the parasite in the cytoplasm of its host cell, referred to as Maurer's clefts, and proposed to generate from the parasitophorous vacuole membrane, are central to the transport of parasite proteins to the red blood cell. They tightly interact with the host cell membrane even upon merozoite release. This interaction together with exported parasite proteins interacting with the host cell sub-membrane skeleton might prevent the premature rupture of the red cell membrane and consequent release of immature merozoites. Maintaining the integrity of the red cell membrane upon its growth is likely crucial for the parasite because it has weakened its host cell membrane by altering the cohesion between the plasma membrane and sub-membrane skeleton *via* the phosphorylation and the recruitment of host cell membrane and skeletal proteins. On the other hand, one can consider that the parasite has prepared its host cell membrane not only for entry but also for egress because reversing the parasite-induced modifications, for example by the activation of phosphatases, would highly facilitate the rupture of the red cell plasma membrane.

The merozoite release, following the engulfment of the infected erythrocyte, relies on an unique site of opening allowing the egress of the first one or two merozoites; the release of the remaining merozoites results from the curling and eversion of the red blood cell membrane. Importantly, the same sequence of events has been observed whether the infected erythrocytes were in suspension or adhering to the substrate (which is the usual status of *P. falciparum* infected erythrocytes because of cytoadherence to the micro-vessel endothelium and to non-infected erythrocytes). The physical parameters of curling and eversion of the red cell membrane emphasized once more the importance of parasite-induced changes to the host cell membrane.

Red blood cell remodelling by the malaria parasite necessitates both efficient export of parasite proteins to the host cell and extensive membrane synthesis. These processes, together with the parasite enzymatic activities, such as proteases, protein kinases and phosphatases, which are crucial for the intra-cellular survival of the parasite and evasion from splenic clearance and host immune response, deserve precise characterization because they are Achilles heels that could be targeted by specific drugs or antibodies.

9. Acknowledgements

We are very grateful to Maryse Lebrun for critical reading of the manuscript and apologize to researchers whose work has not been directly cited in this review because of limiting space. This work was supported by the University Montpellier 2 and the CNRS. XY Yam was supported by the MalParTraining FP6 Marie Curie Action under contract No. MEST-CT-2005-020492. A Mbengue is supported by a PhD fellowship from the French Ministère de l'Education Nationale, de la Recherche et de la Technologie.

10. References

Abkarian, M., Massiera, G., Berry, L., Roques, M., Braun-Breton, C., 2011, A novel mechanism for malaria parasite egress from the red blood cell. Blood,.

Adisa, A., Albano, F.R., Reeder, J., Foley, M., Tilley, L., 2001, Evidence for a role for a *Plasmodium falciparum* homologue of Sec31p in the export of proteins to the surface of malaria parasite-infected erythrocytes. J Cell Sci 114, 3377-3386.

Adisa, A., Rug, M., Foley, M., Tilley, L., 2002, Characterisation of a [delta]-COP homologue in the malaria parasite, *Plasmodium falciparum*. Mol. Biochem. Parasitol. 123, 11-21.

Adisa, A., Rug, M., Klonis, N., Foley, M., Cowman, A.F., Tilley, L., 2003, The Signal Sequence of Exported Protein-1 Directs the Green Fluorescent Protein to the Parasitophorous Vacuole of Transfected Malaria Parasites. J. Biol Chem 278, 6532-6542.

Adisa, A., Frankland, S., Rug, M., Jackson, K., Maier, A.G., Walsh, P., Lithgow, T., Klonis, N., Gilson, P.R., Cowman, A.F., Tilley, L., 2007, Re-assessing the locations of components of the classical vesicle-mediated trafficking machinery in transfected *Plasmodium falciparum*. International Journal for Parasitology 37, 1127-1141.

Aikawa, M., Miller, L., Johnson, J., Rabbege, J., 1978, Erythrocyte entry by malarial parasites. A moving junction between erythrocyte and parasite. The Journal of Cell Biology 77, 72-82.

Aikawa, M., Miller, L.H., Rabbege, J.R., Epstein, N., 1981, Freeze-fracture study on the erythrocyte membrane during malarial parasite invasion. The Journal of Cell Biology 91, 55-62.

Alexandre, J.S.F., Yahata, K., Kawai, S., Torii, M., Kaneko, O., 2011, PEXEL-independent trafficking of *Plasmodium falciparum* SURFIN4.2 to the parasite-infected red blood cell and Maurer's clefts. Parasitology International 60, 313-320.

Allred, D.R., Gruenberg, J.E., Sherman, I.W., 1986, Dynamic rearrangements of erythrocyte membrane internal architecture induced by infection with *Plasmodium falciparum*. Journal of Cell Science 81, 1-16.

An, X., Mohandas, N., 2010, Red cell membrane and malaria. Transfus Clin Biol 17, 197-199.

Arastu-Kapur, S., Ponder, E.L., Fonovic, U.P., Yeoh, S., Yuan, F., Fonovic, M., Grainger, M., Phillips, C.I., Powers, J.C., Bogyo, M., 2008, Identification of proteases that regulate erythrocyte rupture by the malaria parasite *Plasmodium falciparum*. Nature chemical biology 4, 203-213.

Atkinson, C., Aikawa, M., Perry, G., Fujino, T., Bennett, V., Davidson, E., Howard, R., 1988, Ultrastructural localization of erythrocyte cytoskeletal and integral membrane proteins in *Plasmodium falciparum*-infected erythrocytes. Eur J Cell Biol 45, 192-199.

Atkinson, C., Aikawa, M., 1990, Ultrastructure of malaria-infected erythrocytes. Blood Cells 16, 351-368.

Balu, B., Maher, S.P., Pance, A., Chauhan, C., Naumov, A.V., Andrews, R.M., Ellis, P.D., Khan, S.M., Lin, J.W., Janse, C.J., *et al.*, 2011, CCR4-associated factor 1 coordinates the expression of *Plasmodium falciparum* egress and invasion proteins. Eukaryotic Cell 10, 1257-1263.

Bannister, L., Mitchell, G., Butcher, G., Dennis, E., 1986, Lamellar membranes associated with rhoptries in erythrocytic merozoites of *Plasmodium knowlesi*: a clue to the mechanism of invasion. Parasitology 92, 291-303.

Bannister, L., Mitchell, G., 1989, The fine structure of secretion by Plasmodium knowlesi merozoites during red cell invasion. J Protozool 36, 362-367.

Baruch, D.I., Pasloske, B.L., Singh, H.B., Bi, X., Ma, X.C., Feldman, M., Taraschi, T.F., Howard, R.J., 1995, Cloning the *P. falciparum* gene encoding PfEMP1, a malarial variant antigen and adherence receptor on the surface of parasitized human erythrocytes. Cell 82, 77-87.

Baumeister, S., Winterberg, M., Duranton, C., Huber, S.M., Lang, F., Kirk, K., Lingelbach, K., 2006, Evidence for the involvement of *Plasmodium falciparum* proteins in the formation of new permeability pathways in the erythrocyte membrane. Mol Microbiol 60, 493-504.

Behnke, M.S., Khan, A., Wootton, J.C., Dubey, J.P., Tang, K., Sibley, L.D., 2011, Virulence differences in *Toxoplasma* mediated by amplification of a family of polymorphic pseudokinases. Proc. Natl. Acad. Sci. U.S.A 108, 9631-9636.

Besteiro, S., Michelin, A., Poncet, J., Dubremetz, J.F., Lebrun, M., 2009, Export of a *Toxoplasma gondii* rhoptry neck protein complex at the host cell membrane to form the moving junction during invasion. PLoS Pathog 5, e1000309.

Besteiro, S., Dubremetz, J.-F., Lebrun, M., 2011, The moving junction of apicomplexan parasites: a key structure for invasion. Cellular Microbiology 13, 797-805.

Bhattacharjee, S., Hiller, N.L., Liolios, K., Win, J., Kanneganti, T.-D., Young, C., Kamoun, S., Haldar, K., 2006, The Malarial Host-Targeting Signal Is Conserved in the Irish Potato Famine Pathogen. PLoS Pathog 2, e50.

Bietz, S., Montilla, I., Külzer, S., Przyborski, J.M., Lingelbach, K., 2009, Recruitment of human aquaporin 3 to internal membranes in the *Plasmodium falciparum* infected erythrocyte. Mol. Biochem. Parasitol 167, 48-53.

Blisnick, T., Morales Betoulle, M.E., Barale, J.-C., Uzureau, P., Berry, L., Desroses, S., Fujioka, H., Mattei, D., Braun Breton, C., 2000, Pfsbp1, a Maurer's cleft *Plasmodium falciparum* protein, is associated with the erythrocyte skeleton. Mol. Biochem. Parasitol 111, 107-121.

Blisnick, T., Vincensini, L., Barale, J.C., Namane, A., Braun Breton, C., 2005, LANCL1, an erythrocyte protein recruited to the Maurer's clefts during *Plasmodium falciparum* development. Mol. Biochem. Parasitol 141, 39-47.

Blisnick, T., Vincensini, L., Fall, G., Braun-Breton, C., 2006, Protein phosphatase 1, a *Plasmodium falciparum* essential enzyme, is exported to the host cell and implicated in the release of infectious merozoites. Cellular Microbiology 8, 591-601.

Boddey, J.A., Moritz, R.L., Simpson, R.J., Cowman, A.F., 2009, Role of the *Plasmodium* Export Element in Trafficking Parasite Proteins to the Infected Erythrocyte. Traffic 10, 285-299.

Boddey, J.A., Hodder, A.N., Gunther, S., Gilson, P.R., Patsiouras, H., Kapp, E.A., Pearce, J.A., de Koning-Ward, T.F., Simpson, R.J., Crabb, B.S., Cowman, A.F., 2010, An aspartyl protease directs malaria effector proteins to the host cell. Nature 463, 627-631.

Braun-Breton, C., Blisnick, T., Barbot, P., Bulow, R., Pereira da Silva, L., Langsley, G., 1992, *Plasmodium falciparum* and *Plasmodium chabaudi*: characterization of glycosylphosphatidylinositol-degrading activities. Experimental Parasitology 74, 452-462.

Chandramohanadas, R., Davis, P.H., Beiting, D.P., Harbut, M.B., Darling, C., Velmourougane, G., Lee, M.Y., Greer, P.A., Roos, D.S., Greenbaum, D.C., 2009, Apicomplexan parasites co-opt host calpains to facilitate their escape from infected cells. Science 324, 794-797.

Chang, H.H., Falick, A.M., Carlton, P.M., Sedat, J.W., DeRisi, J.L., Marletta, M.A., 2008, N-terminal processing of proteins exported by malaria parasites. Mol. Biochem. Parasitol 160, 107-115.

Charpian, S., Przyborski, J.M., 2008, Protein Transport Across the Parasitophorous Vacuole of Plasmodium falciparum: Into the Great Wide Open. Traffic 9, 157-165.

Cooke, B.M., Buckingham, D.W., Glenister, F.K., Fernandez, K.M., Bannister, L.H., Marti, M., Mohandas, N., Coppel, R.L., 2006, A Maurer's cleft-associated protein is essential for expression of the major malaria virulence antigen on the surface of infected red blood cells. J. Cell Biol. 172, 899-908.

Crabb, B.S., Cooke, B.M., Reeder, J.C., Waller, R.F., Caruana, S.R., Davern, K.M., Wickham, M.E., Brown, G.V., Coppel, R.L., Cowman, A.F., 1997, Targeted Gene Disruption Shows That Knobs Enable Malaria-Infected Red Cells to Cytoadhere under Physiological Shear Stress. Cell 89, 287-296.

Cyrklaff,M., Sanchez, C.P., Killian, N., Bisseye, C., Simpore, J., Frischknecht, F., Lanzer, M., 2011, Hemoglobin S and C interfere with actin remodeling in *Plasmodium falciparum*-infected erythrocytes. Science 2011 Nov 10. [Epub ahead of print]

de Koning-Ward, T.F., Gilson, P.R., Boddey, J.A., Rug, M., Smith, B.J., Papenfuss, A.T., Sanders, P.R., Lundie, R.J., Maier, A.G., Cowman, A.F., Crabb, B.S., 2009, A newly discovered protein export machine in malaria parasites. Nature 459, 945-949.

Dixon, M.W.A., Hawthorne, P.L., Spielmann, T., Anderson, K.L., Trenholme, K.R., Gardiner, D.L., 2008, Targeting of the Ring Exported Protein 1 to the Maurer's Clefts is Mediated by a Two-Phase Process. Traffic 9, 1316-1326.

Dixon, M.W.A., Kenny, S., McMillan, P.J., Hanssen, E., Trenholme, K.R., Gardiner, D.L., Tilley, L., 2011, Genetic ablation of a Maurer's cleft protein prevents assembly of the Plasmodium falciparum virulence complex. Mol Microbiol 81, 982-993.

Dluzewski, A.R., Fryer, P.R., Griffiths, S., Rangachari, K., Wilson, R.J., Gratzer, W.B., 1988, Exclusion of red cell membrane cytoskeleton from the parasitophorous vacuole membrane of the internalised malaria parasite. Cell Biol Int Rep 12, 149.

Dluzewski, A., Fryer, P., Griffiths, S., Wilson, R., Gratzer, W., 1989, Red cell membrane protein distribution during malarial invasion. J Cell Sci 92, 691-699.

Dluzewski, A., Zicha, D., Dunn, G., WB, G., 1995, Origins of the parasitophorous vacuole membrane of the malaria parasite: surface area of the parasitized red cell. Eur J Cell Biol. 68, 446-449.

Duranton, C., Tanneur, V., Lang, C., Brand, V.B., Koka, S., Kasinathan, R.S., Dorsch, M., Hedrich, H.J., Baumeister, S., Lingelbach, K., *et al.*, 2008, A high specificity and affinity interaction with serum albumin stimulates an anion conductance in malaria-infected erythrocytes. Cell Physiol Biochem 22, 395-404.

Dvorak, J.A., Miller, L.H., Whitehouse, W.C., Shiroishi, T., 1975, Invasion of erythrocytes by malaria merozoites. Science 187, 748-750.

Eksi, S., Williamson, K.C., 2011, Protein Targeting to the Parasitophorous Vacuole Membrane of *Plasmodium falciparum*. Eukaryotic Cell 10, 744-752.

El Hajj, H., Lebrun, M., Arold, S.T., Vial, H., Labesse, G., Dubremetz, J.F., 2007, ROP18 is a rhoptry kinase controlling the intracellular proliferation of *Toxoplasma gondii*. PLoS Pathog 3, e14.

Elmendorf, H., Haldar, K., 1994, *Plasmodium falciparum* exports the Golgi marker sphingomyelin synthase into a tubovesicular network in the cytoplasm of mature erythrocytes. J. Cell Biol. 124, 449-462.

Etzion, Z., Perkins, M., 1989, Localization of a parasite encoded protein to erythrocyte cytoplasmic vesicles of Plasmodium falciparum-infected cells. Eur J Cell Biol 48, 174-179.

Fairhurst, R.M., Wellems, T.E., 2006, Modulation of malaria virulence by determinants of *Plasmodium falciparum* erythrocyte membrane protein-1 display. Curr Opin Hematol 13, 124-130.

Ferru, E., Giger, K., Pantaleo, A., Campanella, E., Grey, J., Ritchie, K., Vono, R., Turrini, F., Low, P.S., 2011, Regulation of membrane-cytoskeletal interactions by tyrosine phosphorylation of erythrocyte band 3. Blood 117, 5998-6006.

Fischer, K., Marti, T., Rick, B., Johnson, D., Benting, J., Baumeister, S., Helmbrecht, C., Lanzer, M., Lingelbach, K., 1998, Characterization and cloning of the gene encoding the vacuolar membrane protein EXP-2 from *Plasmodium falciparum*. Mol. Biochem. Parasitol. 92, 47-57.

Frankland, S., Adisa, A., Horrocks, P., Taraschi, T.F., Schneider, T., Elliott, S.R., Rogerson, S.J., Knuepfer, E., Cowman, A.F., Newbold, C.I., Tilley, L., 2006, Delivery of the Malaria Virulence Protein PfEMP1 to the Erythrocyte Surface Requires Cholesterol-Rich Domains. Eukaryotic Cell 5, 849-860.

Frankland, S., Elliott, S.R., Yosaatmadja, F., Beeson, J.G., Rogerson, S.J., Adisa, A., Tilley, L., 2007, Serum Lipoproteins Promote Efficient Presentation of the Malaria Virulence Protein PfEMP1 at the Erythrocyte Surface. Eukaryotic Cell 6, 1584-1594.

Fremount, H.N., Miller, L.H., 1975, Deep vascular schizogony in *Plasmodium fragile*: organ distribution and ultrastructure of erythrocytes adherent to vascular endothelium. The American Journal of Tropical Medicine and Hygiene 24, 1-8.

Frischknecht, F., Lanzer, M., 2008, The Plasmodium falciparum Maurer's clefts in 3D. Mol Microbiol 67, 687-691.

Gehde, N., Hinrichs, C., Montilla, I., Charpian, S., Lingelbach, K., Przyborski, J.M., 2009, Protein unfolding is an essential requirement for transport across the parasitophorous vacuolar membrane of *Plasmodium falciparum*. Mol Microbiol 71, 613-628.

Gilbert, L.A., Ravindran, S., Turetzky, J.M., Boothroyd, J.C., Bradley, P.J., 2007, *Toxoplasma gondii* targets a protein phosphatase 2C to the nuclei of infected host cells. Eukaryotic Cell 6, 73-83.

Gilson, P.R., Crabb, B.S., 2009, Morphology and kinetics of the three distinct phases of red blood cell invasion by *Plasmodium falciparum* merozoites. International Journal for Parasitology 39, 91-96.

Ginsburg, H., Kutner, S., Krugliak, M., Cabantchik, Z.I., 1985, Characterization of permeation pathways appearing in the host membrane of *Plasmodium falciparum* infected red blood cells. Mol. Biochem. Parasitol 14, 313-322.

Glushakova, S., Yin, D., Li, T., Zimmerberg, J., 2005, Membrane transformation during malaria parasite release from human red blood cells. Current biology : CB 15, 1645-1650.

Glushakova, S., Mazar, J., Hohmann-Marriott, M.F., Hama, E., Zimmerberg, J., 2009, Irreversible effect of cysteine protease inhibitors on the release of malaria parasites from infected erythrocytes. Cellular Microbiology 11, 95-105.

Grellier, P., Rigomier, D., Clavey, V., Fruchart, J.C., Schrevel, J., 1991, Lipid traffic between high density lipoproteins and *Plasmodium falciparum*-infected red blood cells. J. Cell Biol. 112, 267-277.

Gruenberg, J., Allred, D., Sherman, I., 1983, Scanning electron microscope-analysis of the protrusions (knobs) present on the surface of *Plasmodium falciparum*-infected erythrocytes. J. Cell Biol. 97, 795-802.

Gruring, C., Heiber, A., Kruse, F., Ungefehr, J., Gilberger, T.-W., Spielmann, T., 2011, Development and host cell modifications of *Plasmodium falciparum* blood stages in four dimensions. Nat Commun 2, 165.

Günther, K., Tümmler, M., Arnold, H.-H., Ridley, R., Goman, M., Scaife, J.G., Lingelbach, K., 1991, An exported protein of *Plasmodium falciparum* is synthesized as an integral membrane protein. Mol. Biochem. Parasitol 46, 149-157.

Haase, S., de Koning-Ward, T.F., 2010, New insights into protein export in malaria parasites. Cellular Microbiology 12, 580-587.

Haldar, K., de Amorim, A., Cross, G., 1989, Transport of fluorescent phospholipid analogues from the erythrocyte membrane to the parasite in Plasmodium falciparum-infected cells. J. Cell Biol. 108, 2183-2192.

Haldar, K., Samuel, B.U., Mohandas, N., Harrison, T., Hiller, N.L., 2001, Transport mechanisms in Plasmodium-infected erythrocytes: lipid rafts and a tubovesicular network. International Journal for Parasitology 31, 1393-1401.

Haldar, K., Kamoun, S., Hiller, N.L., Bhattacharje, S., van Ooij, C., 2006, Common infection strategies of pathogenic eukaryotes. Nat Rev Micro 4, 922-931.

Hanssen, E., Hawthorne, P., Dixon, M.W.A., Trenholme, K.R., McMillan, P.J., Spielmann, T., Gardiner, D.L., Tilley, L., 2008a, Targeted mutagenesis of the ring-exported protein-1 of *Plasmodium falciparum* disrupts the architecture of Maurer's cleft organelles. Mol Microbiol 69, 938-953.

Hanssen, E., Sougrat, R., Frankland, S., Deed, S., Klonis, N., Lippincott-Schwartz, J., Tilley, L., 2008b, Electron tomography of the Maurer's cleft organelles of *Plasmodium falciparum*-infected erythrocytes reveals novel structural features. Mol Microbiol 67, 703-718.

Hanssen, E., Carlton, P., Deed, S., Klonis, N., Sedat, J., DeRisi, J., Tilley, L., 2010, Whole cell imaging reveals novel modular features of the exomembrane system of the malaria parasite, *Plasmodium falciparum*. International Journal for Parasitology 40, 123-134.

Hanzal-Bayer, M.F., Hancock, J.F., 2007, Lipid rafts and membrane traffic. FEBS Lett 22, 2098-2104.

Harrison, T., Samuel, B.U., Akompong, T., Hamm, H., Mohandas, N., Lomasney, J.W., Haldar, K., 2003, Erythrocyte G Protein-Coupled Receptor Signaling in Malarial Infection. Science 301, 1734-1736.

Henrich, P., Kilian, N., Lanzer, M., Cyrklaff, M., 2009, 3-D analysis of the Plasmodium falciparum Maurer's clefts using different electron tomographic approaches. Biotechnology Journal 4, 888-894.

Hiller, N.L., Akompong, T., Morrow, J.S., Holder, A.A., Haldar, K., 2003, Identification of a Stomatin Orthologue in Vacuoles Induced in Human Erythrocytes by Malaria Parasites: A role for microbial raft proteins in Apicomplexan vacuole biogenesis. J. Biol. Chem. 278, 48413-48421.

Hiller, N.L., Bhattacharjee, S., van Ooij, C., Liolios, K., Harrison, T., Lopez-Estrano, C., Haldar, K., 2004, A Host-Targeting Signal in Virulence Proteins Reveals a Secretome in Malarial Infection. Science 306, 1934-1937.

Homewood, C.A., Neame, K.D., 1974, Malaria and the permeability of the host erythrocyte. Nature 252, 718-719.

Kamata, K., Manno, S., Ozaki, M., Takakuwa, Y., 2008, Functional evidence for presence of lipid rafts in erythrocyte membranes: Gsalpha in rafts is essential for signal transduction. American Journal of Hematology 83, 371-375.

Khanna, R., Chang, S.H., Andrabi, S., Azam, M., Kim, A., Rivera, A., Brugnara, C., Low, P.S., Liu, S.C., Chishti, A.H., 2002, Headpiece domain of dematin is required for the stability of the erythrocyte membrane. Proc. Natl. Acad. Sci. U.S.A 99, 6637-6642.

Kilejian, A., 1979, Characterization of a protein correlated with the production of knob-like protrusions on membranes of erythrocytes infected with *Plasmodium falciparum*. Proc. Natl. Acad. Sci U.S.A 76, 4650-4653.

Kilejian, A., Rashid, M.A., Parra, M., Yang, Y.F., 1991, Sequence of the knob protein of *Plasmodium falciparum* recognized by a monoclonal antibody. Mol. Biochem. Parasitol 48, 231-233.

Kirk, K., 2001, Membrane Transport in the Malaria-Infected Erythrocyte. Physiol. Rev. 81, 495-537.

Klales, A.M., Chakrabarti, B., Vitelli, V., Mahadevan, L., Manoharan, V., 2007. Physics of the curling ribbons. In: American Physical Society communication, APS March Meeting, March5-9, 2007.

Knuepfer, E., Rug, M., Klonis, N., Tilley, L., Cowman, A.F., 2005a, Trafficking determinants for PfEMP3 export and assembly under the Plasmodium falciparum-infected red blood cell membrane. Mol Microbiol 58, 1039-1053.

Knuepfer, E., Rug, M., Klonis, N., Tilley, L., Cowman, A.F., 2005b, Trafficking of the major virulence factor to the surface of transfected *P. falciparum*-infected erythrocytes. Blood 105, 4078-4087.

Koshino, I., Takakuwa, Y., 2009, Disruption of lipid rafts by lidocaine inhibits erythrocyte invasion by *Plasmodium falciparum*. Experimental Parasitology 123, 381-383.

Koussis, K., Withers-Martinez, C., Yeoh, S., Child, M., Hackett, F., Knuepfer, E., Juliano, L., Woehlbier, U., Bujard, H., Blackman, M.J., 2009, A multifunctional serine protease primes the malaria parasite for red blood cell invasion. EMBO J 28, 725-735.

Külzer, S., Rug, M., Brinkmann, K., Cannon, P., Cowman, A., Lingelbach, K., Blatch, G.L., Maier, A.G., Przyborski, J.M., 2010, Parasite-encoded Hsp40 proteins define novel mobile structures in the cytosol of the *P. falciparum*-infected erythrocyte. Cellular Microbiology 12, 1398-1420.

Lalle, M., Currà, C., Ciccarone, F., Pace, T., Cecchetti, S., Fantozzi, L., Ay, B., Breton, C.B., Ponzi, M., 2011, Dematin, a Component of the Erythrocyte Membrane Skeleton, Is Internalized by the Malaria Parasite and Associates with *Plasmodium* 14-3-3. J Biol Chem 286, 1227-1236.

Lanzer, M., Wickert, H., Krohne, G., Vincensini, L., Braun Breton, C., 2006, Maurer's clefts: A novel multi-functional organelle in the cytoplasm of *Plasmodium falciparum*-infected erythrocytes. International Journal for Parasitology 36, 23-36.

Lauer, S.A., Rathod, P.K., Ghori, N., Haldar, K., 1997, A Membrane Network for Nutrient Import in Red Cells Infected with the Malaria Parasite. Science 276, 1122-1125.

Lauer, S., VanWye, J., Harrison, T., McManus, H., Samuel, B.U., Hiller, N.L., Mohandas, N., Haldar, K., 2000, Vacuolar uptake of host components, and a role for cholesterol and sphingomyelin in malarial infection. EMBO J 19, 3556-3564.

Lew, V.L., 2011, Malaria: surprising mechanism of merozoite egress revealed. Current biology : CB 21, R314-316.

Lingelbach, K.R., 1993, *Plasmodium falciparum*: A Molecular View of Protein Transport from the Parasite into the Host Erythrocyte. Experimental Parasitology 76, 318-327.

Lingelbach, K., Joiner, K., 1998, The parasitophorous vacuole membrane surrounding Plasmodium and Toxoplasma: an unusual compartment in infected cells. J Cell Sci 111, 1467-1475.

Maier, A.G., Cooke, B.M., Cowman, A.F., Tilley, L., 2009, Malaria parasite proteins that remodel the host erythrocyte. Nat Rev Micro 7, 341-354.

Marti, M., Good, R.T., Rug, M., Knuepfer, E., Cowman, A.F., 2004, Targeting Malaria Virulence and Remodeling Proteins to the Host Erythrocyte. Science 306, 1930-1933.

Mercier, C., Adjogble, K.D.Z., Däubener, W., Delauw, M.-F.-C., 2005, Dense granules: Are they key organelles to help understand the parasitophorous vacuole of all apicomplexa parasites? International Journal for Parasitology 35, 829-849.

Mikkelsen, R.B., Kamber, M., Wadwa, K.S., Lin, P.S., Schmidt-Ullrich, R., 1988, The role of lipids in *Plasmodium falciparum* invasion of erythrocytes: a coordinated biochemical and microscopic analysis. Proc. Natl. Acad. Sci. U.S.A 85, 5956-5960.

Mordue, D.G., Desai, N., Dustin, M., Sibley, L.D., 1999, Invasion by *Toxoplasma gondii* Establishes a Moving Junction That Selectively Excludes Host Cell Plasma Membrane Proteins on the Basis of Their Membrane Anchoring. J Exp Med 190, 1783-1792.

Murphy, S.C., Samuel, B.U., Harrison, T., Speicher, K.D., Speicher, D.W., Reid, M.E., Prohaska, R., Low, P.S., Tanner, M.J., Mohandas, N., Haldar, K., 2004, Erythrocyte detergent-resistant membrane proteins: their characterization and selective uptake during malarial infection. Blood 103, 1920-1928.

Murphy, S.C., Harrison, T., Hamm, H.E., Lomasney, J.W., Mohandas, N., Haldar, K., 2006a, Erythrocyte G Protein as a Novel Target for Malarial Chemotherapy. PLoS Med 3, e528.

Murphy, S.C., Hiller, N.L., Harrison, T., Lomasney, J.W., Mohandas, N., Haldar, K., 2006b, Lipid rafts and malaria parasite infection of erythrocytes (Review). Molecular Membrane Biology 23, 81 - 88.

Nguitragool, W., Bokhari, A.A., Pillai, A.D., Rayavara, K., Sharma, P., Turpin, B., Aravind, L., Desai, S.A., 2011, Malaria parasite clag3 genes determine channel-mediated nutrient uptake by infected red blood cells. Cell 145, 665-677.

Nunes, M.C., Goldring, J.P., Doerig, C., Scherf, A., 2007, A novel protein kinase family in *Plasmodium falciparum* is differentially transcribed and secreted to various cellular compartments of the host cell. Mol Microbiol 63, 391-403.

Nyalwidhe, J., Lingelbach, K., 2006, Proteases and chaperones are the most abundant proteins in the parasitophorous vacuole of Plasmodium falciparum infected erythrocytes. PROTEOMICS 6, 1563-1573.

Pachlatko, E., Rusch, S., Müller, A., Hemphill, A., Tilley, L., Hanssen, E., Beck, H.-P., 2010, MAHRP2, an exported protein of *Plasmodium falciparum*, is an essential component of Maurer's cleft tethers. Mol Microbiol 77, 1136-1152.

Pantaleo, A., Ferru, E., Carta, F., Mannu, F., Giribaldi, G., Vono, R., Lepedda, A.J., Pippia, P., Turrini, F., 2010, Analysis of changes in tyrosine and serine phosphorylation of red cell membrane proteins induced by *P. falciparum* growth. Proteomics 10, 3469-3479.

Papakrivos, J., Newbold, C.I., Lingelbach, K., 2005, A potential novel mechanism for the insertion of a membrane protein revealed by a biochemical analysis of the *Plasmodium falciparum* cytoadherence molecule *Pf*EMP-1. Mol Microbiol 55, 1272-1284.

Pei, X., An, X., Guo, X., Tarnawski, M., Coppel, R., Mohandas, N., 2005, Structural and Functional Studies of Interaction between *Plasmodium falciparum* Knob-associated Histidine-rich Protein (KAHRP) and Erythrocyte Spectrin. J Biol Chem 280, 31166-31171.

Pei, X., Guo, X., Coppel, R., Bhattacharjee, S., Haldar, K., Gratzer, W., Mohandas, N., An, X., 2007, The ring-infected erythrocyte surface antigen (RESA) of *Plasmodium falciparum* stabilizes spectrin tetramers and suppresses further invasion. Blood 110, 1036-1042.

Petter, M., Haeggstrom, M., Khattab, A., Fernandez, V., Klinkert, M., Wahlgren, M., 2007, Variant proteins of the *Plasmodium falciparum* RIFIN family show distinct subcellular localization and developmental expression patterns. Mol. Biochem. Parasitol 156, 51 - 61.

Przyborski, J.M., Miller, S.K., Pfahler, J.M., Henrich, P.P., Rohrbach, P., Crabb, B.S., Lanzer, M., 2005, Trafficking of STEVOR to the Maurer's clefts in *Plasmodium falciparum*-infected erythrocytes. EMBO J 24, 2306-2317.

Przyborski, J.M., 2008, The Maurer's clefts of *Plasmodium falciparum*: parasite-induced islands within an intracellular ocean. Trends Parasitol 24, 285-288.

Roggwiller, E., Betoulle, M.E., Blisnick, T., Braun Breton, C., 1996, A role for erythrocyte band 3 degradation by the parasite gp76 serine protease in the formation of the parasitophorous vacuole during invasion of erythrocytes by *Plasmodium falciparum*. Mol. Biochem. Parasitol 82, 13-24.

Rowe, J.A., Claessens, A., Corrigan, R.A., Arman, M., 2009, Adhesion of *Plasmodium falciparum*-infected erythrocytes to human cells: molecular mechanisms and therapeutic implications. Expert Rev. Mol. Med. 11, e16.

Rug, M., Prescott, S.W., Fernandez, K.M., Cooke, B.M., Cowman, A.F., 2006, The role of KAHRP domains in knob formation and cytoadherence of *P falciparum*-infected human erythrocytes. Blood 108, 370-378.

Russo, I., Babbitt, S., Muralidharan, V., Butler, T., Oksman, A., Goldberg, D.E., 2010, Plasmepsin V licenses *Plasmodium* proteins for export into the host erythrocyte. Nature 463, 632-636.

Saeij, J.P., Boyle, J.P., Coller, S., Taylor, S., Sibley, L.D., Brooke-Powell, E.T., Ajioka, J.W., Boothroyd, J.C., 2006, Polymorphic secreted kinases are key virulence factors in toxoplasmosis. Science 314, 1780-1783.

Samuel, B.U., Mohandas, N., Harrison, T., McManus, H., Rosse, W., Reid, M., Haldar, K., 2001, The Role of Cholesterol and Glycosylphosphatidylinositol-anchored Proteins of Erythrocyte Rafts in Regulating Raft Protein Content and Malarial Infection. J. Biol. Chem. 276, 29319-29329.

Sargeant, T., Marti, M., Caler, E., Carlton, J., Simpson, K., Speed, T., Cowman, A., 2006, Lineage-specific expansion of proteins exported to erythrocytes in malaria parasites. Genome Biology 7, R12.

Saridaki, T., Fröhlich, K.S., Braun-Breton, C., Lanzer, M., 2009, Export of PfSBP1 to the Plasmodium falciparum Maurer's Clefts. Traffic 10, 137-152.

Spielmann, T., Gardiner, D.L., Beck, H.-P., Trenholme, K.R., Kemp, D.J., 2006a, Organization of ETRAMPs and EXP-1 at the parasite-host cell interface of malaria parasites. Mol Microbiol 59, 779-794.

Spielmann, T., Hawthorne, P.L., Dixon, M.W.A., Hannemann, M., Klotz, K., Kemp, D.J., Klonis, N., Tilley, L., Trenholme, K.R., Gardiner, D.L., 2006b, A Cluster of Ring Stage-specific Genes Linked to a Locus Implicated in Cytoadherence in *Plasmodium falciparum* Codes for PEXEL-negative and PEXEL-positive Proteins Exported into the Host Cell Mol. Biol. Cell 17, 3613-3624.

Spycher, C., Rug, M., Klonis, N., Ferguson, D.J.P., Cowman, A.F., Beck, H.-P., Tilley, L., 2006, Genesis of and Trafficking to the Maurer's Clefts of Plasmodium falciparum-Infected Erythrocytes. Mol. Cell. Biol. 26, 4074-4085.

Spycher, C., Rug, M., Pachlatko, E., Hanssen, E., Ferguson, D., Cowman, A.F., Tilley, L., Beck, H.-P., 2008, The Maurer's cleft protein MAHRP1 is essential for trafficking of PfEMP1 to the surface of Plasmodium falciparum-infected erythrocytes. Mol Microbiol 68, 1300-1314.

Staines, H.M., Ellory, J.C., Kirk, K., 2001, Perturbation of the pump-leak balance for Na+ and K+ in malaria-infected erythrocytes. American Journal of Physiology - Cell Physiology 280, C1576-C1587.

Tamez, P.A., Bhattacharjee, S., van Ooij, C., Hiller, N.L., LlinÃ¡s, M., Balu, B., Adams, J.H., Haldar, K., 2008, An Erythrocyte Vesicle Protein Exported by the Malaria Parasite Promotes Tubovesicular Lipid Import from the Host Cell Surface. PLoS Pathog 4, e1000118.

Tilley, L., Hanssen, E., 2008, A 3D view of the host cell compartment in P. falciparum-infected erythrocytes. Transfusion Clinique et Biologique 15, 72-81.

Tonkin, C.J., Pearce, J.A., McFadden, G.I., Cowman, A.F., 2006, Protein targeting to destinations of the secretory pathway in the malaria parasite *Plasmodium falciparum*. Current Opinion in Microbiology 9, 381-387.

Torii, M., Adams, J.H., Miller, L.H., Aikawa, M., 1989, Release of merozoite dense granules during erythrocyte invasion by Plasmodium knowlesi. Infect. Immun. 57, 3230-3233.

Trager, W., Rudzinska, M.A., C., B.P., 1966, The fine structure of *Plasmodium falciparum* and its host erythrocytes in natural malarial infections in man*. Bull World Health Organ 35, 883-885.

Trelka, D.P., Schneider, T.G., Reeder, J.C., Taraschi, T.F., 2000, Evidence for vesicle-mediated trafficking of parasite proteins to the host cell cytosol and erythrocyte surface membrane in *Plasmodium falciparum* infected ertythrocytes. Mol. Biochem. Parasitol 106, 131-145.

van Ooij, C., Tamez, P., Bhattacharjee, S., Hiller, N.L., Harrison, T., Liolios, K., Kooij, T., Ramesar, J., Balu, B., Adams, J., *et al.*, 2008, The Malaria Secretome: From Algorithms to Essential Function in Blood Stage Infection. PLoS Pathog 4, e1000084.

Vincensini, L., Richert, S., Blisnick, T., Van Dorsselaer, A., Leize-Wagner, E., Rabilloud, T., Braun Breton, C., 2005, Proteomic Analysis Identifies Novel Proteins of the Maurer's Clefts, a Secretory Compartment Delivering *Plasmodium falciparum* Proteins to the Surface of Its Host Cell. Mol Cell Proteomics 4, 582-593.

von Heijne, G., 1985, Signal sequences : The limits of variation. Journal of Molecular Biology 184, 99-105.

Waller, K.L., Cooke, B.M., Nunomura, W., Mohandas, N., Coppel, R.L., 1999, Mapping the binding domains involved in the interaction between the *Plasmodium falciparum* knob-associated histidine-rich protein (KAHRP) and the cytoadherence ligand *P. falciparum* erythrocyte membrane protein 1 (PfEMP1). J Biol Chem 274, 23808-23813.

Waller, K.L., Nunomura, W., Cooke, B.M., Mohandas, N., Coppel, R.L., 2002, Mapping the domains of the cytoadherence ligand *Plasmodium falciparum* erythrocyte membrane protein 1 (PfEMP1) that bind to the knob-associated histidine-rich protein (KAHRP). Mol. Biochem. Parasitol 119, 125-129.

Ward, G., Miller, L., Dvorak, J., 1993, The origin of parasitophorous vacuole membrane lipids in malaria-infected erythrocytes. J Cell Sci 106, 237-248.

Waterkeyn, J.G., Wickham, M.E., Davern, K.M., Cooke, B.M., Coppel, R.L., Reeder, J.C., Culvenor, J.G., Waller, R.F., Cowman, A.F., 2000, Targeted mutagenesis of *Plasmodium falciparum* erythrocyte membrane protein 3 (*Pf*EMP3) disrupts cytoadherence of malaria-infected red blood cells. EMBO J 19, 2813-2823.

Wickert, H., Wissing, F., Andrews, K.T., Stich, A., Krohne, G., Lanzer, M., 2003, Evidence for trafficking of PfEMP1 to the surface of *P. falciparum*-infected erythrocytes via a complex membrane network. Eur J Cell Biol 82, 271-284.

Wickert, H., Gottler, W., Krohne, G., Lanzer, M., 2004, Maurer's cleft organization in the cytoplasm of *Plasmodium falciparum*-infected erythrocytes: new insights from three-dimensional reconstruction of serial ultrathin sections. Eur J Cell Biol 83, 567-582.

Wickert, H., Krohne, G., 2007, The complex morphology of Maurer's clefts: from discovery to three-dimensional reconstructions. Trends in Parasitology 23, 502-509.

Wickham, M.E., Rug, M., Ralph, S.A., Klonis, N., McFadden, G.I., Tilley, L., Cowman, A.F., 2001, Trafficking and assembly of the cytoadherence complex in *Plasmodium falciparum*-infected human erythrocytes. EMBO J 20, 5636-5649.

Wickham, M.E., Culvenor, J.G., Cowman, A.F., 2003, Selective inhibition of a two-step egress of malaria parasites from the host erythrocyte. J Biol Chem 278, 37658-37663.

Winter, G., Kawai, S., Haeggström, M., Kaneko, O., von Euler, A., Kawazu, S.-i., Palm, D., Fernandez, V., Wahlgren, M., 2005, SURFIN is a polymorphic antigen expressed on *Plasmodium falciparum* merozoites and infected erythrocytes. J Exp Med 201, 1853-1863.

Yeoh, S., O'Donnell, R.A., Koussis, K., Dluzewski, A.R., Ansell, K.H., Osborne, S.A., Hackett, F., Withers-Martinez, C., Mitchell, G.H., Bannister, L.H., *et al.*, 2007, Subcellular Discharge of a Serine Protease Mediates Release of Invasive Malaria Parasites from Host Erythrocytes. Cell 131, 1072-1083.

Zuccala, E.S., Baum, J., 2011, Cytoskeletal and membrane remodelling during malaria parasite invasion of the human erythrocyte. British Journal of Haematology 154, 680-689.

Part 4

Current Trends in Malaria Diagnosis

9

Current Issues in Clinical and Laboratory Diagnosis in Malaria

Adeola Orogade
Ahmadu Bello University Teaching Hospital, Shika Zaria Nigeria

Diagnosis is not the end, but the beginning of practice. ~Martin H. Fischer

1. Introduction

Malaria is a protozoan infection (Najera &Hempel, 2006 as cited in Okwa & Ibidapo, 2010) with protean manifestations in the human species (Mohaptra, 2002; Murthy, 2000; Talib, 1996) causing nearly one million deaths mainly in African children and decreasing gross domestic product by as much as 1.3% in countries with high disease rates (World Health Organization [WHO], 2010). Approximately half of the world's population is at risk of malaria and in 2008; malaria was present in 108 countries and territories of the world (WHO, 2010). The most specific at risk population groups include young children in stable transmission areas, non immune pregnant women, semi immune pregnant women irrespective of HIV status, people with HIV/AIDS, international travelers to malaria endemic from non endemic areas as well as immigrants from endemic areas and their children living in non endemic areas returning to their home countries to visit friends and relatives (WHO, 2010).

Making a diagnosis requires careful clinical examination and laboratory investigation. Whereas malaria could be over diagnosed in endemic areas, (Ammah et al, 1999; Gwer et al, 2007; Hussain et al, 2009; Rehlis & Kurczewska, 2001; Rougemont et al, 2003; Smith et al, 1994;) in the non endemic areas a high index of suspicion is usually required (Berrang –Ford et al, 2008). However, in the most vulnerable: neonates, under fives, (Dzeing-Ella et al 2005) pregnant women, the elderly and non immune(Sengoz inan et al,2010) who may develop potential life threatening complications of *falciparum* malaria, it is important in most cases to make a rapid, accurate diagnosis to ensure prompt treatment. WHO recommends that before giving treatment, clinical malaria should be confirmed by parasite –based diagnosis. Treatment given solely on the basis of symptoms (presumptive diagnosis and treatment) should only be considered when a parasitological diagnosis is not possible. In 2008, 33 of 43 malaria endemic countries in the African region and 45 out of 63 countries in other regions were reported to have developed a policy of parasitological testing of suspected malaria cases in persons of all ages. However, policy development has not matched actual practice. Parasitological test for suspected malaria cases is carried out in less than 20% of individuals living in 21 of the highest disease burden countries.(WHO, 2010).

Moreover, the field of malaria diagnosis is rapidly expanding and bringing to fore hitherto unidentified issues both clinically and in the laboratory. Malaria, once thought to be rare in the newborn (Molyneux, 1989) has in recent times been increasingly reported (Falade et al, 2007; Ibanesebor, 1995; Kamwendo et al, 2002; Lamikanra,1993; Lehner & Andrews, 1988; Muktar et al, 2006; Olowu et al, 2000; Opare,2010; Runsewe –Abiodun et al, 2006; Sowunmi et al, 1996) Incidences range from 0.3 to 33%in these areas (Fisher, 2003) and has brought into question the extent of protection for the baby in the face of maternal placental infections such as HIV. Malaria infection is also described in the first 6 months of life which may be clinically indistinguishable from common bacterial and viral infections (Orogade, 2006).The use of clinical algorithms proposed for malaria diagnosis and their role as predictors for morbidity and mortality are being investigated (Tabitha et al, 2005). With the introduction of rapid diagnostic tests (RDTs) for diagnosis in malaria, there should be less need for presumptive diagnosis based solely on clinical features in high burden areas. However, there is a growing need to monitor and assess the performance of the RDTs in face of varied availability of RDTs and their low specificity and sensitivity in mixed malaria parasite infections. This chapter reviews these current issues in malaria diagnosis and discusses their implication for prompt malaria identification and treatment which are key aspects of the WHO policy and strategy for global malaria control.

2. Clinical features in malaria

2.1 Newborn

2.1.1 Prevalence of congenital malaria

Congenital malaria is defined as the presence of malaria parasites in the peripheral smear of the newborn within the first week of life (Mc Gregory, 1986). It had been thought to be rare due to the known effectiveness of placental barrier but recent reports from malaria endemic areas of incidence in small numbers were made. In a national multicenter study carried out to determine the epidemiology of congenital malaria in Nigeria (Falade et al, 2007), 1,875 babies were assessed within the first 4 hours of life for parasitemia using freshly prepared Giemsa kept at pH 7.2 to stain conventional thick and methanol fixed thin blood smears. A prevalence of 5.1% of patent parasitemia was obtained. It was observed that the mean parasite density in these neonates was low (8-200/µl) as was also reported in an earlier study by Mc Guiness et al (1998). In about two thirds of these babies with parasitemia observed in the first 4 hours of life there was spontaneous parasite clearance by the second day of life, while 33.7% of them persisted and babies became symptomatic within the first 3 days postpartum.

2.1.2 Relationship between malaria in pregnancy and congenital malaria

Antepartum maternal and placental parasitemia have been identified as consistent risk factors for congenital malaria (Orogade et al 2004,2008). Neonates in these studies who had peripartum malaria parasitemia had a 20 fold increased risk of infection. In Papua New Guinea, Lehner et al(1990) observed that where there was a maternal antepartum parasitaemia of 29.4%, there were corresponding cord and neonatal blood parasitemia of 14.6% and 7.7%. They found a significant correlation between anti malarial IgG antibodies in paired maternal and cord blood which indicated transplacental transfer. Using the PCR methods, Kamwenedo et al (2002) also working in Malawi had demonstrated that cord blood genotypes were a subset of the maternal and placental blood. An issue of current interest relating to the integrity of the placenta has been the role of HIV infection. In several recent studies (Steketee,2004; Ticconi et al, 2003; van Ejik et al, 2003; Verhoeff et al, 1999;), it has been found that HIV impaired the ability of pregnant women to control malaria parasitemia. Results from these studies showed that HIV-infected women experienced consistently higher prevalence of peripheral and placental malaria (summary relative risk = 1.58 and 1.66, respectively), higher parasite densities, and more febrile illnesses, severe anemia, and adverse birth outcomes when compared with HIV-uninfected women, particularly in multigravidae. Thus, HIV alters the typical gravidity-specific pattern of malaria risk by shifting the burden from primarily primigravidae and secundigravidae to all pregnant women.

2.1.3 Implication for malaria prophylaxis in pregnancy

Maternal, especially perinatal malaria is a significant risk factor for congenital malaria. Intermittent preventive therapy (IpT) is recommended by WHO for pregnant women and infants in areas of high transmission in Sub Saharan Africa with stable malaria transmission who are particularly vulnerable to the consequences of malaria. This prophylaxis when adequately taken as two doses at least one month apart substantially reduces both maternal and neonatal morbidity and mortality related to malaria. However, the progress report on malaria prevention (WHO, 2010) indicates that coverage with Intermittent Preventive treatment for pregnant women (IPTp) has remained far below the target levels. Thirty three out of 43 endemic countries in Africa had adopted the IPTp programme by 2009. Only 55% of all women attending antenatal clinics received the second dose of IPTp and since not all women attend antenatal clinic, household surveys in some countries report 2.4% to 62% with an overall weighted average of 12% received the second dose of therapy. This presents a picture that calls for urgent action to reduce maternal malaria and its consequences.

2.1.4 Major clinical features in congenital malaraia

The major clinical features in congenital are fever within the first 24 hours of life, refusal to suck and anaemia (Orogade et al, 2008). Fever is the most consistent feature while some other studies have described hepatosplenomegaly, jaundice, irritability. These are indistinguishable from features commonly seen in neonatal septicaemia. The implication of this is that every febrile neonate born to a mother who is epidemiologically vulnerable for malaria should be screened for malaria as well as other bacterial and viral infections.

2.2 Zero – Five months

2.2.1 Trend of malaria parasitaemia with age

There have been variable findings in prevalence of malaria parasitemia in this age group, ranging from 0% in children less than 3 months (Okwa, 2000) to 17.2 % in the first six months of life (Orogade, 2006) and 27.1% in a similar series by Afolabi et al (2001). Age specific parasite rates showed a sharp drop in frequency of parasitemia from first to second week of life (Orogade, 2006), but this gradually increases with age till the sixth month of life. This initial sharp drop has been attributed to spontaneous clearance of parasites which occurs in some babies at this time. It is noteworthy that about one fifth of all parasitemia occurs in the first month of life. The neonatal age group in this study formed a large burden of the disease prevalence. Mothers who were gravida 1-2, who did not utilize chemoprophylaxis in pregnancy and had education ranging from none to primary school level were important as risk factors for malaria parasitemia in this age group. These same risk factors have also been identified especially in malaria endemic regions where women in their first two pregnancies who develop maternal parasitemia have been identified as high risk for maternal anaemia and fetal complications such as fetal wastages, still births, premature deliveries and low birth weight in the newborn babies. In this study parasitemia documented in the first week of life would likely have resulted from congenital acquisition as prevalence of 9.31% obtained closely compares to the recent congenital malaria reports

There is an average low mean parasite density rate of 64.82 ± 50.61/μL (Orogade, 2006)and this does not vary with age groups, $\chi 2$ (Bartlett's test) = 6.09, p=0.29. The mean Haematocrit is also significantly lower than controls low at 35.62 ± 7.09.%. Analysis of variants revealed a significant positive correlation between the mean haematocrit and malaria parasitemia.

Use of malaria prevention was 93.6% and this had a significant impact on reduction of parasitemia. Of the methods used for malaria prevention, window/door net screening and insecticides sprays were the most common. Less than half of mothers used bednets for their babies and only 7(2.8%)of these were insecticide treated bednets. Other non conventional methods used were local chemicals (*ota pia-pia*) sprayed on floors and walls in the rooms where the children slept. This apparently significantly reduced parasitemia where it was used one and half fold. Of all the babies seen only 47.4% were being exclusive breast fed.

Beyond the neonatal period, the use of malaria prevention methods in particular *ota pia-pia* were significant for protection against malaria. *Ota pia-pia* which was used in 13.37% of cases seems to have been quite effective. This is a locally prepared chemical which when sprayed on floors and walls in the rooms are effective anti vector agents. However, the exact chemical compositions of these chemicals are yet to be fully analyzed and the safety of their use is not documented. Moreso, their potential harmful effects to the newborn and infant are unknown. Insecticide treated bednets have been introduced in Nigeria as an effective measure of malaria prophylaxis. However Orogade (2006) revealed a very poor utilization of this proven effective measure. Bednets, which has been a preventive measure of long standing use was utilized for less than half of the babies. There was rather more common use of window/door net screens as well as insecticide sprays which have also been known and in use for several years but which are not as effective.

There was low educational status in more than a third of the mothers and this affects how well informed the mothers would be especially about health preventive matters. This less popular use of bednets as well as the level of health information the mothers may comprehend could explain the poor use of treated bednets. Socioeconomic status of families, though not investigated in this study has been found to be a reflection of the choice of malaria preventive measures, in this region. Socioeconomic status determines the economic power to sustain the preventive measure chosen, so cheaper, locally made and available means would be more acceptable.

2.2.2 Clinical effects of parasitemia

The major clinical symptoms apart from fever were cough, diarrhea generalized rash, excessive crying and vomiting (Afolabi, 2001; Orogade, 2006). All these symptoms are non specific but had about one half to two fold occurrence in children with malaria than in others without malaria parasitemia. Fever however seems to be the most constant factor even in the older infant and children. The babies had a low mean temperature of 37.7°C ± 0.58 and respiratory distress with respiratory rate of 45.66 ± 21.6 cycles/minute. Dehydration, palmar pallor, jaundice and hepatomegaly were the commonest signs though not of significant relationship. Palmar pallor is not a good indicator of anaemia $\chi2 = 1.24$, $p= 0.264$. The children with parasitemia had relatively low grade fever with mean temperatures of 37.7 ± 0.58 and tachycardia, mean pulse rate of 137.67 ± 9.94..Overall most of the clinical features were non-specific and could not be attributable to only malaria. Malaria in the children aged 0-5 months though the prevalences and parasite densities are lower, yet it produces significant morbidity in the children. Prevention of malaria in the pregnant women by chemoprophylaxis is still an area that requires focus and advocacy and public enlightenment on the use of insecticide treated nets for more widespread use is needed.

2.3 Six months – Five years

2.3.1 Clinical features of complicated and uncomplicated malaria

In the areas of stable malaria transmission, this group of children are the most affected in morbidity and mortality. Reporting the findings of severe malaria in Gabonese children, children Dzeing-Ella et al (2005) observed that most children with severe malaria are under 5 years old. Commonest features were anaemia, respiratory distress, cerebral malaria hypoglycaemia. Anaemia was commoner in children under 18 months of age, while cerebral malaria was commoner above 18 months. Poor prognostic factors were coma, hyperlactaemia and hypoglycaemia. Another study reporting uncomplicated malaria in febrile under 5 years children (Ikeh & Teclaire, 2008) showed prevalences of about 52.2% and the most common presentation was fever. Most of the children within this age group at are various levels of developing immunity and yet have parasite rates that could range from 80-90%. This explains their potential to develop severe malaria.

2.3.2 Use of clinical algorithms and predictors for malaria morbidity and mortality

Development of clinical algorithms were initially done as guidelines to ensure that the young child at risk of potentially fatal diseases were identified and received prompt attention and commenced some management at the community level. In this guideline, the Integrated Management of Childhood Diseases [IMCI], children under 5 years of age, living in areas of high malaria endemicity were to be treated for malaria if they presented to a health facility with fever, temp >37. 5°C. Studies by Tabitha et al (2005) found in a study that using a set of symptoms and signs with highest sensitivity and specificity and comparing these to parasitemia, a significant proportion of patients would have been sent home untreated. This tendency increased with increasing age. In situations as alluded to by the report of Khan et al (2005), the other issue was that often there were co-morbidities in febrile illness in some communities. Simply using algorithms for treatment of malaria might also lead to delay in treatment of other equally life threatening infections like Enteric fever which was commonly observed in their study. Algorithms on the one hand may lead to wastefulness of treatment supplies and on the other hand endanger lives for other possibly life threatening conditions.

2.4 School aged 5-12years

2.4.1 Asymptomatic malaria parasitemia and its implication for malaria control

The school aged child in an area of high endemicity typically has malaria parasite prevalence rates of up to 75%. Despite this high rates of parasitemia, theses children largely remain asymptomatic, having developed sufficient immunity which is both antiparastic and antitoxic to keep them from having clinical infection (Bruce Chwatt et al as cited by Orogade et al, 2002). In their study, Orogade et al (2002) also observed that these asymptomatic children had high levels of gametocytaemia (65%). Possible association between asymptomatic parasitemia and the utilization of vector control measures were analyzed. Vector control measure utilization was strongly related and inversely associated with the rates of ASMP. The estimation of ASMP is therefore recommended for use as an index for evaluation of malaria vector control programmes.

3. Laboratory diagnosis in malaria

3.1 Role of presumptive versus laboratory diagnosis for treatment

The policy and strategies for Malaria control by the WHO hinges on Malaria prevention, diagnosis and treatment. Diagnosis of malaria has been a challenge in both endemic and non endemic countries alike: the former having overdiagnosis with consequences of wastage of resources for treatment, excessive drug pressure and antimalarial drug resistance and the latter under diagnosis or even missed diagnosis which in some cases lead to malaria mortality. Gwer et al (2007) in an over view of problems associated with overdiagnosis in severe malaria identified the unavailability and unreliable parasitological confirmation of parasitemia as the greatest challenge in endemic countries.

The commonest symptom of malaria is fever and the subject of how many febrile episodes in susceptible populations in endemic areas even in the face of detectable parasitemia is attributable to malaria has been of immense research. Mc Guiness et al (1998) proposed some clinical case definitions for malaria in southern Ghana. Using logistic regression to model fever risk as continuous function of parasite density, fever attributable to malaria was defined by season and age groups. It was concluded that attributable fever was 51% and 22% in wet and dry seasons respectively for infants while in the children older than one year, it was higher in both seasons: 89% and 36% respectively. They also observed a lower estimated parasite density threshold for initiation of a febrile episode in infants than the older child. In another study Rougement et al (1991) working in Niger, West Africa investigated parasitemia based on 3 criteria of febrile episodes: the duration, intensity and possibility of a non malarial cause. The proportion of febrile cases attributable to parasitemia ranged from 0 to 0.92 but there was no association between parasitemia and low intensity fevers, or fever of greater than 3 days duration in the presence of an obvious non malaria cause. They however also found highly significant relationship between parasitemia and fever in the high transmission season. It seems from these studies that making a diagnosis by clinical case definitions based on epidemiological factors may be a useful tool in areas where laboratory facilities are not always available or reliable.

However, Valerie et al (2010) again observed from studies done over 20years that there was a growing decline in malaria transmission in East Africa and a subsequent proportion of fever associated with Plasmodium falciparum. They concluded that the decline provides evidence for policy change from presumptive antimalarial therapy to laboratory diagnosis before treatment (Valerie et al 2009, 2010). Much has gone into training of personnel for laboratory diagnosis and as Ngasala et al (2008) reported on the impact of training in clinical and microscopy diagnosis of childhood malarial on prescription and health outcome: microscopy reduces prescription but there is great variation in accuracy of readings. With this observation, the caution by English et al (2009) might be only apt that rapid universal policy change that abandons presumptive antimalarial treatment for African children might be premature and in fact cause more harm than good.

3.2 Comparisons between rapid diagnostic tests and microscopy in malaria

The gold standard for malaria parasite identification and quantification has been the microscopic examination of thick and fixed thin blood smears using Giemsa stain. In cases of anticipated low malaria parasite densities, care should be taken to maintain the pH of the stain around 7 and a freshly prepared stain achieves better results (Orogade et al, 2008). Other techniques utilised to enhance microscopy include the acridine orange fluorescent technique (Keiser el al, 2002; Lowe et al, 1996; Nicholas, 1997). This has proved to be quite useful but requires the additional requirements of fluorescent microscopy. Maintenance of a good quality, effective microscopy service involves the provision of high quality supplies, reagents, microscopes as well as technical competence and an adequate work environment to prepare usable blood films (Coleman et al, 2002; Durrheim et al, 1997, Kachur et al, 1998; Kain et al, 1998; Kilan et al, 2000; Omeara et al, 2005 as cited in Bell et al, 2006).

Obstacles to lab diagnosis of malaria as have been reported in Mali (Dolo et al, 2010) are the same experience in most developing countries where malaria is endemic. These includeunderuse of laboratory diagnosis by clinicians, absence of qualified laboratory facilities in some locations, and poor continuous professional education of laboratory technicians.

Introduction of Rapid Diagnostic tests was intended to fill the need for accuracy, speed and reliability which standard microscopy has fallen short of. These are antigen detecting rapid diagnostic tests which detect the histidine rich protein 2(HRP_2) and Plasmodium lactate dehydrogenase(pLDH) which are usually produced during the erythrocytic cycle. Several studies have evaluated the effectiveness of these tests compared with microscopy and the results have consistently shown high sensitivity and specificity but inability to differentiate mixed infections (Chinkhumba, 2010; Gatti et al, 2007; Tomas et al, 2001). However the successful implementation of RDT has been bedevilled by poor product performance, inadequate methods to determine the quality of products and a lack of emphasis and capacity to deal with these.(Bell et al 2006) Another group (Christopher et al, 2008) described the limitations of RDTs as having: all or none test results, inability to diagnose non falciparum malaria, variable heat stability and safety risks related to blood sampling (especially HIV and hepatitis B). Also of equal concern is that negative RDT results are often ignored and patients are treated anyway.

3.3 Provision of centralised rapid diagnostic test centres for more efficient diagnosis

To ascertain some degree of quality assurance and uniformity of results there is need to develop centralised RDT centres. These centres serve for purchase, transport, storage of RDTs kits as well as provide training for personnel that administer the tests at community level. It could serve as a reference laboratory since there are more highly skilled personnel and results of tests could be ascertained. Church et al (2003), describe such a centre which has supported and facilitated the RDT programme. Bastiaens et al (2011) have described results of researches carried on at such centres which showed improved diagnosis of malaria when government policy changed to implementation of testing before treatment in malaria. However, Derua et al (2011), describe in their study the perception of the users and health service providers which were dissimilar. Whereas the clinicians and patients were satisfied with the overall performance of the labs, the laboratory personnel expressed dissatisfaction over working conditions and some details of laboratory procedures. This signal is worth more investigation across regional centres so that the efforts gained would not be undermined. There is also noted that there is need to integrate these services into existing healthcare services to ensure sustainability in the long run.

3.4 Newer microscopic techniques

Due to the limitations of the rapid diagnostic tests already noted, the RDTs are not the end in malaria diagnosis. Using Polymerase chain reaction (PCR) techniques some of the limitations have been overcome. Myjak et al (2002), describe PCR techniques that have been utilised to enhance malaria diagnosis in mixed infections and especially in patients with low parasite densities, while Patsoula et al (2003) reported a single step PCR based method to differentiate mixed infections and Ahmet et al (2010) have used nested PCR and Real-Time PCR for detection of *Plasmodium vivax*.

Reliable enumeration of malaria parasites in thick blood film using digital analysis is also described by Frean (2009).

3.5 Other non specific laboratory tests in malaria diagnosis

Some workers have identified some other non malaria haematological indicators of the diagnosis and course of malaria (Ida E et al, 2007). Such include low levels of thrombocyte, leucocytes and coagulation factors II- VII-X as well as raised levels of C-reactive protein, lactate dehydrogenase and bilirubin. It is suggested that these could serve as markers of active disease as well as for monitoring during treatment and especially so when malaria parasites are difficult to identify.

4. Conclusion

- There has been tremendous increase in research in malaria diagnosis in the last decade.
- There should be an increased awareness and identification of congenital, neonatal and early infancy malaria especially in endemic areas. This also calls for closer monitoring and care of the pregnant woman at risk of malaria infection
- Clinical algorithms for malaria diagnosis are not sensitive enough for predicting morbidity or mortality.

- Reliance on rapid diagnostic tests should be put into context. Areas with mixed malaria parasite infection would need some other confirmatory tests while in other areas, uncertain distribution of reagents and trained personnel could limit the effectiveness of RDTs in diagnosis.

5. References

Afolabi,L; Salako, A; Mafe, A; Ovwigho, U; Rabiu, A; Sanyaolu, N &Ibrahim, M. (2001). Malaria in the first 6 months of life in urban African Infants with anemia. *The American Journal of Tropical Medicine and Hygiene,* Vol. 65, No. 6, pp. 822-827

Ahmet, G; Fadime, E. & Ismail S. (2010). Detection of Plasmodium vivax by NestedPCR and Real-Time PCR. *Korean Journal of Parasitology*, Vol. 48, No.2, (June 2010) DOI:10.3347/kjp.2010.48.2.99 pp. 99-103

Ammah, A; Nkuo-Akenji, T; Ndip, R; Deas, J. (1999). An update on concurrent malaria and typhoid fever inCameroon. *Transactions of The Royal Society Of Tropical Medicine And Hygiene,* Vol. 93, No. 2, (Mar-Apr 1999), pp.127-129

Bastiaens, G; Schaftenaar, E; Ndaro, A; Keuter, M; Bousema, T. & Shekalaghe S. (2011).Malaria diagnostic testing and treatment practices in three different Plasmodium falciparum transmission settings in Tanzania: before and after a government policy change, In: *Malaria Journal* 2011, Available from http://www.malariajournal.com/content/10/1/76.

Bell, D; Wongsrichanalai, C & Barnwell, J. (2006) Ensuring quality and access for malaria diagnosis: how can it be achieved? In: *Evaluating Diagnostics Review 2006,* Available from www.nature.com/reviews/micro

Berrang –Ford, L; MacLean, J; Gyorkos, T; Ford, J. & Ogden N. (2008). Climate change and Malaria in Canada: a systems approach, In: *Interdisciplinary Perspectives on Infectious Diseases.* Vol. 2009, Article ID 385487, doi:10.1155/2009/385487

Chinkhumba, J; Skarbinski, J; Chilima, B; Campbell, C; Ewing, V; Joaquin, M; Sande, J; Ali,D; Mathanga, D. (2010). Comparative field performance and adherence to test results of four malaria rapid diagnostic tests among febrile patients more than five years of age in Blantyre, Malawi. 2010. In: *Malaria Journal* 2010. Available from http://www. malariajournal.com/content

Christopher,J; Hopkins, H; Ansah, E; Leslie, T & Reyburn, H.(2008). Opportunities and threats in targeting Antimalarials for the AMFm: the Role of Diagnostics. Discussion paper prepared for the Consultative Forum on AMFm- the Affordable Medicine Facility- malaria Available at www.rrf.org

Church, D; Lichenfeld, A; Elsayed, S; Kuhn, & Gregson D. (2003). *Archives of Pathology &Laboratory Medicine,* Vol. 127, (June 2003)

Derua, Y; Ishengoma, D; Rwegoshora, R; Tenu, F; MAssaga, J; Mboera, L; & Magesa, M. (2011). Users' and health service providers' perception on quality of laboratory malaria diagnosis in Tanzania. In: *Malaria Journal*. Available from http://www.malariajournal.com/content/10/1/78

Dolo, A; Diallo, M; Saye, R; Konare, A; Ouattra, A; Poudiougo, B; Kouyate, B; Minta, D.&Doumbo, O. (2010). Obstacles to laboratory diagnosis of malaria in Mali-perspectives. *Medicine Tropicale,* Vol. 70, (2010), pp. 158-162

English, M; Reyburn, H; Goodman, C. & Snow, R. (2009). Abandoning presumptive antimalarial treatment for febrile children aged less than five years—A case of running before we can walk? *PLoS Medicine,* Vol. 6, No.1, (2009) e1000015.doi:10.1371/journal.pmed.1000015

Falade, C; Mokuolu, O; Okafor H, Orogade,A et al. (2007).Epidemiology of congenitalmalaria in Nigeria: a multicentre study. *Tropical Medicine and International Health,* Vol. 12, No. 11,(2007), pp.1-9

Gay- Andrieu, F; Adehossi, E; Lacroix, Veronique; Gagara, M; Ibrahim, L; Kourna, among H;Boureima, H. (2005).Epidemiological, clinical and Biological features of malaria children in Niamey, Niger. In: *Malaria Journal.* Available at: http://www.malariajournal.com/content/4/1/10

Gatti, S; Gramegna, M; Bisoffi, Z; Raglio, A; Gulletta, M; Klersy, C; Bruno, A; Maserati, R;Madama, S; Scaglia, M.& THE GISPI STUDY GROUP. (2007). A comparison of three diagnostic techniques for malaria: a rapid diagnostic test (NOWH Malaria), PCR and microscopy. *Annals of Tropical Medicine & Parasitology,* Vol. 101, No. 3, (2007), pp.195–204

Gwer, S; Newton C. & Berkley J. (2007). Overdiagnosis and co-morbidities of severe malaria in African children: a guide for clinicians. *American Journal of Tropical Medicine and Hygiene,* Vol.77, No. 6, Suppl, (December 2007), pp. 6-13

Hussain, N; Echoga, A.& Iwarere O.(2009). Pattern of malaria presentation and treatment at Obiesan Naval Medical Centre, Lagos- Nigeria. *European Journal of Scientific Research,* Vol. 27, No.1, (2009), pp. 120-127, ISSN1450-216X

Ibhanesebhor, S. (1995). Clinical characteristics of neonatal malaria. *Journal of Tropical Paediatrics,* Vol. 41, (1995), pp. 330–333

Ida, E; Lasse, S; Vestergaard, Kirsten, M; Antia, M. & Bygbjerg I. (2007). Laboratory indicators of the diagnosis and course of imported Malaria. *Scandinavian Journal of Infectious Diseases,* Vol. 39, (2007), pp. 707-713

Ikeh, E; Teclaire, N. (2008). Prevalence of malaria parasitaemia and associated factors in febrile under-5 children seen in Primary Health care centres in Jos, North Central Nigeria. *Nigeria Postgraduate Medical Journal, Vol.* 15, No. 2, pp.65-69

John, A. (2009). Reliable enumeration of malaria parasites in thick blood films using digital image analysis. In: *Malaria Journal,* (2009), 8:218 doi:10.1186/1475-2875-8-218

Keiser, J; Utzinger, J; Premji, Z; Yamagata, Y & Singer B. (2002). Acridine Orange for malaria, the Diagnosis: its diagnostic performance; its promotion and implementation in Tanzania and implications for malaria control. *Annals of Tropical Medicine and Parsitology,* Vol. 96, No. 7, pp. 643-654

Kamwendo, D; Dzinjalamala, F; Snounou, G. et al.(2002). Plasmodium falciparum: PCR detection and genotyping of isolates from peripheral, placental, and cord blood of pregnant Malawian women and their infants. *Transactions of The Royal Society Of Tropical Medicine And Hygiene,* Vol. 96, (2002), pp. 145–149.

Khan, A; Mekan, S; Abbas, Z & Smego, R. (2005). Concurrent malaria and enteric fever in Pakistan. *Singapore Medical Journal,* Vol. 46, No.11, (2005), pp. 635-638

Lamikanra, O. (1993). A study of malaria parasitaemia in pregnant women, placentae, cord blood and newborn babies in Lagos, Nigeria. *West African Journal of Medicine,* Vol. 12, (1993), pp. 213–217.

Lehner, J; & Andrews, C. (1988). Congenital malaria in Papua New Guinea. *Transactions of The Royal Society Of Tropical Medicine And Hygiene,* Vol.82, (1988), pp. 822–826.

Lowe, B; Jeffa, N; New, L; Pedersen, C; Engbaek, K& Marsh, K (1996). Acridine orange fluorescence techniques as alternatives to traditional Giemsa staining for the diagnosis of malaria in developing countries. *Transactions of The Royal Society Of Tropical Medicine And Hygiene,* Vol. 90, No.1, (1996), pp. 34-36

Mc Gregor, I. (1986). Congenitally acquired malaria. *Post Graduate Doctor, Vol.* 2, (1986), pp. 52-56

Mc Guinness, D; Koram, K; Bennett, S; Wagner, G; Nkrumah, F, Riley E. (1998). Clinical case definitions for malaria: clinical malaria associated with very low parasite rates in African infants. *Transactions of The Royal Society Of Tropical Medicine And Hygiene*, Vol. 92, No.5, (1998), pp. 527-531

Mohapatra, M; Padhiary, K; Mishra, D; Sethy, G. (2002). Atypical manifestations of Plasmodium vivax malaria. *Indian Journal of Malariology*, Vol.39, No. 1-2, (Mar-Jun 2002), pp. 18-25

Molyneux, M.(1989) Malaria- clinical features in children. *Journal of the Royal Society ofMedicine*, Vol. 82, Supplement No. 17, (1989), pp. 35

Murthy, G; Sahay, R; Srinivasan, V; Upadhaya, A; Shantaram, V; Gayatri, K. (2000). Clinical profile of falciparum malaria in a tertiary care hospital. *Journal of the Indian Medical Association*, Vol. 98, No. 4, (Apr 2000), pp. 160-162, 169.

Mukhtar, M; Lesi, F; Iroha, E; Egri-Okwaji M& Mafe A. (2006). Congenital malaria among inborn babies at a tertiary centre in Lagos. *Nigeria Journal of Tropical Pediatrics*, Vol. 52, (2006), pp. 19–23

Myjak P ; Nahorski, W; Pieniazek, N; Pietkiewicz, H. Usefulness of PCR for Diagnosis of Imported Malaria in Poland. *European Journal of Clinical Microbiology & Infectious Diseases, Vol. 21,* (2002), pp. 215–218 DOI 10.1007/s10096-001-0690-0

Ngasala, B; Mubi, M; Warsame, M; Petzold, M; Massele, A; Gustafsson, L; Tomson, G; Premji, Z.& Bjorkman A. (2008). Impact of training in clinical and microscopy diagnosis of childhood malaria on antimalarial drug prescription and health outcome at primary health care level in Tanzania: A randomized controlled trial. *Malaria Journal,(* 2008), **7**:199 doi:10.1186/1475-2875-7-199

Okwa,O. (2000). The status of malaria among infants aged 0-5 years in Lagos State, Nigeria. *Nigeria Quarterly Journal of Hospital Medicine,*Vol. 10, No.2, (2000), pp. 87-89

Okwa, O.& Ibidapo, A. (2010). The Malaria situation, perception of cause and treatment in a Nigerian University. *Journal of Medicine and Medical Sciences,*Vol. 1, No.6, (July 2010), pp. 213-222 Available from: http://www.interesjournals.org/JMMS

Olowu, A; Sowunmi, A & Abohweyere, A. (2000). Congenital malaria in a hyperendemic area: a revisit. *African Journal of Medicine & Medical Science, Vol.* 29, (2000), pp. 211–213

Orogade, A; Falade, C; Okafor, H; Mokuolu, O; Mamman, A; Tagbo, A; Ogunkunle, O; Ernest, K; Callahan, M.& Hamer, D. (2008). Clinical and laboratory features of congenital malaria in Nigeria. *Journal of Pediatric Infectious Diseases, Vol.* 3, (2008), pp. 181–187

Orogade, A. (2006). Malaria in febrile under six months old children in North Western Nigeria. *Proceedings of 27th African Health Congress,* Durban, South Africa,2006

Orogade, A. (2004). Neonatal Malaria in a mesodermic Malaria area of Northern Nigeria. *Annals of African Medicine,* Vol. 3, No. 4, (2004), pp. 170 – 173

Orogade, A; Ogala, W & Aikhionbare, H. (2002) Asymptomatic Malaria Parasitaemia- a suitable index for evaluating Malaria Vector Control measures. *Nigerian Journal of Paediatrics.*, Vol. 29, No.2, (July 2010), pp. 23-26

Patsoula, E; Spanakos,G; Sofianatou, D; Parara, M;& Vakalis N. (2003). A single step, PCR – based method for detection and differenciation of Plasmodium vivax and P. Falciparum. *Annals of Tropical Medicine & Parasitology*, Vol. 97, No. 1, pp. 15-21

Rehlis, N. & Kurczewska M. (2001). Analysis of different clinical critaeria in malaria patients in Papua New Guinea. *Wiadomości Parazytologiczne,*Vol.47, No.3, (2001), pp. 371-376

Rougemont, P; Brenner, M; Moret, M; Breslow, N; Dumbo, M; Dolo, A; Soula, G; & Perrin M. (2003). Epidemilogical basis for clinical diagnosis of childhood malaria in endemic zone in West Africa. *The Lancet,* Vol. 338, Issue 8778, (23 November 1991), pp. 1292-1295

Runsewe-Abiodun, I; Ogunfowora, O; & Fetuga, B. (2006). Neonatal malaria in Nigeria – a 2 year review. *Bio Medical Centrale Pediatrics, Vol.* 6, (2006), pp. 19.

Sekene, B; Karine, B; Phillipe, P; Phillipe B & Jean D. (2002). Contribution of nonspecific laboratory Test to the diagnosis of malaria in febrile travelers returning from value Endemic areas:of hypocholesterlemia. *Journal of Travel Medicine,* Vol. 9, (2002), pp. 117-121

Sengoz Inan, A; Erdem, I; Ozturkengin, D et al. (2010) Malaria: evaluation of 40 cases. *Turkish Society for Parasitology, Vol.* 34, No.3, pp. 147-151

Schellenberg, J. & Hayes R. (1994). Attributable fraction estimates and case definitions for malaria in endemic areas. *Statistics in Medicine,* Vol. 13, No.22, (Nov 30 1994), pp. 2345-58.

Steketee R,W; Ter Kuile, F; Parise, M; Verhoeff, F; Udhayakumar, V; Newman, R;, Van eijk, A.& Rogerson, S. (2004). The burden of co-infection with human immunodeficiency virus type 1 and malaria in pregnant women in sub-Saharan Africa. *The American Journal of Tropical Medicine and Hygiene,* Vol. 71, (2 suppl) (2004), pp. 41-54

Sowunmi, A; Ilesanmi, J; Akindele et al. (1996). Placental falciparum infection and outcome of pregnancy in Nigerian mothers from an endemic area. *Journal of Obstetrics & Gynecology, Vol.* 16, (1996), pp. 211–216.

Tabitha, W; Mwangi; Mohammed, M; Dayo, H; Snow, R.& Marsh K. (2005).Clinical algorithms for malaria diagnosis lack utility among people of different age groups. *Tropical Medicine and International Health,* Vol. 10, No. 6, (June 2005) pp. 530–536

Talib, S; Gaikwad, A.& Jirwankar, P. (1996). Protean manifestations of malaria--(multi organ dysfunction syndrome), Vol. 39, No. 5, (Dec 1996), pp. 473-476.

Ticconi, C; Mapfumo, M; Dorrucci, M; Naha, N; Tarira, E; Pietropolli, A& Rezza, G.(2003). Effect of maternal HIV and malaria infection on pregnancy and perinatal outcome in Zimbabwe. *Journal of Acquired Immune Deficiency Syndromes & Human Retrovirology,* Vol. 34, (2003), pp. 289-294.

Tomas, J; Martin, P; Grobusch2 & Gundel H. (2001). Evaluation of a Dipstick Test for the Rapid Diagnosis of Imported Malaria Among Patients Presenting Within the Network TropNetEurop. *Scandinavian Journal of Infectious Diseases, Vol* 33, (2001), pp. 752–754

Valérie, D; Christian, L; Hassan, M; Deo, Mtasiwa; Marcel, T. & Blaise, G. (2009). Time To Move from Presumptive Malaria Treatm ent to Laboratory-Confirmed Diagnosis and Treatment in African Children with Fever. *PLoS Medicine,* Vol. 6, No.1, e1000015. doi:10.1371/journal.pmed.1000015

Valérie, D; Christian, L. & Blaise, G. (2010). Reduction in the proportion of fevers associated with Plasmodium falciparum parasitaemia in Africa: a systematic review. In: *Malaria Journal* 2010Available from: http://www.malariajournal.com/content/9/1/240

van Eijk A; Ayisi, J; ter Kuile, F; Misore, A; Otieno, J; Rosen, D; Kager,P; Steketee, R;Nahlen, B. (2003). HIV increases the risk of malaria in women of all gravidities in Kisumu, Kenya. *AIDS,* Vol. 17, (2003), pp. 595-603.

Verhoeff, F; Brabin,B; Hart, C;, Chimsuku, L; Kazembe,P. & Broadhead, RL. (1999) malariaIncreased prevalence of malaria in HIV-infected pregnant women and its implications for control.*Tropical Medicine and International Health,*Vol.4, (1999), pp. 5-12.

World Health Organization [WHO], (2010). World Malaria Report. Available from: http://www.who.int/malaria/world_malaria_report_2010

Part 5

Malaria Immunology

10

The Immunology of Malaria

Sam M. Kinyanjui
KEMRI-Wellcome Trust Research Programme, Kilifi, Kenya

1. Introduction

The main impetus for trying to understand immunity to malaria is the need to develop effective malaria vaccines. Despite years of knowing that humans can be immune to malaria the mechanisms underlying this immunity are yet to be properly understood. This is, in part, attributable to the complexity of the malaria parasite and its life cycle resulting in a complex parasite-host relation. The outcome of a malaria infection is a consequence of interactions between host, parasite and environmental factors. As such attempts to correlate outcome with a single immunological parameter often results in spurious associations that do not hold in different circumstances. This situation is exacerbated by the lack of natural animal models for human malaria from which observations could reliably be extrapolated. Consequently, much of our understanding of malaria immunity is based on extrapolation of in vitro observations or deduced from phenomenological observations.

As is the case with immunity to other infections, immunity to malaria is the result of a combination of genetic resistance, non-adaptive immunity, and acquired or adaptive immunity. This chapter will mainly focus on immunity to *Plasmodium falciparum* malaria because it accounts for largest proportion of disease and practically all malaria mortality.

2. Genetic resistance to malaria

Population genetics studies suggest that a large proportion of the variability in malaria incidence among people residing in a malaria endemic area may be attributable to genetic factors (Mackinnon *et al* 2005). This indicates that in addition to the well known genetic variations in red cell components there are a number of other genetic variations, albeit with less obvious phenotype, that also affect susceptibility to malaria. The discovery of these variations has accelerated in the recent while thanks to advances in molecular biology techniques especially the capacity to do high throughput DNA sequencing (Williams 2009).

2.1 Protection against malaria by haemoglobinopathies and other red cell mutations

Haldane in 1949 was the first to hypothesize that certain red cell mutations reached unexpectedly high prevalence in malaria endemic areas because these mutations protect against malaria and hence confer survival advantage over non-carriers (Haldane 1949, Piel *et al* 2010, Weatherall 1997). This hypothesis has since been confirmed through a number of studies that have reported over 80% protection against severe malaria among sickle cell heterozygotes (Hill *et al* 1991, Williams *et al* 2005b) and haemoglobin C homozygotes (Modiano *et al* 2001) and between 40-60% protection among α+ thalassaemia heterozygotes (Allen *et al* 1997, Wambua *et al* 2006, Williams *et al* 2005d). Interestingly, when thalassaemia and sickle cell are co-inherited the protection provided by each trait separately was lost (Penman *et al* 2009, Williams *et al* 2005c). Mutations that affect other components of the red cell have also been shown to provide protection against malaria. Although some studies suggest that only hemizygote Glucose-6-Phosphate Dehydrogenase (G6PD) deficient male are protected against malaria (Guindo *et al* 2007) other studies found that female homozygotes also enjoy significant protection against malaria (Clark *et al* 2009, Ruwende *et al* 1995).

The mechanisms by which haemoglobinopathies protect against malaria are poorly understood. Decreased parasite invasion and growth, possibly due to altered membrane characteristics and physiology in abnormal cells has been reported (Senok *et al* 1997). The susceptibility of G6PD deficient and thalassaemic cells to oxidative damage which in turn kills the parasite inside has been cited as a possible explanation for their protection against malaria (Friedman 1978, Golenser and Chevion 1989, Mendez *et al* 2011) At the same time, infected abnormal red cells exhibit reduced cytoadherence and rosetting, two phenomena that have been implicated in pathogenesis of cerebral malaria (Carlson *et al* 1994, Cholera *et al* 2008, Fairhurst *et al* 2005).

However, protection by haemoglobinopathies might not be entirely passive; a study by Williams et al (2005) found that protection by sickle cell trait against all forms of clinical malaria increased with age over the first ten years of life suggesting that the mechanisms cited above may interact with age-acquired immunity to enhance protection against malaria (Williams *et al* 2005a). Indeed, increased phagocytosis of infected mutant cells has been observed in the presence of otherwise normal parasite growth (Ayi *et al* 2004, Gallo *et al* 2009, Yuthavong *et al* 1990) further supporting the idea of synergy between natural and active immunity.

2.2 Other genetic polymorphisms that influence susceptibility to malaria

In addition to red cell polymorphism, several other genetic polymorphisms have also been implicated in natural resistance to malaria. The majority of these are in DNA regions that encode or control the encoding of components of the immune system and cellular adhesion proteins (Lopez *et al* 2010). The latter are important with regard to malaria as they have been implicated in the adherence of malaria infected red cells in the microvasculature of organs such as the brain; a process that contributes to the pathology of malaria. While some of these polymorphisms such as class 1 HLA-Bw53 allele have large effects; about 40% protection against severe malarial anaemia and cerebral malaria (Hill *et al* 1991), the others have subtle effect and are difficult to detect except in very large studies. The relationship between genetic polymorphisms and susceptibility to malaria is complex. Different polymorphism have varying influence on different syndromes of malaria some affect susceptibility to severe but not mild malaria or asymptomatic infection. Furthermore, the association with susceptibility to malaria for some polymorphism is only evident in one geographic region (West Africa only in the case of HLABw53 allele) but absent in other regions (Hill *et al* 1991). Although this could reflect some methodological difference in studies done in different regions, it also suggests that other unidentified genetic and environmental factors may modify the association between a known polymorphism and malaria outcome. Table 1 lists out some of the polymorphism identified so far, and illustrates that a large number of genes are involved in determining susceptibility to malaria.

Functions	Gene (Protein)
Major Histocompatibility complex antigens	HLA-B53, HLA-DRB1
Pro-inflammatory cytokine and cytokine receptors	Interferon alpha receptor 1 (IFNαR1); interferon gamma and interferon gamma receptor (IFN-γR & IFNγR); Tumor Necrotic Factor alpha (TNF-α); Interleukin 1α, 1β ,4 and 12b (IL-1α/β, 4, & 12b)
Anti-inflammatory cytokines	Interleukin 10 (IL-10)
B-cell function regulation	Interleukin 4 (IL-4), TNFSF5 (CD40L)
Complement pathway components	Complement receptor 1 (CR1); Mannose Binding Lectin 2 (MBL2)
Nitric oxide (NO) pathway (immunoregulatory and microbicidal)	Nitric oxide synthase 2A (NOS2A)
Components of innate immunity	Toll-like receptors 1, 4, 9 (TLR1, TLR4, TLR9)
Macrophage receptor for antibodies	Fc gama receptor 2A and 3B (FcγRIIA & FcγRIIIB)
Blood cells development	Stem Cell Growth Factor (SCGF)
Blood Group antigens	Groups A, O, B
Acute Phase proteins	Haptoglobin
Cellular Adhesion Molecules	Thrombospondin receptor (CD36), Intercellular adhesion molecule1 (ICAM1); Platelet-endothelial cell adhesion molecule (PECAM)
Chromosomal region with immune genes cluster	Chromosome 5 region 5q31-q33

Table 1. Genes Reported to Be Associated with Susceptibility to Malaria

3. Innate and acquired immunity

Decreasing frequency and severity of malaria episodes with age among endemic populations is the best indicator that people do acquire immunity to malaria following repeated exposure. However, because both the truly protective immune response to malaria and those that simply reflect exposure to malaria increase concurrently with age, many putative in vitro measure of "immunity" to malaria show no correlation with protection against malaria. As such disentangling protective responses from non-protective ones in the complex milieu of responses provoked by malaria parasites is a major objective of malaria immunity studies. Unfortunately, differences in study methodology, polymorphism of target antigens or epitopes and other factors, such as variation in transmission in different study settings and even microvariations in transmission within a given study setting makes it difficult to develop a consistent picture of the efficacy of a given natural or vaccine-induced immune response in protecting against malaria (Bejon *et al* 2009, Kinyanjui *et al* 2009, Marsh and Kinyanjui 2006).

3.1 Natural history of acquired immunity to malaria

As shown in figure 1, in areas of stable malaria transmission, the majority of severe disease and death due to malaria occur mainly in children but parasite prevalence continue to rise well beyond childhood (Roca-Feltrer *et al* 2010, Snow *et al* 1997, Snow *et al* 1994). This has led to the suggestion that acquisition of immunity to malaria may be biphasic with immunity to disease being acquired before immunity to infection. Observations from experimental infection studies lend support to this suggestion. Records from malariotherapy in the 1940s which involved deliberate infection of syphilis patients with malaria so that the fever induced can kill syphilis spirochetes, show that in most patients, fever and high parasitaemia occurred in the first 25 days after which a low-density asymptomatic infection persisted for many months (Collins and Jeffery 1999b). More recently some modelling have suggested that immunity to severe disease may develop after only one or two episodes of disease (Gupta *et al* 1999a, Gupta *et al* 1999b). In reality, there is an overlap between the two phases of immunity otherwise anti-disease immunity acting in the absence of anti-parasite immunity would not prevent the parasites from multiplying and eventually overwhelming the patient. Furthermore, the risk of disease is proportional to parasite density (Rougemont *et al* 1991, Smith *et al* 1994) therefore immune mechanisms that clear parasites will also reduce the risk of disease.

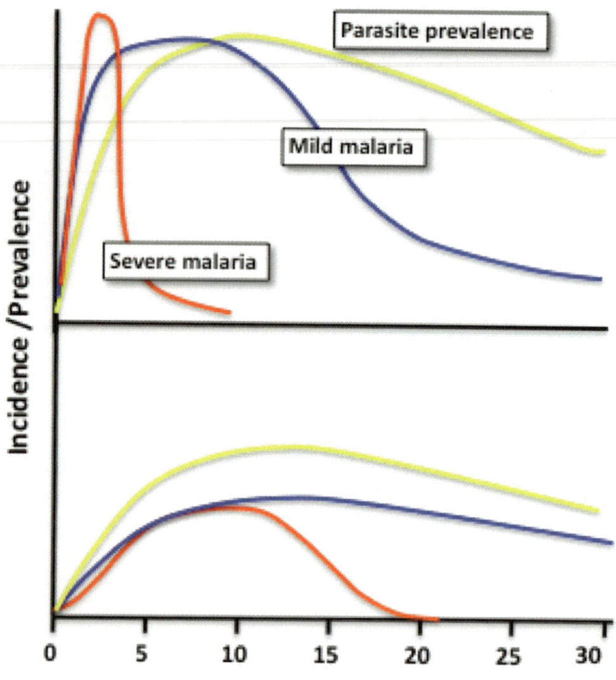

Fig. 1. A typical age pattern for incidence of severe and mild malaria and prevalence of asymptomatic malaria infection in an area of high (upper graph) and low (lower graph) malaria transmission

3.2 Strain specificity of malaria immunity

It has been suggested that the reason why immunity to malaria takes so long to acquire is because malaria is transmitted as a construct of many independent "strains" and one needs to accumulate immunity to all the circulating strains (Gupta and Day 1994, Gupta and Hill 1995). The observations in malariotherapy that infection with a given strain gave considerably more protection against re-infection by the same strain than by a different strain (Collins and Jeffery 1999a, Jeffery 1966) points to strain-specific immunity. However, unlike in the laboratory where cloned lines can be physically separated, maintaining such a population structure in the field despite sexual mixing is difficult (Babiker *et al* 1994, Hill and Babiker 1995, Ranford-Cartwright *et al* 1993). Nonetheless a number of models suggest that efficient immunity responses directed against a polymorphic antigenic determinant could constrain parasite populations into discrete non-overlapping strains with respect to that antigen (Gupta and Hill 1995, Recker *et al* 2008, Recker *et al* 2004).

Immune responses against the variant parasite antigens (VSA) exported to the surface of infected red cells, of which PfEMP1 is the best characterised, are an example of immunity that might be sufficiently efficient to structure malaria parasite population into "strains". These antigens are highly polymorphic and undergo clonal antigenic variation (Brannan *et al* 1994, Recker *et al* 2011, Roberts *et al* 1992). Antibodies to VSA provide variant-specific protection against malaria (Bull *et al* 1999, Bull *et al* 1998, Marsh *et al* 1989, Newbold *et al* 1992). The number of VSA variants against which an individual has antibodies increases with age (Bull *et al* 1998, Iqbal *et al* 1993, Reeder *et al* 1994). Thus, acquisition of immunity to malaria might, in part, involve the accumulation of antibodies against the circulating repertoire of VSA variants. It is thought that the variation of these antigens serve as an parasite immune evasion mechanism and therefore the need to avoid the generation of cross-reactive responses might provide the selection pressure necessary to maintain the circulation of distinct variants within a parasite population (Gupta and Hill 1995, Recker *et al* 2008, Recker *et al* 2004).

4. Immune effector mechanisms in malaria immunity

Although both cellular and humoral immunity are thought to be involved in malaria immunity, the relative importance of each in protection against malaria is not yet well established. In particular much of the data on cellular immunity comes from animal models. However, many of these animals are poor models of human malaria. Furthermore, data from different animal species and between different strains of same species often vary considerably making it difficult to generate definitive conclusion regarding immune effector mechanisms in malaria.

4.1 CD8+ T-cells (CTL)

CD8+ T cells are also referred to as cytotoxic T-cells (CTL) because they can kill infected cells directly by various cytotoxicity mechanisms. Because hepatocytes express class 1 HLA, the receptor for CD8+ T cells, the liver stage of malaria parasites is thought to be capable of inducing CTL responses. The role of CTL in the protection against malaria was first demonstrated in the classical experiments involving the immunization of animals and human with irradiated sporozoites. Such immunization resulted in complete, though short-lived, immunity (Clyde 1975, Nussenzweig *et al* 1967, Rieckmann *et al* 1974). Adoptive transfer of CTL and CTL depletion experiments in animals showed that although high levels of anti-sporozoite antibodies were observed in the immunized subjects, the protection observed was mediated by CTL (Schofield *et al* 1987, Suss *et al* 1988, Weiss *et al* 1988). The fact that adoptively transferred CTL pre-primed with *P. berghei* failed to protect against infection by *P. yoelii* indicates that protection by CTL is species-specific (Romero *et al* 1989). Later studies showed that CTL mediate their protection by preventing parasite development in the liver (Rodrigues 1991). Although CTL can kill parasites by perforin-mediated lysis and FAS-induced apoptosis of infected cells (Kagi *et al* 1994, Lowin *et al* 1994), depletion of FasL and perforin did not affect CD8+ mediated-protection against *P yoelii* infection in mice suggesting that the protection is probably cytokine-mediated (Morrot and Zavala 2004). Indeed, The importance of the cytokine pathway in which IFN-γ stimulates the host cell to kill the parasites through nitric oxide (NO) production has been demonstrated in mice (Schofield *et al* 1987).

Indirect evidence for CTL protection against malaria in humans is borne in the association between some class 1 HLA alleles and protection against malaria (Hill *et al* 1991). Over 30 peptides on the sporozoites and liver stage antigens of malaria parasites have now been identified as epitopes for human CTL (Aidoo and Udhayakumar 2000, Aidoo *et al* 1995, Bottius *et al* 1996) Some of these epitopes exhibit extensive polymorphism generated by non-synonymous mutations, an indication that they are under some sort of selection possibly by host immunity (Hughes and Hughes 1995, Lockyer *et al* 1989, Schofield 1989).

4.2 Cytokine response to malaria – Role of innate immunity and CD4+ T-cells

Malaria disease is characterised by production of a wide range of cytokines. Studies suggest that these come from both the innate arm and the adaptive arm of the immune system. Because parasites multiply very rapidly, it is likely that the innate arm mediates early cytokines responses against malaria. An early interferon gamma (IFN-γ) response has been shown to be important in protecting against development of severe disease symptoms (Cabantous *et al* 2005, D'Ombrain *et al* 2008, Perlaza *et al* 2011) as has the ability of one's cells to produce TNF-α or INF-γ upon stimulation with live parasites in vitro (Robinson *et al* 2009). Natural killer cells (NK) have been implicated as the source of early proinflammatory responses such as IFN-γ and TNF-α against malaria parasites (Artavanis-Tsakonas and Riley 2002, Korbel *et al* 2005) while other studies point to γδT–cells and αβT-cells (D'Ombrain *et al* 2008, Horowitz *et al* 2010). However, the relative contribution of each type of cells is debatable. Activation of innate immunity depends on broad recognition of pathogens. This recognition is driven by receptors that recognise pathogen associated molecular patterns (PAMPs). Among the best characterised of these pattern recognition receptors are Toll-like receptors (TLR), of which ten have been described in man so far. Upon recognition of PAMPs, TRLs induce a signalling cascade leading to secretion of proinflammatory cytokines, chemokines, and interferons. Malaria parasite glycophosphoinostol (GPI) has been shown to interact with TLR2 and to some extent TLR4 (Franklin *et al* 2009, Gowda 2007, Krishnegowda *et al* 2005). While some studies suggest that haemozoin, a product of haemoglobin digestion by malaria parasites interacts with TLR9 (Coban *et al* 2005), other studies suggest that haemozoin is immunologically inert and it's the parasite DNA that it complexes with that interact with TRLs to induce a proinflammatory response (Parroche *et al* 2007). It is also possible that malaria parasites can induce the innate immune system through interaction between other non-TLR receptors and AT-rich parasite DNA fragments (Sharma *et al* 2011).

Subsequent to the innate responses that mediate early resistance to malaria infection, the adaptive immunity takes over with CD4+ T-cells becoming the main producers of cytokines. Traditionally mature CD4+ T-cells are placed in two groups that are associated with distinct cytokine profiles. Production of interferon alpha/gamma (INF-α/γ), lymphotoxin-α (TNF-β), interleukin-12 (IL-12) defines type 1 helper cells (Th1) and is associated with a strong cell-mediated immunity while production of IL-4, 5, 6, 9, 10 and 13 define type 2 (Th2) which are associated with antibody production. However, because some T-cells and non-T-cells can produce both Th1 and Th2 cytokines, it may be more appropriate to talk of a type 1 (TR1) or a type 2 response (TR2) (Clerici and Shearer 1994). In malaria, the TR1/TR2 dichotomy is most evident in the mouse-*P. chabaudi* model (Langhorne *et al* 1989, Taylor-Robinson and Phillips 1993). In this model, TR1 dominates the early response of mice to acute *P. chabaudi* infection and parasite killing is mediated by INF-γ, tumour necrosis factor (TNF-α) and nitric oxide (NO) secreted by activated Th1 CD4+, macrophages, and natural killer cells. In *P. berghei* and *P. yoelii* models, TR1 response induced through sporozoites vaccination have been shown to provide strong protection against challenge infections (Oliveira *et al* 2008, Purcell *et al* 2008). On the other hand, a shift towards TR2 leads to less symptomatic chronic infections (Clerici and Shearer 1994). Along with inhibiting both INF-γ and TNF-α, type 2 cytokines also stimulate B-cells to secrete of antibodies (Fell and Smith 1998, Pretolani and Goldman 1997, Taylor-Robinson 1995). The dual anti-parasite/ pathogenetic nature of TR1 is also evident in *P. berghei* infections (Hirunpetcharat *et al* 1999, Rudin *et al* 1997). Other murine-malaria models display variable tendencies towards either type of responses during acute and chronic infections (Taylor-Robinson and Smith 1999).

The distinction between type 1 and 2 responses is less clear in human malaria. Increased IFN-γ is associated with the resolution of parasitaemia in acute malaria episodes (Winkler *et al* 1998) and a delay in re–infection (Luty *et al* 1999) while reduced levels accompany hyper-parasitaemia in children (Winkler *et al* 1999). Similarly, levels of type 1 response were lower among Malawian malaria patients than among patients of other disease, with a reverse trend being observed for the type 2 responses (Jason *et al* 2001). INF-γ levels were found to be higher in pregnant women who did not have placental malaria than in those who did (Moore *et al* 1999). These observations argue for a possible anti-parasite role of TR1 in humans. Furthermore CD4+ secreted IL-2 and TNF–α are associated with the protection provided by the experimental vaccine RTS'S (Lumsden *et al* 2011). On the other hand, IL-10 and IL-4, both type 2 cytokines, have been associated with protection against malarial anaemia (Biemba *et al* 2000, Kurtzhal *et al* 1998). Although reduced secretion of INF-γ by immune T-cells in response to malaria led to the conclusion that reduced pathology in immune individuals may be attributable to down-regulation of TR1 cytokines (Chizzolini *et al* 1990), Winkler et al (1999) observed a striking increase in type 1 cytokines in immune adults (Winkler *et al* 1999). It is likely that efficient immunity to malaria requires a balance in between TR1 and TR2.

4.3 Regulatory T cells

There is now an increasing recognition of the role played by a third population of CD4+ T-cells in malaria immunity (Walther *et al* 2009). This cells, designated regulatory T-cells (Tregs), additionally express CD25 and FOXP3 cellular markers and mediate their actions through immunomodulatory cytokines IL-10 and TGF-β. Studies in mouse models suggest that these cytokines help reduce immunopathology by suppressing proinflammatory cytokines (Nie *et al* 2007) although if induced too early in an infection they may suppress the protective effects of the proinflammatory cytokines and allow the parasite to multiply uncontrollably (Walther *et al* 2005). In humans, TGF–β, which appears to interact with Tregs, is associated with increased risk of clinical disease and a high parasite growth in vivo (Todryk *et al* 2008). As such a fine balance between the symptom-suppressing effects of Tregs and the parasite-suppressing effect of symptom-inducing cytokines is needed for an optimal outcome following malaria infection (Berretta *et al* 2011).

5. Humoral responses in malaria

5.1 Evidence for involvement in protection against malaria

There is no doubt that humoral responses are important in protection against malaria. Direct evidence for this comes from passive transfer experiments both in animal models (Groux and Gysin 1990) and humans. In a series of experiments carried out in the early 1960s by Cohen, Macgregor, and Carrington intra-muscular administration of purified IgG from malaria immune African adults into Gambian and East African children suffering from clinical malaria caused a marked drop in parasitaemia within five days. IgG from Europeans without prior exposure to malaria did not show this parasitocidal effect; indicating that the antibodies from Africans were malaria-specific (Cohen *et al* 1961, McGregor 1963). Similar results were obtained in more recent transfer experiments that used African immune serum to treat Thai malaria patients (Druilhe and al 1997, Sabchareon *et al* 1991). In addition, Edozien et al (1962) showed that antibodies that protected against malaria could be obtained from cord blood thus demonstrating that the passively acquired maternal immunity against malaria in infant, is at least in part, antibody–mediated (Edozien *et al* 1962).

Strong, albeit indirect, evidence for the protective efficacy of antimalarial antibodies comes from classical longitudinal studies where a person's history of malaria disease during a follow-up period is assessed for association with levels of antibodies to various malaria antigens at the beginning of the follow-up period. Using this approach a number of antibody responses to various antigens, some of which listed in figure 2, have been shown in to be associated with protection against malaria. Two shortcomings of this approach are the assumptions that all those who did not get an malaria episode during the follow-up are immune and that the levels of antibodies measured at the beginning of the follow-up period last through the period and any failure to see protection reflects lack of protection by the antibodies. (Bejon *et al* 2010, Kinyanjui *et al* 2009). However, the presence of variation of exposure even within limited geographic region (Bejon *et al* 2010) means that some people may fail to get an episode during follow-up simply because they were not exposed rather than because they are immune. In addition, humoral responses to malaria have been found to be short-lived (Kinyanjui *et al* 2003) as such even people with protective levels at the beginning of a follow-up might have non-protective levels by the time they encounters the next infection.

5.2 Mechanisms by which antibodies protect against malaria

In vitro, antibodies from immune individuals have been shown to inhibit sporozoites invasion of hepatocytes (Dent *et al* 2008, Fidock *et al* 1997, Pasquetto *et al* 1997), prevent merozoites invasion of red blood cells (Haynes *et al* 2002, Tham *et al* 2009, Vande Waa *et al* 1984), depress parasite growth (Crompton *et al* 2010, Dent *et al* 2008, McCallum *et al* 2008, Wilson *et al* 2010), and promote parasite phagocytosis by macrophages (Druilhe and Khusmith 1987, Groux *et al* 1990). Furthermore, immune serum can disrupt rosettes (Carlson *et al* 1994, Vigan-Womas *et al* 2010) and the binding of infected erythrocytes to endothelial cell ligands (Iqbal *et al* 1993, Ricke *et al* 2000, Udeinya *et al* 1983), two phenomena which, as earlier indicated, have been implicated in the pathogenesis of severe malaria.

However, it is not clear how well in vitro antibody activities correlate with effector mechanisms in vivo. Malaria literature is replete with reports of lack of a correlation between antimalarial antibody titres measured in vitro and malaria protection (Erunkulu *et al* 1992, Marsh *et al* 1989, Thelu *et al* 1991) This is because the majority of malaria antibodies are probably directed against cellular debris released when schizonts burst and are of little consequence with regard to protection.

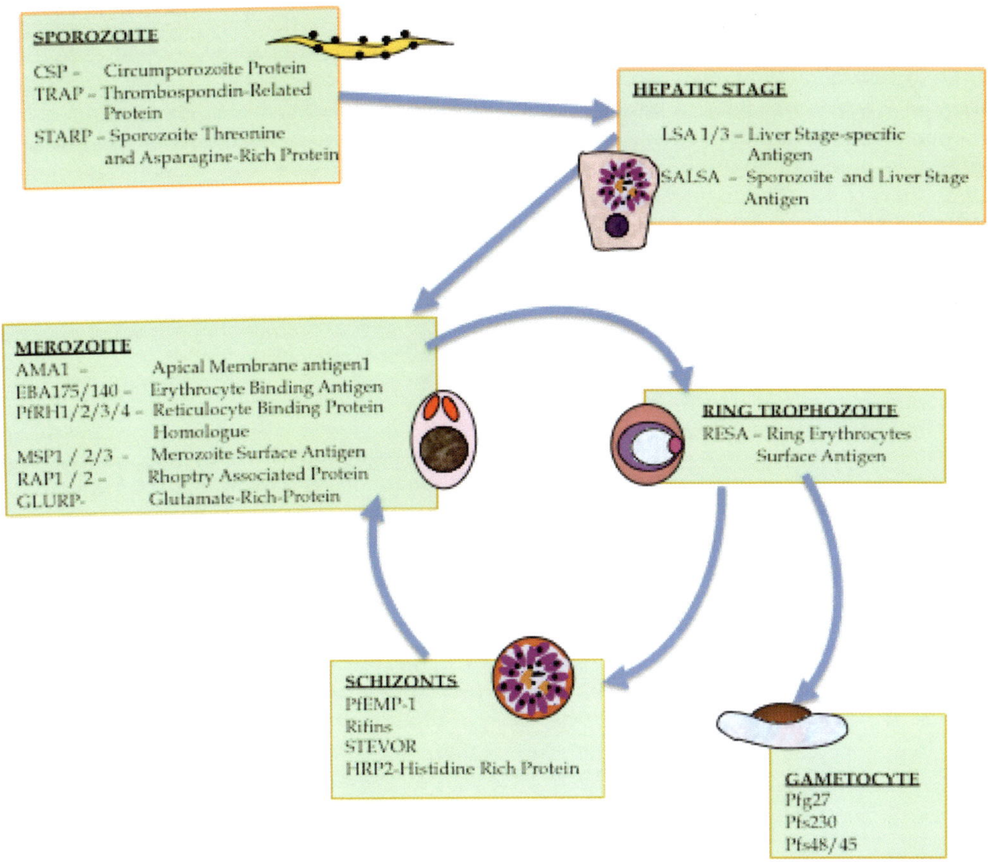

Fig. 2. Malaria antigens associated with various stages of the parasite that are thought to be targets for immune responses.

Under a variety of in vitro situations, malaria antibodies are often ineffective against parasites in the absence of effector cells and may even promote parasite growth (Galamo *et al* 2009, Shi *et al* 1999). Despite exhibiting potent anti-parasitic activity in vivo, the antibodies used in the transfer experiments in Thailand showed no activity in vitro except in presence of monocytes (Bouharoun-Tayoun *et al* 1990, Sabchareon *et al* 1991). Conversely, antibodies that do not protect in vivo were unable to interact with monocytes in vitro (Groux and Gysin 1990). Thus it has been suggested that the ability of antibodies to cooperate with effector cells may be more important than their quantity (Bouharoun Tayoun and Druilhe 1992). It has been noted that humoral responses to malaria show pronounced skewing towards cytophilic antibodies IgG1 and IgG3 subclasses, unlike responses to other pathogens where IgG1 and IgG2 dominate (Ferrante and Rzepczyk 1997). This bias has been reported severally in responses against ring-infected erythrocyte surface antigen (RESA) (Beck *et al* 1995, Dubois *et al* 1993), merozoites surface antigens (MSA1/2) (Rzepczyk *et al* 1997, Taylor *et al* 1995) and schizont antigens (Nguer *et al* 1997, Piper *et al* 1999, Thelu *et al* 1991).

This skew towards cytophilic antibodies, which need to bind to effector cells before they can mediate any action against antigens, could explain the failure of malaria antibodies to exert anti-parasitic activity on their own. In vitro work has shown that while cytophilic antibodies cooperate with monocytes in inhibiting parasites, non-cytophilic subclasses antagonise this cooperation (Bouharoun Tayoun and Druilhe 1992). Data from field studies indicate that young children and non-immune adults have a high proportion of non-cytophilic antibodies (Wahlgren *et al* 1983), while cytophilic antibodies are associated with protection against infection (Aribot *et al* 1996, Ferreira *et al* 1996, Salimonu *et al* 1982) and better prognosis during acute malaria episodes (Sarthou *et al* 1997). Taken together, these data suggests that acquisition of immunity to malaria may involve a shift in responses from non-cytophilic to cytophilic antibodies (Bouharoun Tayoun and Druilhe 1992).

5.3 Antibody dependent cellular inhibition (ADCI)

An interesting observation in the transfer experiments was the failure of passively transferred antibodies to completely eradicate all the parasites. This may have parallels in the failure of otherwise highly immune individuals to eliminate chronic low-grade infections. One proposal is that the parasites that escaped the transferred immunity comprised "strains" of parasites against which the antibodies lacked specificity. Two arguments against this are that the antibodies from immune African adults are expected to be directed against multiple antigens, which should help overcome restriction by the strain-specificity of responses to individual antigens, and more importantly, the same antibodies were subsequently shown to be effective against the breakthrough parasites. A density dependent mechanism designated antibody dependent cellular inhibition (ADCI), has been proposed to explain the interaction between cytophilic antibody and monocytes (Druilhe and Perignon 1997). This interaction causes the monocytes to release mediators that reversibly inhibit the growth of parasite ring stages. The amount of inhibiting mediators released is proportional to the ratio of merozoites to monocytes, which explains why the drop in parasitaemia following injection of immune IgG was proportional to the initial parasitaemia. Decline of either antibody levels, or numbers of monocytes or merozoites reverses inhibition and the parasite population flares up. A further implication of the hypothesis is that since the inhibiting mediators are non-specific, this mechanism does not select for particular parasite variants. However, the huge in drop parasitaemia seen in the transfer experiment is more consistent with a parasitocidal rather than the parasitostatic effect implied by ADCI and other antibody-mediated mechanisms cannot be excluded.

5.4 Longevity of antibody responses to malaria antigens

Among people living in endemic areas, levels of antibodies to many malaria antigens vary with the seasonality of malaria transmission, often being higher during periods of high malaria transmission than at the end of a low transmission season (Cavanagh *et al* 1998, Giha *et al* 1998, Nebie *et al* 2008). Second, levels of antibodies to malaria antigens often tend to be higher in individuals who also have malaria parasites at the time when their antibodies are measured than in those without parasites (al-Yaman *et al* 1995, Bull *et al* 2002, Kinyanjui *et al* 2004). These phenomena are typically seen in young children, probably because adults typically have much higher antibody levels that take longer to decay appreciably even in the absence of an infection [(Fruh *et al* 1991, Riley *et al* 1993, Taylor *et al* 1998). These observations and those from other longitudinal studies where malaria antibodies fell from relatively high levels to low levels within a few weeks of treatment of a clinical episode (Branch *et al* 1998, Fonjungo *et al* 1999, Fruh *et al* 1991) suggest that antibody responses to many malaria antigens are relatively short-lived. The preponderance of IgG3 subclass, which has a shorter half-life than the other IgG subclasses, might, in part, explain the brevity of antimalarial antibody responses. However, detailed kinetics studies on the decay of antimalarial antibodies suggest that even the other subclasses decline at a rate that is faster than can be explained by normal catabolic decay (Kinyanjui *et al* 2003). This brevity of circulating antibody responses might explain the rapid re-infection seen among individuals living in endemic areas after malaria treatment.

6. Mechanisms of immune evasion by malaria parasites

Like other parasites, malaria parasites are not passive partners in the interaction with the host immune system. The immune system exerts a strong selective pressure on malaria parasites. They have therefore over time evolved a number of mechanisms to evade the immune system.

Polymorphism is a common feature of many malaria antigens and is generated through recombination during fertilization or clonal antigenic variation (Anders and Smythe 1989, Borst *et al* 1995). The circumsporozoite protein (CSP) (Dame *et al* 1984, Lockyer *et al* 1989) and thrombospondin–related adhesive protein (TRAP) (Robson *et al* 1998) on the surface of sporozoites all have regions of extensive polymorphism as does the major merozoite antigens; merozoite surface proteins (MSP-2 & MSP-2) (Cooper 1993, Felger *et al* 1994), ring stage erythrocyte surface antigen (RESA) (Perlmann *et al* 1984) and the apical membrane antigen-1 (AMA-1) (Verra and Hughes 1999).

The antigens inserted by mature parasites on to the surface of the host red cells, which include PfEMP1, rifins, and STEVOR, not only exhibit extensive polymorphism between isolates from different patients, they also under go clonal variation so that each new generation of parasites exhibits different variant from the previous one (Bachmann *et al* 2011, Baruch *et al* 1995, Blythe *et al* 2004, Chen *et al* 1998, Cheng *et al* 1998, Niang *et al* 2009). In many instances, there is little immunological cross reactivity between different polymorphic variants of the same antigens meaning that encounter with parasites bearing one variant does not generate protection against infections bearing a different variant.

Some of the proteins in the parasite have not evolved a high level of polymorphism instead parasites escapes immune responses directed against these proteins through functional redundancy. In other words, the parasites are able to utilise more than one protein to achieve the same function. This is particularly the case for proteins involved in essential functions such as invasion of the red cell. The erythrocyte binding ligand (EBL) and the reticulocyte binding homologues (RH) protein families, (Adams *et al* 2001, Reiling *et al* 2010, Triglia *et al* 2009) both involved in invasion, consist of four and five closely related, but not identical, proteins respectively. Blocking invasion mediated by one of these protein results in a shift toward invasion pathways mediated by the other proteins (Lobo *et al* 2006, Lopaticki *et al* 2011, Persson *et al* 2008).

There is some evidence to suggest that apart from escaping immune recognition, malaria parasites can actively subvert the immune system and may direct it towards less effective responses. Some malaria antigens such as glycosylphosphatidylinositol (GPI) contain sections of tandem amino acid repeats in their structure. Such polymeric structures can cross-link B-cell antigen receptors and induce T-cell independent antibody production that is characterised by IgM dominance and poor affinity maturation and memory cells induction (Garcia de Vinuesa *et al* 1999). Besides being short-lived and ineffective, T-cell independent responses can also thwart protective responses to adjacent critical epitopes through epitopic inhibition (Schofield 1991). Disruption of splenic architecture, which prevents the formation of germinal centres and that could also lead to T-cell independent responses, has been observed in animal malaria model (Achtman *et al* 2003). Malaria parasites have been shown to prevent the maturation of dendritic cells through binding of infected red cells to dendritic cells using parasite generated variant surface antigens (Urban *et al* 1999, Urban *et al* 2001). However, other studies suggest that dendritic cell inhibition could also be mediated through other interactions not involving surface antigens (Elliott *et al* 2007). Furthermore, studies in mouse models suggest that the parasite –induced defect in maturation does not necessarily affect dendritic cells ability to induce protection in vivo (Pouniotis *et al* 2004). Recently it has been suggested that malaria parasite use the activation of regulatory T cells that suppress antiparasite cytokines production as a way of escaping the immune system. Mice whose T regulatory cells are depleted can survive infection with a lethal strain of *P. yoelii* and exhibit increased T-cell responsiveness to parasite antigens compared to normal mice (Hisaeda *et al* 2004).

7. Conclusions

Although research has contributed significantly in our understanding of immunity towards malaria, there are still considerable gaps in our knowledge. Closing these gaps in order to facilitate the development of malaria vaccines remains one of the major goals of tropical diseases research. Two areas are key to developing a comprehensive picture of the interaction between the malaria parasites and the immune system: first there is need to standardise current methods for studying immunity to malaria in order to address the numerous inconsistencies concerning the efficacy of various response to malaria often encountered in the literature. Second there is need to take advantage of the advances in molecular biology in studying immunity to malaria for example use of high throughput sequencing and DNA and protein microarray technology to facilitate the simultaneous study of the large range of responses evoked by a malaria infection or the development transgenic animal and parasite models that approximate better to malaria infections in human.

8. References

Achtman, AH, Khan, M, MacLennan, IC and Langhorne, J (2003). *Plasmodium chabaudi* chabaudi infection in mice induces strong B cell responses and striking but temporary changes in splenic cell distribution. *J Immunol* 171(1): 317-324

Adams, JH, Blair, PL, Kaneko, O and Peterson, DS (2001). An expanding ebl family of *Plasmodium falciparum*. *Trends Parasitol* 17(6): 297-299

Aidoo, I and Udhayakumar, I (2000). Field studies of cytotoxic T lymphocytes in malaria infections: implications for malaria vaccine development. *Parasitol. Today* 16(2): 50-56.

Aidoo, M, Lalvani, A, Allsopp, CE, Plebanski, M, Meisner, SJ, Krausa, P, Browning, M, Morris-Jones, S, Gotch, F, Fidock, DA and et al. (1995). Identification of conserved antigenic components for a cytotoxic T lymphocyte-inducing vaccine against malaria. *Lancet* 345(8956): 1003-1007.

al-Yaman, F, Genton, B, Anders, R, Taraika, J, Ginny, M, Mellor, S and Alpers, MP (1995). Assessment of the role of the humoral response to *Plasmodium falciparum* MSP2 compared to RESA and SPf66 in protecting Papua New Guinean children from clinical malaria. *Parasite Immunol* 17(9): 493-501

Allen, SJ, O'Donnell, A, Alexander, ND, Alpers, MP, Peto, TE, Clegg, JB and Weatherall, DJ (1997). alpha+-Thalassemia protects children against disease caused by other infections as well as malaria. *Proc. Natl. Acad. Sci. USA* 94(26): 14736-14741.

Anders, RF and Smythe, JA (1989). Polymorphic antigens in *Plasmodium falciparum*. *Blood* 74(6): 1865-1875.

Aribot, G, Rogier, C, Sarthou, J, Trape, J, Balde, A, Druilhe, P and Roussilhon, C (1996). Pattern of immunoglobulin isotype response to *Plasmodium falciparum* blood-stage antigens in individuals living in a holoendemic area of Senegal (Dielmo, west Africa). *Am. J. Trop. Med. Hyg. 1996 May; 54(5): 449-57*

Artavanis-Tsakonas, K and Riley, EM (2002). Innate immune response to malaria: rapid induction of IFN-gamma from human NK cells by live *Plasmodium falciparum*-infected erythrocytes. *J Immunol* 169(6): 2956-2963

Ayi, K, Turrini, F, Piga, A and Arese, P (2004). Enhanced phagocytosis of ring-parasitized mutant erythrocytes: a common mechanism that may explain protection against falciparum malaria in sickle trait and beta-thalassemia trait. *Blood* 104(10): 3364-3371

Babiker, H, Ranford-Cartwright, L, Currie, D, Charlwood, J, Billingsley, P, Teuscher, T and Walliker, D (1994). Random mating in a natural population of the malaria parasite *Plasmodium falciparum*. *Parasitology. 1994 Nov; 109 (Pt 4): 413-21*

Bachmann, A, Predehl, S, May, J, Harder, S, Burchard, GD, Gilberger, TW, Tannich, E and Bruchhaus, I (2011). Highly co-ordinated var gene expression and switching in clinical *Plasmodium falciparum* isolates from non-immune malaria patients. *Cell Microbiol* 13(9): 1397-1409

Baruch, DI, Pasloske, BL, Singh, HB, Bi, X, Ma, XC, Feldman, M, Taraschi, TF and Howard, RJ (1995). Cloning the *P. falciparum* gene encoding PfEMP1, a malarial variant antigen and adherence receptor on the surface of parasitized human erythrocytes. *Cell* 82(1): 77-87

Beck, H, Felger, I, Genton, B, Alexander, N, al-Yaman, F, Anders, R and Alpers, M (1995). Humoral and cell-mediated immunity to the *Plasmodium falciparum* ring-infected erythrocyte surface antigen in an adult population exposed to highly endemic malaria. *Infect. Immun. 1995 Feb; 63(2): 596-600*

Bejon, P, Warimwe, G, Mackintosh, CL, Mackinnon, MJ, Kinyanjui, SM, Musyoki, JN, Bull, P and Marsh, K (2009). Immunity to febrile malaria in children: an analysis that distinguishes immunity from lack of exposure. *Infect Immun*

Bejon, P, Williams, TN, Liljander, A, Noor, AM, Wambua, J, Ogada, E, Olotu, A, Osier, FH, Hay, SI, Farnert, A and Marsh, K (2010). Stable and unstable malaria hotspots in longitudinal cohort studies in Kenya. *PLoS Med* 7(7): e1000304

Berretta, F, St-Pierre, J, Piccirillo, CA and Stevenson, MM (2011). IL-2 contributes to maintaining a balance between CD4+Foxp3+ regulatory T cells and effector CD4+ T cells required for immune control of blood-stage malaria infection. *J Immunol* 186(8): 4862-4871

Biemba, G, Gordeuk, VR, Thuma, P and Weiss, G (2000). Markers of inflammation in children with severe malarial anaemia. *Trop. Med. Int. Health.* 5(4): 256-262.

Blythe, JE, Surentheran, T and Preiser, PR (2004). STEVOR--a multifunctional protein? *Mol Biochem Parasitol* 134(1): 11-15

Borst, P, Bitter, W, McCulloch, R, Van-Leeuwen, F and Rudenko, G (1995). Antigenic variation in malaria. *Cell* 82(July): 1-4

Bottius, E, BenMohamed, L, Brahimi, K, Gras, H, Lepers, JP, Raharimalala, L, Aikawa, M, Meis, J, Slierendregt, B, Tartar, A, Thomas, A and Druilhe, P (1996). A novel *Plasmodium falciparum* sporozoite and liver stage antigen (SALSA) defines major B, T helper, and CTL epitopes. *J. Immunol* 156(8): 2874-2884.

Bouharoun Tayoun, H and Druilhe, P (1992). Antibodies in falciparum malaria: what matters most, quantity or quality? *Mem. Inst. Oswaldo. Cruz. 1992; 87 Suppl 3: 229-34*

Bouharoun-Tayoun, H, Attanath, P, Sabchareon, A, Chongsuphajaisiddhi, T and Druilhe, P (1990). Antibodies that protect humans against *Plasmodium falciparum* blood stages do not on their own inhibit parasite growth and invasion in vitro, but act in cooperation with monocytes. *J. Exp. Med.* 172(6): 1633-1641.

Branch, O, Udhayakumar, V, Hightower, A, Oloo, A, Hawley, W, Nahlen, B, Bloland, P, Kaslow, D and Lal, A (1998). A longitudinal investigation of IgG and IgM antibody responses to the merozoite surface protein-1 19-kiloDalton domain of *Plasmodium falciparum* in pregnant women and infants: associations with febrile illness, parasitemia, and anemia. *Am. J. Trop. Med. Hyg. 1998 Feb; 58(2): 211-9*

Brannan, L, Turner, C and Phillips, R (1994). Malaria parasites undergo antigenic variation at high rates in vivo. *Proc. Roy. Soc. Lond. B. Biol. Sci. 1994 Apr 22; 256(1345): 71-5*

Bull, PC, Lowe, BS, Kaleli, N, Njuga, F, Kortok, M, Ross, A, Ndungu, F, Snow, RW and Marsh, K (2002). *Plasmodium falciparum* Infections Are Associated with Agglutinating Antibodies to Parasite-Infected Erythrocyte Surface Antigens among Healthy Kenyan Children. *J Infect Dis* 185(11): 1688-1691

Bull, PC, Lowe, BS, Kortok, M and Marsh, K (1999). Antibody recognition of *Plasmodium falciparum* erythrocyte surface antigens in Kenya: evidence for rare and prevalent variants. *Infect Immun* 67(2): 733-739

Bull, PC, Lowe, BS, Kortok, M, Molyneux, CS, Newbold, CI and Marsh, K (1998). Parasite antigens on the infected red cell surface are targets for naturally acquired immunity to malaria. *Nat. Med.* 4(3): 358-360

Cabantous, S, Poudiougou, B, Traore, A, Keita, M, Cisse, MB, Doumbo, O, Dessein, AJ and Marquet, S (2005). Evidence that interferon-gamma plays a protective role during cerebral malaria. *J Infect Dis* 192(5): 854-860

Carlson, J, Nash, G, Gabutti, V, al Yaman, F and Wahlgren, M (1994). Natural protection against severe *Plasmodium falciparum* malaria due to impaired rosette formation. *Blood. 1994 Dec 1; 84(11): 3909-14*

Cavanagh, DR, Elhassan, IM, Roper, C, Robinson, VJ, Giha, H, Holder, AA, Hviid, L, Theander, TG, Arnot, DE and McBride, JS (1998). A longitudinal study of type-specific antibody responses to *Plasmodium falciparum* merozoite surface protein-1 in an area of unstable malaria in Sudan. *J Immunol* 161(1): 347-359

Chen, Q, Barragan, A, Fernandez, V, Sundstrom, A, Schlichtherle, M, Sahlen, A, Carlson, J, Datta, S and Wahlgren, M (1998). Identification of *Plasmodium falciparum* erythrocyte membrane protein 1 (PfEMP1) as the rosetting ligand of the malaria parasite *P. falciparum*. *J Exp Med* 187(1): 15-23

Cheng, Q, Cloonan, N, Fischer, K, Thompson, J, Waine, G, Lanzer, M and Saul, A (1998). stevor and rif are *Plasmodium falciparum* multicopy gene families which potentially encode variant antigens. *Mol. Biochem. Parasitol.* 97(1-2): 161-176.

Chizzolini, C, Grau, GE, Geinoz, A and Schrijvers, D (1990). T lymphocyte interferon-gamma production induced by *Plasmodium falciparum* antigen is high in recently infected non-immune and low in immune subjects. *Clin. Exp. Immunol.* 79(1): 95-99.

Cholera, R, Brittain, NJ, Gillrie, MR, Lopera-Mesa, TM, Diakite, SA, Arie, T, Krause, MA, Guindo, A, Tubman, A, Fujioka, H, Diallo, DA, Doumbo, OK, Ho, M, Wellems, TE and Fairhurst, RM (2008). Impaired cytoadherence of *Plasmodium falciparum*-infected erythrocytes containing sickle hemoglobin. *Proc Natl Acad Sci U S A* 105(3): 991-996

Clark, TG, Fry, AE, Auburn, S, Campino, S, Diakite, M, Green, A, Richardson, A, Teo, YY, Small, K, Wilson, J, Jallow, M, Sisay-Joof, F, Pinder, M, Sabeti, P, Kwiatkowski, DP and Rockett, KA (2009). Allelic heterogeneity of G6PD deficiency in West Africa and severe malaria susceptibility. *Eur J Hum Genet* 17(8): 1080-1085

Clerici, M and Shearer, GM (1994). The Th1-Th2 hypothesis of HIV infection: new insights. *Immunol Today* 15(12): 575-581.

Clyde, DF (1975). Immunization of man against falciparum and vivax malaria by use of attenuated sporozoites. *Am. J. Trop. Med. Hyg.* 24(3): 397-401.

Coban, C, Ishii, KJ, Kawai, T, Hemmi, H, Sato, S, Uematsu, S, Yamamoto, M, Takeuchi, O, Itagaki, S, Kumar, N, Horii, T and Akira, S (2005). Toll-like receptor 9 mediates innate immune activation by the malaria pigment hemozoin. *J Exp Med* 201(1): 19-25

Cohen, S, McGregor, I and S, C (1961). Gama-Globulin and acquired immunity to huma malaria. *Nature* 192(November 25): 735-737

Collins, WE and Jeffery, GM (1999a). A retrospective examination of secondary sporozoite- and trophozoite- induced infections with *Plasmodium falciparum*: development of parasitologic and clinical immunity following secondary infection. *Am. J. Trop. Med. Hyg.* 61(1 Suppl): 20-35.

Collins, WE and Jeffery, GM (1999b). A retrospective examination of sporozoite- and trophozoite-induced infections with *Plasmodium falciparum*: development of parasitologic and clinical immunity during primary infection. *Am. J. Trop. Med. Hyg.* 61(1 Suppl): 4-19.

Cooper, JA (1993). Merozoite Surface Antigen-1 of Plasmodium. *Parasitol. Today* 9(2): 50 - 54

Crompton, PD, Miura, K, Traore, B, Kayentao, K, Ongoiba, A, Weiss, G, Doumbo, S, Doumtabe, D, Kone, Y, Huang, CY, Doumbo, OK, Miller, LH, Long, CA and Pierce, SK (2010). In vitro growth-inhibitory activity and malaria risk in a cohort study in mali. *Infect Immun* 78(2): 737-745

D'Ombrain, MC, Robinson, LJ, Stanisic, DI, Taraika, J, Bernard, N, Michon, P, Mueller, I and Schofield, L (2008). Association of early interferon-gamma production with immunity to clinical malaria: a longitudinal study among Papua New Guinean children. *Clin Infect Dis* 47(11): 1380-1387

Dame, JB, Williams, JL, McCutchan, TF, Weber, JL, Wirtz, RA, Hockmeyer, WT, Maloy, WL, Haynes, JD, Schneider, I, Roberts, D and et al. (1984). Structure of the gene encoding the immunodominant surface antigen on the sporozoite of the human malaria parasite *Plasmodium falciparum*. *Science* 225(4662): 593-599.

Dent, AE, Bergmann-Leitner, ES, Wilson, DW, Tisch, DJ, Kimmel, R, Vulule, J, Sumba, PO, Beeson, JG, Angov, E, Moormann, AM and Kazura, JW (2008). Antibody-mediated growth inhibition of *Plasmodium falciparum*: relationship to age and protection from parasitemia in Kenyan children and adults. *PLoS One* 3(10): e3557

Druilhe, P and al, e (1997). In vivo veritas: lessons from immunoglobulin-transfer experiments in malaria patients.

Druilhe, P and Khusmith, S (1987). Epidemiological correlation between levels of antibodies promoting merozoite phagocytosis of *Plasmodium falciparum* and malaria-immune status. *Infect. Immun.* 55(4): 888-891.

Druilhe, P and Perignon, J (1997). A hypothesis about the chronicity of malaria infection. *Parasitol. Today* 13(9): 353-355

Dubois, B, Deloron, P, Astagneau, P, Chougnet, C and Lepers, J (1993). Isotypic analysis of *Plasmodium falciparum*-specific antibodies and their relation to protection in Madagascar. *Infect. Immun. 1993 Oct; 61(10): 4498-500*

Edozien, J, Gilles, H and Udeozo, I (1962). Adult and cord blood gammaglobulin and immunity to malaria in Nigerians. *Lancet* 2: 951-955

Elliott, SR, Spurck, TP, Dodin, JM, Maier, AG, Voss, TS, Yosaatmadja, F, Payne, PD, McFadden, GI, Cowman, AF, Rogerson, SJ, Schofield, L and Brown, GV (2007). Inhibition of dendritic cell maturation by malaria is dose dependent and does not require *Plasmodium falciparum* erythrocyte membrane protein 1. *Infect Immun* 75(7): 3621-3632

Erunkulu, OA, Hill, AV, Kwiatkowski, DP, Todd, JE, Iqbal, J, Berzins, K, Riley, EM and Greenwood, BM (1992). Severe malaria in Gambian children is not due to lack of previous exposure to malaria. *Clin. Exp. Immunol.* 89(2): 296-300.

Fairhurst, RM, Baruch, DI, Brittain, NJ, Ostera, GR, Wallach, JS, Hoang, HL, Hayton, K, Guindo, A, Makobongo, MO, Schwartz, OM, Tounkara, A, Doumbo, OK, Diallo, DA, Fujioka, H, Ho, M and Wellems, TE (2005). Abnormal display of PfEMP-1 on erythrocytes carrying haemoglobin C may protect against malaria. *Nature* 435(7045): 1117-1121

Felger, I, Tavul, L, Kabintik, S, Marshall, V, Genton, B, Alpers, M and Beck, H (1994). *Plasmodium falciparum*: extensive polymorphism in merozoite surface antigen 2 alleles in an area with endemic malaria in Papua New Guinea. *Exp. Parasitol. 1994 Sep; 79(2): 106-16*

Fell, A and Smith, N (1998). Immunity to asexual blood stages of Plasmodium: Is resistance to acute malaria adaptive or innate. *Parasitol. Today* 14(9): 364-368

Ferrante, A and Rzepczyk, C (1997). Atypical IgG subclass antibody responses to *Plasmodium falciparum* asexual stage antignes. *Parasitol. Today* 13(4): 145 - 148

Ferreira, M, Kimura, E, De, S, JM and Katzin, A (1996). The isotype composition and avidity of naturally acquired anti-*Plasmodium falciparum* antibodies: differential patterns in clinically immune Africans and Amazonian patients. *Am. J. Trop. Med. Hyg. 1996 Sep; 55(3): 315-23*

Fidock, D, Pasquetto, V, Gras, H, Badell, E, Eling, W, Ballou, W, Belghiti, J, Tartar, A and Druilhe, P (1997). *Plasmodium falciparum* sporozoite invasion is inhibited by naturally acquired or experimentally induced polyclonal antibodies to the STARP antigen. *Eur. J. Immunol. 1997 Oct; 27(10): 2502-13*

Fonjungo, PN, Elhassan, IM, Cavanagh, DR, Theander, TG, Hviid, L, Roper, C, Arnot, DE and McBride, JS (1999). A longitudinal study of human antibody responses to *Plasmodium falciparum* rhoptry-associated protein 1 in a region of seasonal and unstable malaria transmission. *Infect Immun* 67(6): 2975-2985

Franklin, BS, Parroche, P, Ataide, MA, Lauw, F, Ropert, C, de Oliveira, RB, Pereira, D, Tada, MS, Nogueira, P, da Silva, LH, Bjorkbacka, H, Golenbock, DT and Gazzinelli, RT (2009). Malaria primes the innate immune response due to interferon-gamma induced enhancement of toll-like receptor expression and function. *Proc Natl Acad Sci U S A* 106(14): 5789-5794

Friedman, MJ (1978). Erythrocytic mechanism of sickle cell resistance to malaria. *Proc. Natl. Acad. Sci. USA* 75(4): 1994-1997.

Fruh, K, Doumbo, O, Muller, HM, Koita, O, McBride, J, Crisanti, A, Toure, Y and Bujard, H (1991). Human antibody response to the major merozoite surface antigen of *Plasmodium falciparum* is strain specific and short-lived. *Infect. Immun.* 59(4): 1319-1324.

Galamo, CD, Jafarshad, A, Blanc, C and Druilhe, P (2009). Anti-MSP1 block 2 antibodies are effective at parasite killing in an allele-specific manner by monocyte-mediated antibody-dependent cellular inhibition. *J Infect Dis* 199(8): 1151-1154

Gallo, V, Schwarzer, E, Rahlfs, S, Schirmer, RH, van Zwieten, R, Roos, D, Arese, P and Becker, K (2009). Inherited glutathione reductase deficiency and *Plasmodium falciparum* malaria--a case study. *PLoS One* 4(10): e7303

Garcia de Vinuesa, C, O'Leary, P, Sze, DM, Toellner, KM and MacLennan, IC (1999). T-independent type 2 antigens induce B cell proliferation in multiple splenic sites, but exponential growth is confined to extrafollicular foci. *Eur J Immunol* 29(4): 1314-1323

Giha, HA, Theander, TG, Staalso, T, Roper, C, Elhassan, IM, Babiker, H, Satti, GM, Arnot, DE and Hviid, L (1998). Seasonal variation in agglutination of *Plasmodium falciparum*-infected erythrocytes. *Am. J. Trop. Med. Hyg.* 58(4): 399-405

Golenser, J and Chevion, M (1989). Oxidant stress and malaria: host-parasite interrelationships in normal and abnormal erythrocytes. *Semin. Hematol.* 26(4): 313-325.

Gowda, DC (2007). TLR-mediated cell signaling by malaria GPIs. *Trends Parasitol* 23(12): 596-604

Groux, H and Gysin, J (1990). Opsonization as an effector mechanism in human protection against asexual blood stages of *Plasmodium falciparum*: functional role of IgG subclasses. *Res. Immunol. 1990 Jul-Aug; 141(6): 529-42*

Groux, H, Perraut, R, Garraud, O, Poingt, JP and Gysin, J (1990). Functional characterization of the antibody-mediated protection against blood stages of *Plasmodium falciparum* in the monkey Saimiri sciureus. *Eur J. Immunol* 20(10): 2317-2323.

Guindo, A, Fairhurst, RM, Doumbo, OK, Wellems, TE and Diallo, DA (2007). X-linked G6PD deficiency protects hemizygous males but not heterozygous females against severe malaria. *PLoS Med* 4(3): e66

Gupta, S and Day, KP (1994). A strain theory of malaria transmission. *Parasitol Today* 10(12): 476 - 481

Gupta, S and Hill, AV (1995). Dynamic interactions in malaria: host heterogeneity meets parasite polymorphism. *Proc Biol Sci* 261(1362): 271-277

Gupta, S, Snow, RW, Donnelly, C and Newbold, C (1999a). Acquired immunity and postnatal clinical protection in childhood cerebral malaria. *Proc. R. Soc. Lond. B. Biol. Sci.* 266(1414): 33-38.

Gupta, S, Snow, RW, Donnelly, CA, Marsh, K and Newbold, C (1999b). Immunity to non-cerebral severe malaria is acquired after one or two infections. *Nat. Med.* 5(3): 340-343.

Haldane, J (1949). The rate of mutation of human genes. *Hereditas Supplement* 35: 267-273

Haynes, JD, Moch, JK and Smoot, DS (2002). Erythrocytic malaria growth or invasion inhibition assays with emphasis on suspension culture GIA. *Methods Mol Med* 72: 535-554

Hill, AV, Allsopp, CE, Kwiatkowski, D, Anstey, NM, Twumasi, P, Rowe, PA, Bennett, S, Brewster, D, McMichael, AJ and Greenwood, BM (1991). Common west African HLA antigens are associated with protection from severe malaria. *Nature* 352(6336): 595-600.

Hill, W and Babiker, H (1995). Estimation of numbers of malaria clones in blood samples. *Proc. R. Soc. Lond. B. Biol. Sci. 1995 Dec 22; 262(1365): 249-57*

Hirunpetcharat, C, Finkelman, F, Clark, IA and Good, MF (1999). Malaria parasite-specific Th1-like T cells simultaneously reduce parasitemia and promote disease. *Parasite Immunol* 21(6): 319-329.

Hisaeda, H, Maekawa, Y, Iwakawa, D, Okada, H, Himeno, K, Kishihara, K, Tsukumo, S and Yasutomo, K (2004). Escape of malaria parasites from host immunity requires CD4+ CD25+ regulatory T cells. *Nat Med* 10(1): 29-30

Horowitz, A, Newman, KC, Evans, JH, Korbel, DS, Davis, DM and Riley, EM (2010). Cross-talk between T cells and NK cells generates rapid effector responses to *Plasmodium falciparum*-infected erythrocytes. *J Immunol* 184(11): 6043-6052

Hughes, M and Hughes, A (1995). Natural selection on Plasmodium surface proteins. *Mol. Biochem. Parasitol. 1995 Apr; 71(1): 99-113*

Iqbal, J, Perlmann, P and Berzins, K (1993). Serological diversity of antigens expressed on the surface of erythrocytes infected with *Plasmodium falciparum. Trans. Roy. Soc. Trop. Med. Hyg. 1993 Sep-Oct; 87(5): 583-8*

Jason, J, Archibald, LK, Nwanyanwu, OC, Bell, M, Buchanan, I, Larned, J, Kazembe, PN, Dobbie, H, Parekh, B, Byrd, MG, Eick, A, Han, A and Jarvis, WR (2001). Cytokines and malaria parasitemia. *Clin Immunol* 100(2): 208-218

Jeffery, GM (1966). Epidemiological significance of repeated infections with homologous and heterologous strains and species of Plasmodium. *Bull. World. Health. Organ.* 35(6): 873-882

Kagi, D, Vignaux, F, Ledermann, B, Burki, K, Depraetere, V, Nagata, S, Hengartner, H and Golstein, P (1994). Fas and perforin pathways as major mechanisms of T cell-mediated cytotoxicity. *Science* 265(5171): 528-530.

Kinyanjui, SM, Bejon, P, Osier, FH, Bull, PC and Marsh, K (2009). What you see is not what you get: implications of the brevity of antibody responses to malaria antigens and transmission heterogeneity in longitudinal studies of malaria immunity. *Malar J* 8: 242

Kinyanjui, SM, Bull, P, Newbold, CI and Marsh, K (2003). Kinetics of antibody responses to *Plasmodium falciparum*-infected erythrocyte variant surface antigens. *J Infect Dis* 187(4): 667-674

Kinyanjui, SM, Mwangi, T, Bull, PC, Newbold, CI and Marsh, K (2004). Protection against clinical malaria by heterologous immunoglobulin G antibodies against malaria-infected erythrocyte variant surface antigens requires interaction with asymptomatic infections. *J Infect Dis* 190(9): 1527-1533

Korbel, DS, Newman, KC, Almeida, CR, Davis, DM and Riley, EM (2005). Heterogeneous human NK cell responses to *Plasmodium falciparum*-infected erythrocytes. *J Immunol* 175(11): 7466-7473

Krishnegowda, G, Hajjar, AM, Zhu, J, Douglass, EJ, Uematsu, S, Akira, S, Woods, AS and Gowda, DC (2005). Induction of proinflammatory responses in macrophages by the glycosylphosphatidylinositols of *Plasmodium falciparum*: cell signaling receptors, glycosylphosphatidylinositol (GPI) structural requirement, and regulation of GPI activity. *J Biol Chem* 280(9): 8606-8616

Kurtzhal, JA, Adabayeri, V, Goka, BQ, Akanmori, BD, Oliver-Commey, JO, Nkrumah, FK, Behr, C and Hviid, L (1998). Low plasma concentrations of interleukin 10 in severe malarial anaemia compared with cerebral and uncomplicated malaria. *Lancet* 351: 1768-1772

Langhorne, J, Gillard, S, Simon, B, Slade, S and Eichmann, K (1989). Frequencies of CD4+ T cells reactive with *Plasmodium chabaudi* chabaudi: distinct response kinetics for cells with Th1 and Th2 characteristics during infection. *Int Immunol* 1(4): 416-424

Lobo, CA, Rodriguez, M, Struchiner, CJ, Zalis, MG and Lustigman, S (2006). Associations between defined polymorphic variants in the PfRH ligand family and the invasion pathways used by *P. falciparum* field isolates from Brazil. *Mol Biochem Parasitol* 149(2): 246-251

Lockyer, M, Marsh, K and Newbold, C (1989). Wild isolates of *Plasmodium falciparum* show extensive polymorphism in T cell epitopes of the circumsporozoite protein. *Mol. Biochem. Parasitol. 1989 Dec; 37(2): 275-80*

Lopaticki, S, Maier, AG, Thompson, J, Wilson, DW, Tham, WH, Triglia, T, Gout, A, Speed, TP, Beeson, JG, Healer, J and Cowman, AF (2011). Reticulocyte and erythrocyte binding-like proteins function cooperatively in invasion of human erythrocytes by malaria parasites. *Infect Immun* 79(3): 1107-1117

Lopez, C, Saravia, C, Gomez, A, Hoebeke, J and Patarroyo, MA (2010). Mechanisms of genetically-based resistance to malaria. *Gene* 467(1-2): 1-12

Lowin, B, Hahne, M, Mattmann, C and Tschopp, J (1994). Cytolytic T-cell cytotoxicity is mediated through perforin and Fas lytic pathways. *Nature* 370(6491): 650-652.

Lumsden, JM, Schwenk, RJ, Rein, LE, Moris, P, Janssens, M, Ofori-Anyinam, O, Cohen, J, Kester, KE, Heppner, DG and Krzych, U (2011). Protective immunity induced with the RTS,S/AS vaccine is associated with IL-2 and TNF-alpha producing effector and central memory CD4 T cells. *PLoS One* 6(7): e20775

Luty, AJ, Lell, B, Schmidt-Ott, R, Lehman, LG, Luckner, D, Greve, B, Matousek, P, Herbich, K, Schmid, D, Migot-Nabias, F, Deloron, P, Nussenzweig, RS and Kremsner, PG (1999). Interferon-gamma responses are associated with resistance to reinfection with *Plasmodium falciparum* in young African children. *J. Infect. Dis.* 179(4): 980-988.

Mackinnon, MJ, Mwangi, TW, Snow, RW, Marsh, K and Williams, TN (2005). Heritability of malaria in Africa. *PLoS Med* 2(12): e340

Marsh, K and Kinyanjui, S (2006). Immune effector mechanisms in malaria. *Parasite Immunol* 28(1-2): 51-60

Marsh, K, Otoo, L, Hayes, R, Carson, D and Greenwood, B (1989). Antibodies to blood stage antigens of *Plasmodium falciparum* in rural Gambians and their relation to protection against infection. *Trans. Roy. Soc. Trop. Med. Hyg. 1989 May-Jun; 83(3): 293-303*

McCallum, FJ, Persson, KE, Mugyenyi, CK, Fowkes, FJ, Simpson, JA, Richards, JS, Williams, TN, Marsh, K and Beeson, JG (2008). Acquisition of growth-inhibitory antibodies against blood-stage *Plasmodium falciparum*. *PLoS One* 3(10): e3571

McGregor, IA (1963). Treatment of East African *P. falciparum* malaria with west African human globulin. *Trans. Roy. Soc. Trop. Med. Hyg.* 57: 170-175

Mendez, D, Linares, M, Diez, A, Puyet, A and Bautista, JM (2011). Stress response and cytoskeletal proteins involved in erythrocyte membrane remodeling upon *Plasmodium falciparum* invasion are differentially carbonylated in G6PD A-deficiency. *Free Radic Biol Med* 50(10): 1305-1313

Modiano, D, Luoni, G, Sirima, BS, Simpore, J, Verra, F, Konate, A, Rastrelli, E, Olivieri, A, Calissano, C, Paganotti, GM, D'Urbano, L, Sanou, I, Sawadogo, A, Modiano, G and Coluzzi, M (2001). Haemoglobin C protects against clinical *Plasmodium falciparum* malaria. *Nature* 414(6861): 305-308

Moore, JM, Nahlen, BL, Misore, A, Lal, AA and Udhayakumar, V (1999). Immunity to placental malaria. I. Elevated production of interferon- gamma by placental blood mononuclear cells is associated with protection in an area with high transmission of malaria. *J. Infect. Dis.* 179(5): 1218-1225.

Morrot, A and Zavala, F (2004). Effector and memory CD8+ T cells as seen in immunity to malaria. *Immunol Rev* 201: 291-303

Nebie, I, Tiono, AB, Diallo, DA, Samandoulougou, S, Diarra, A, Konate, AT, Cuzin-Ouattara, N, Theisen, M, Corradin, G, Cousens, S, Ouattara, AS, Ilboudo-Sanogo, E and Sirima, BS (2008). Do antibody responses to malaria vaccine candidates influenced by the level of malaria transmission protect from malaria? *Trop Med Int Health* 13(2): 229-237

Newbold, C, Pinches, R, Roberts, D and Marsh, K (1992). *Plasmodium falciparum*: the human agglutinating antibody response to the infected red cell surface is predominantly variant specific. *Exp. Parasitol. 1992 Nov; 75(3): 281-92*

Nguer, C, Diallo, T, Diouf, A, Tall, A, Dieye, A, Perraut, R and Garraud, O (1997). *Plasmodium falciparum*- and merozoite surface protein 1-specific antibody isotype balance in immune Senegalese adults. *Infect. Immun. 1997 Nov; 65(11): 4873-6*

Niang, M, Yan Yam, X and Preiser, PR (2009). The *Plasmodium falciparum* STEVOR multigene family mediates antigenic variation of the infected erythrocyte. *PLoS Pathog* 5(2): e1000307

Nie, CQ, Bernard, NJ, Schofield, L and Hansen, DS (2007). CD4+ CD25+ regulatory T cells suppress CD4+ T-cell function and inhibit the development of *Plasmodium berghei*-specific TH1 responses involved in cerebral malaria pathogenesis. *Infect Immun* 75(5): 2275-2282

Nussenzweig, RS, Vanderberg, J, Most, H and Orton, C (1967). Protective immunity produced by the injection of x-irradiated sporozoites of *Plasmodium berghei*. *Nature* 216(111): 160-162.

Oliveira, GA, Kumar, KA, Calvo-Calle, JM, Othoro, C, Altszuler, D, Nussenzweig, V and Nardin, EH (2008). Class II-restricted protective immunity induced by malaria sporozoites. *Infect Immun* 76(3): 1200-1206

Parroche, P, Lauw, FN, Goutagny, N, Latz, E, Monks, BG, Visintin, A, Halmen, KA, Lamphier, M, Olivier, M, Bartholomeu, DC, Gazzinelli, RT and Golenbock, DT (2007). Malaria hemozoin is immunologically inert but radically enhances innate responses by presenting malaria DNA to Toll-like receptor 9. *Proc Natl Acad Sci U S A* 104(6): 1919-1924

Pasquetto, V, Fidock, DA, Gras, H, Badell, E, Eling, W, Ballou, WR, Belghiti, J, Tartar, A and Druilhe, P (1997). *Plasmodium falciparum* sporozoite invasion is inhibited by naturally acquired or experimentally induced polyclonal antibodies to the STARP antigen. *Eur J. Immunol* 27(10): 2502-2513.

Penman, BS, Pybus, OG, Weatherall, DJ and Gupta, S (2009). Epistatic interactions between genetic disorders of hemoglobin can explain why the sickle-cell gene is uncommon in the Mediterranean. *Proc Natl Acad Sci U S A* 106(50): 21242-21246

Perlaza, BL, Sauzet, JP, Brahimi, K, BenMohamed, L and Druilhe, P (2011). Interferon-gamma, a valuable surrogate marker of *Plasmodium falciparum* pre-erythrocytic stages protective immunity. *Malar J* 10(1): 27

Perlmann, H, Berzins, K, Wahlgren, M, Carlsson, J, Bjorkman, A, Patarroyo, ME and Perlmann, P (1984). Antibodies in malarial sera to parasite antigens in the membrane of erythrocytes infected with early asexual stages of *Plasmodium falciparum*. *J. Exp. Med.* 159(6): 1686-1704.

Persson, KE, McCallum, FJ, Reiling, L, Lister, NA, Stubbs, J, Cowman, AF, Marsh, K and Beeson, JG (2008). Variation in use of erythrocyte invasion pathways by *Plasmodium falciparum* mediates evasion of human inhibitory antibodies. *J Clin Invest* 118(1): 342-351

Piel, FB, Patil, AP, Howes, RE, Nyangiri, OA, Gething, PW, Williams, TN, Weatherall, DJ and Hay, SI (2010). Global distribution of the sickle cell gene and geographical confirmation of the malaria hypothesis. *Nat Commun* 1: 104

Piper, KP, Roberts, DJ and Day, KP (1999). *Plasmodium falciparum*: analysis of the antibody specificity to the surface of the trophozoite-infected erythrocyte. *Exp. Parasitol.* 91(2): 161-169

Pouniotis, DS, Proudfoot, O, Bogdanoska, V, Apostolopoulos, V, Fifis, T and Plebanski, M (2004). Dendritic cells induce immunity and long-lasting protection against blood-stage malaria despite an in vitro parasite-induced maturation defect. *Infect Immun* 72(9): 5331-5339

Pretolani, M and Goldman, M (1997). IL-10: a potential therapy for allergic inflammation? *Immunol Today* 18(6): 277-280.

Purcell, LA, Wong, KA, Yanow, SK, Lee, M, Spithill, TW and Rodriguez, A (2008). Chemically attenuated Plasmodium sporozoites induce specific immune responses, sterile immunity and cross-protection against heterologous challenge. *Vaccine* 26(38): 4880-4884

Ranford-Cartwright, L, Balfe, P, Carter, R and Walliker, D (1993). Frequency of cross-fertilization in the human malaria parasite *Plasmodium falciparum. Parasitology. 1993 Jul; 107 (Pt 1): 11-8*

Recker, M, Arinaminpathy, N and Buckee, CO (2008). The effects of a partitioned var gene repertoire of *Plasmodium falciparum* on antigenic diversity and the acquisition of clinical immunity. *Malar J* 7: 18

Recker, M, Buckee, CO, Serazin, A, Kyes, S, Pinches, R, Christodoulou, Z, Springer, AL, Gupta, S and Newbold, CI (2011). Antigenic variation in *Plasmodium falciparum* malaria involves a highly structured switching pattern. *PLoS Pathog* 7(3): e1001306

Recker, M, Nee, S, Bull, PC, Kinyanjui, S, Marsh, K, Newbold, C and Gupta, S (2004). Transient cross-reactive immune responses can orchestrate antigenic variation in malaria. *Nature* 429(6991): 555-558

Reeder, J, Rogerson, S, al, Y, F, Anders, R, Coppel, R, Novakovic, S, Alpers, M and Brown, G (1994). Diversity of agglutinating phenotype, cytoadherence, and rosette-forming characteristics of *Plasmodium falciparum* isolates from Papua New Guinean children. *Am. J. Trop. Med. Hyg. 1994 Jul; 51(1): 45-55*

Reiling, L, Richards, JS, Fowkes, FJ, Barry, AE, Triglia, T, Chokejindachai, W, Michon, P, Tavul, L, Siba, PM, Cowman, AF, Mueller, I and Beeson, JG (2010). Evidence that the erythrocyte invasion ligand PfRh2 is a target of protective immunity against *Plasmodium falciparum* malaria. *J Immunol* 185(10): 6157-6167

Ricke, CH, Staalsoe, T, Koram, K, Akanmori, BD, Riley, EM, Theander, TG and Hviid, L (2000). Plasma antibodies from malaria-exposed pregnant women recognize variant surface antigens on *Plasmodium falciparum*-infected erythrocytes in a parity-dependent manner and block parasite adhesion to chondroitin sulfate A. *J. Immunol* 165(6): 3309-3316.

Rieckmann, KH, Carson, PE, Beaudoin, RL, Cassells, JS and Sell, KW (1974). Letter: Sporozoite induced immunity in man against an Ethiopian strain of *Plasmodium falciparum. Trans. Roy. Soc. Trop. Med. Hyg.* 68(3): 258-259

Riley, E, Morris, J, S, Blackman, M, Greenwood, B and Holder, A (1993). A longitudinal study of naturally acquired cellular and humoral immune responses to a merozoite surface protein (MSP1) of *Plasmodium falciparum* in an area of seasonal malaria transmission. *Parasite. Immunol. 1993 Sep; 15(9): 513-24*

Roberts, D, Craig, A, Berendt, A, Pinches, R, Nash, G, Marsh, K and Newbold, C (1992). Rapid switching to multiple antigenic and adhesive phenotypes in malaria. *Nature. 1992 Jun 25; 357(6380): 689-92*

Robinson, LJ, D'Ombrain, MC, Stanisic, DI, Taraika, J, Bernard, N, Richards, JS, Beeson, JG, Tavul, L, Michon, P, Mueller, I and Schofield, L (2009). Cellular tumor necrosis factor, gamma interferon, and interleukin-6 responses as correlates of immunity and risk of clinical *Plasmodium falciparum* malaria in children from Papua New Guinea. *Infect Immun* 77(7): 3033-3043

Robson, KJ, Dolo, A, Hackford, IR, Doumbo, O, Richards, MB, Keita, MM, Sidibe, T, Bosman, A, Modiano, D and Crisanti, A (1998). Natural polymorphism in the thrombospondin-related adhesive protein of *Plasmodium falciparum*. *Am. J. Trop. Med. Hyg.* 58(1): 81-89.

Roca-Feltrer, A, Carneiro, I, Smith, L, Schellenberg, JR, Greenwood, B and Schellenberg, D (2010). The age patterns of severe malaria syndromes in sub-Saharan Africa across a range of transmission intensities and seasonality settings. *Malar J* 9: 282

Romero, P, Maryanski, J, Corradin, G, Nussenzweig, R, Nussenzweig, V and Zavala, F (1989). Cloned cytotoxic T cells recognize an epitope in the circumsporozoite protein and protect against malaria. *Nature. 1989 Sep 28; 341(6240): 323-6*

Rougemont, A, Breslow, N, Brenner, E, Moret, A, Dumbo, O, Dolo, A, Soula, G and Perrin, L (1991). Epidemiological basis for clinical diagnosis of childhood malaria in endemic zone in West Africa [see comments] CM: Comment in: Lancet 1991 Dec 21-28;338(8782-8783):1601. Comment in: Lancet 1992 Mar 14;339(8794):690; discussion 690-1. Comment in: Lancet 1992 Mar 14;339(8794):691. *Lancet. 1991 Nov 23; 338(8778): 1292-5*

Rudin, W, Favre, N, Bordmann, G and Ryffel, B (1997). Interferon-gamma is essential for the development of cerebral malaria. *Eur. J. Immunol. 1997 Apr; 27(4): 810-5*

Ruwende, C, Khoo, S, Snow, R, Yates, S, Kwiatkowski, D, Gupta, S, Warn, P, Allsopp, C, Gilbert, S, Peschu, N and et, a (1995). Natural selection of hemi- and heterozygotes for G6PD deficiency in Africa by resistance to severe malaria. *Nature. 1995 Jul 20; 376(6537): 246-9*

Rzepczyk, CM, Hale, K, Woodroffe, N, Bobogare, A, Csurhes, P, Ishii, A and Ferrante, A (1997). Humoral immune responses of Solomon Islanders to the merozoite surface antigen 2 of *Plasmodium falciparum* show pronounced skewing towards antibodies of the immunoglobulin G3 subclass. *Infect. Immun.* 65(3): 1098-1100.

Sabchareon, A, Burnouf, T, Ouattara, D, Attanath, P, Bouharoun-Tayoun, H, Chantavanich, P, Foucault, C, Chongsuphajaisiddhi, T and Druilhe, P (1991). Parasitologic and clinical human response to immunoglobulin administration in falciparum malaria. *Am. J. Trop. Med. Hyg. 1991 Sep; 45(3): 297-308*

Salimonu, LS, Williams, AI and Osunkoya, BO (1982). IgG subclass levels in malaria-infected Nigerians. *Vox Sang* 42(5): 248-251

Sarthou, J, Angel, G, Aribot, G, Rogier, C, Dieye, A, Toure, B, A, Diatta, B, Seignot, P and Roussilhon, C (1997). Prognostic value of anti-*Plasmodium falciparum*-specific immunoglobulin G3, cytokines, and their soluble receptors in West African patients with severe malaria. *Infect. Immun. 1997 Aug; 65(8): 3271-6*

Schofield, L (1989). T cell immunity to malaria sporozoites. *Exp. Parasitol. 1989 Apr; 68(3): 357-64*

Schofield, L (1991). On the function of repetitive domain in protein antigen of Plasmodium and eukaryotic parasites. *Parasitol. Today* 7(5): 99-105

Schofield, L, Villaquiran, J, Ferreira, A, Schellekens, H, Nussenzweig, R and Nussenzweig, V (1987). Gamma interferon, CD8+ T cells and antibodies required for immunity to malaria sporozoites. *Nature. 1987 Dec 17-23; 330(6149): 664-6*

Senok, AC, Nelson, EA, Li, K and Oppenheimer, SJ (1997). Thalassaemia trait, red blood cell age and oxidant stress: effects on *Plasmodium falciparum* growth and sensitivity to artemisinin. *Trans. Roy. Soc. Trop. Med. Hyg.* 91(5): 585-589.

Sharma, S, Deoliveira, RB, Kalantari, P, Parroche, P, Goutagny, N, Jiang, Z, Chan, J, Bartholomeu, DC, Lauw, F, Hall, JP, Barber, GN, Gazzinelli, RT, Fitzgerald, KA and Golenbock, DT (2011). Innate Immune Recognition of an AT-Rich Stem-Loop DNA Motif in the *Plasmodium falciparum* Genome. *Immunity* 35(2): 194-207

Shi, YP, Udhayakumar, V, Oloo, AJ, Nahlen, BL and Lal, AA (1999). Differential effect and interaction of monocytes, hyperimmune sera, and immunoglobulin G on the growth of asexual stage *Plasmodium falciparum* parasites. *Am. J. Trop. Med. Hyg.* 60(1): 135-141.

Smith, T, Schellenberg, J and Hayes, R (1994). Attributable fraction estimates and case definitions for malaria in endemic areas. *Statistics in Medicine* 13: 2345-2358

Snow, R, Omumbo, J, Lowe, B, Molyneux, C, Obiero, J, Palmer, A, Weber, M, Pinder, M, Nahlen, B, Obonyo, C, Newbold, C, Gupta, S and Marsh, K (1997). Relation between severe malaria morbidity in children and level of *Plasmodium falciparum* transmission in Africa [see comments] CM: Comment in: Lancet 1997 Jun 7;349(9066):1636-7. *Lancet. 1997 Jun 7; 349(9066): 1650-4*

Snow, RW, Bastos de Azevedo, I, Lowe, BS, Kabiru, EW, Nevill, CG, Mwankusye, S, Kassiga, G, Marsh, K and Teuscher, T (1994). Severe childhood malaria in two areas of markedly different falciparum transmission in east Africa. *Acta Trop* 57(4): 289-300.

Suss, G, Eichmann, K, Kury, E, Linke, A and Langhorne, J (1988). Roles of CD4- and CD8-bearing T lymphocytes in the immune response to the erythrocytic stages of *Plasmodium chabaudi. Infect. Immun.* 56(12): 3081-3088.

Taylor, R, Smith, D, Robinson, V, McBride, J and Riley, E (1995). Human antibody response to *Plasmodium falciparum* merozoite surface protein 2 is serogroup specific and predominantly of the immunoglobulin G3 subclass. *Infect. Immun. 1995 Nov; 63(11): 4382-8*

Taylor, RR, Allen, SJ, Greenwood, BM and Riley, EM (1998). IgG3 antibodies to *Plasmodium falciparum* merozoite surface protein 2 (MSP2): increasing prevalence with age and association with clinical immunity to malaria. *Am. J. Trop. Med. Hyg.* 58(4): 406-413.

Taylor-Robinson, A (1995). Regulation of immunity to malaria: Valuablc lessons learned from murine models. *Parasitol. Today* 11(9): 341

Taylor-Robinson, A and Smith, E (1999). A role for cytokines in potentiation of malaria vaccines through immunological modulation of blood stage infections. *Immunol. Rev.* 171: 105-124

Taylor-Robinson, AW and Phillips, RS (1993). Protective CD4+ T-cell lines raised against *Plasmodium chabaudi* show characteristics of either Th1 or Th2 cells. *Parasite Immunol* 15(6): 301-310

Tham, WH, Wilson, DW, Reiling, L, Chen, L, Beeson, JG and Cowman, AF (2009). Antibodies to reticulocyte binding protein-like homologue 4 inhibit invasion of *Plasmodium falciparum* into human erythrocytes. *Infect Immun* 77(6): 2427-2435

Thelu, J, Sheick-Zakiuddin, I, Boudin, C, Peyron, F, Picot, S and Ambroise-Thomas, P (1991). Development of natural immunity in *Plasmodium falciparum* malaria: study of antibody response by Western immunoblotting. *J. Clin. Microbiol. 1991 Mar; 29(3): 510-8*

Todryk, SM, Bejon, P, Mwangi, T, Plebanski, M, Urban, B, Marsh, K, Hill, AV and Flanagan, KL (2008). Correlation of memory T cell responses against TRAP with protection from clinical malaria, and CD4 CD25 high T cells with susceptibility in Kenyans. *PLoS One* 3(4): e2027

Triglia, T, Tham, WH, Hodder, A and Cowman, AF (2009). Reticulocyte binding protein homologues are key adhesins during erythrocyte invasion by *Plasmodium falciparum*. *Cell Microbiol* 11(11): 1671-1687

Udeinya, I, Miller, L, McGregor, I and Jensen, J (1983). *Plasmodium falciparum* strain-specific antibody blocks binding of infected erythrocytes to amelanotic melanoma cells. *Nature. 1983 Jun 2-8; 303(5916): 429-31*

Urban, BC, Ferguson, DJ, Pain, A, Willcox, N, Plebanski, M, Austyn, JM and Roberts, DJ (1999). *Plasmodium falciparum*-infected erythrocytes modulate the maturation of dendritic cells [see comments]. *Nature* 400(6739): 73-77

Urban, BC, Mwangi, T, Ross, A, Kinyanjui, S, Mosobo, M, Kai, O, Lowe, B, Marsh, K and Roberts, DJ (2001). Peripheral blood dendritic cells in children with acute *Plasmodium falciparum* malaria. *Blood* 98(9): 2859-2861

Vande Waa, JA, Jensen, JB, Akood, MA and Bayoumi, R (1984). Longitudinal study on the in vitro immune response to *Plasmodium falciparum* in Sudan. *Infect. Immun.* 45(2): 505-510.

Verra, F and Hughes, AL (1999). Natural selection on apical membrane antigen-1 of *Plasmodium falciparum*. *Parassitologia* 41(1-3): 93-95.

Vigan-Womas, I, Lokossou, A, Guillotte, M, Juillerat, A, Bentley, G, Garcia, A, Mercereau-Puijalon, O and Migot-Nabias, F (2010). The humoral response to *Plasmodium falciparum* VarO rosetting variant and its association with protection against malaria in Beninese children. *Malar J* 9: 267

Wahlgren, M, Berzins, K, Perlmann, P and Persson, M (1983). Characterization of the humoral immune response in *Plasmodium falciparum* malaria. II. IgG subclass levels of anti-*P. falciparum* antibodies in different sera. *Clin-Exp-Immunol. 1983 Oct; 54(1): 135-42*

Walther, M, Jeffries, D, Finney, OC, Njie, M, Ebonyi, A, Deininger, S, Lawrence, E, Ngwa-Amambua, A, Jayasooriya, S, Cheeseman, IH, Gomez-Escobar, N, Okebe, J, Conway, DJ and Riley, EM (2009). Distinct roles for FOXP3 and FOXP3 CD4 T cells in regulating cellular immunity to uncomplicated and severe *Plasmodium falciparum* malaria. *PLoS Pathog* 5(4): e1000364

Walther, M, Tongren, JE, Andrews, L, Korbel, D, King, E, Fletcher, H, Andersen, RF, Bejon, P, Thompson, F, Dunachie, SJ, Edele, F, de Souza, JB, Sinden, RE, Gilbert, SC, Riley, EM and Hill, AV (2005). Upregulation of TGF-beta, FOXP3, and CD4+CD25+ regulatory T cells correlates with more rapid parasite growth in human malaria infection. *Immunity* 23(3): 287-296

Wambua, S, Mwangi, TW, Kortok, M, Uyoga, SM, Macharia, AW, Mwacharo, JK, Weatherall, DJ, Snow, RW, Marsh, K and Williams, TN (2006). The effect of alpha+-thalassaemia on the incidence of malaria and other diseases in children living on the coast of Kenya. *PLoS Med* 3(5): e158

Weatherall, DJ (1997). Thalassaemia and malaria, revisited. *Ann. Trop. Med. Parasitol.* 91(7): 885-890.

Weiss, W, Sedegah, M, Beaudoin, R, Miller, L and Good, M (1988). CD8+ T cells (cytotoxic/suppressors) are required for protection in mice immunized with malaria sporozoites. *Proc. Natl. Acad. Sci. USA. 1988 Jan; 85(2): 573-6*

Williams, TN (2009). Human genetic resistance to malaria. *Adv Exp Med Biol* 634: 243-253

Williams, TN, Mwangi, TW, Roberts, DJ, Alexander, ND, Weatherall, DJ, Wambua, S, Kortok, M, Snow, RW and Marsh, K (2005a). An immune basis for malaria protection by the sickle cell trait. *PLoS Med* 2(5): e128

Williams, TN, Mwangi, TW, Wambua, S, Alexander, ND, Kortok, M, Snow, RW and Marsh, K (2005b). Sickle cell trait and the risk of *Plasmodium falciparum* malaria and other childhood diseases. *J Infect Dis* 192(1): 178-186

Williams, TN, Mwangi, TW, Wambua, S, Peto, TE, Weatherall, DJ, Gupta, S, Recker, M, Penman, BS, Uyoga, S, Macharia, A, Mwacharo, JK, Snow, RW and Marsh, K (2005c). Negative epistasis between the malaria-protective effects of alpha+-thalassemia and the sickle cell trait. *Nat Genet* 37(11): 1253-1257

Williams, TN, Wambua, S, Uyoga, S, Macharia, A, Mwacharo, JK, Newton, CR and Maitland, K (2005d). Both heterozygous and homozygous alpha+ thalassemias protect against severe and fatal *Plasmodium falciparum* malaria on the coast of Kenya. *Blood* 106(1): 368-371

Wilson, DW, Crabb, BS and Beeson, JG (2010). Development of fluorescent *Plasmodium falciparum* for in vitro growth inhibition assays. *Malar J* 9: 152

Winkler, S, Willheim, M, Baier, K, Schmid, D, Aichelburg, A, Graninger, W and Kremsner, PG (1998). Reciprocal regulation of Th1- and Th2-cytokine-producing T cells during clearance of parasitemia in *Plasmodium falciparum* malaria. *Infect. Immun.* 66(12): 6040-6044.

Winkler, S, Willheim, M, Baier, K, Schmid, D, Aichelburg, A, Graninger, W and Kremsner, PG (1999). Frequency of cytokine-producing T cells in patients of different age groups with *Plasmodium falciparum* malaria. *J. Infect. Dis.* 179(1): 209-216.

Yuthavong, Y, Bunyaratvej, A and Kamchonwongpaisan, S (1990). Increased susceptibility of malaria-infected variant erythrocytes to the mononuclear phagocyte system. *Blood* 16: 602-604

11

Using Population Genetics to Guide Malaria Vaccine Design

Alyssa E. Barry[1,2], James Beeson[3], John C. Reeder[3,4], Freya J.I. Fowkes[3] and Alicia Arnott[3]
[1]*Walter and Eliza Hall Institute for Medical Research,*
[2]*Department of Medical Biology, University of Melbourne,*
[3]*Burnet Institute,*
[4]*Monash University,*
Australia

1. Introduction

A broadly effective malaria vaccine is a missing component of the practical tools needed to control and eventually eliminate malaria. For more than 50 years malaria researchers have been searching for a strategy that provides long lasting protection against a broad range of parasite strains. Many different approaches have been tested including whole parasite and subunit vaccines composed of one or more parasite surface proteins that are naturally targeted by the host immune response.

Candidates in the malaria vaccine pipeline include surface exposed proteins from each of the morphologically distinct developmental stages of the parasite lifecycle within the human host. Many of these antigens have undergone rigorous developmental and preclinical testing as subunit vaccines [1] but only a few have reached advanced clinical trials: one reason being a lack of funding to carry all promising vaccine candidates to trial [2]. For candidates that have reached Phase II clinical trials in malaria endemic areas, there has been variable success. This is not surprising given that the malaria parasite is a complex and rapidly evolving organism that can quickly adapt to its ever-changing environment and effectively evade human immune responses. Limited understanding of the precise mechanisms and minimal requirements for antimalarial immunity has also hampered vaccine progress [3]. Moreover, the high degree of diversity of parasite surface antigens [4] and the allelic-specificity of the immune response [5, 6] is likely to have contributed significantly to the variable success of malaria vaccines. However genetic diversity is often overlooked in vaccine design with most vaccines formulated on the basis of a single strain. It is now increasingly recognized that to be effective against the worldwide parasite population, a malaria vaccine may need to contain multiple variants of the target antigen [7].

Many studies have investigated the genetic diversity of vaccine antigens that are circulating in natural parasite populations but very little of this knowledge has been applied to malaria vaccine design. Typically, alleles from one or two reference strains (3D7 or FVO) are used in vaccine formulations, but this only partially represents the diversity of alleles circulating in the parasite population (Figure 1 [8]). Moreover, if vaccine alleles are found at low frequencies, the power to measure the success of vaccine trials is limited. This chapter reviews the current state of knowledge of the genetic diversity of leading malaria vaccine candidates, including those for both major human malaria parasites, *Plasmodium falciparum* and *Plasmodium vivax.* We examine the relevance of this diversity to malaria vaccines currently in development and how to use this information in determining which alleles should be used to provide broad coverage against the majority of parasite strains. Using leading candidate vaccine antigens as examples, we outline how population genetic tools can be used to characterise genetic diversity and the distribution of alleles and to define potentially immunologically relevant subgroups of alleles and polymorphisms. Finally, we make recommendations for the design of the next generation of malaria vaccines.

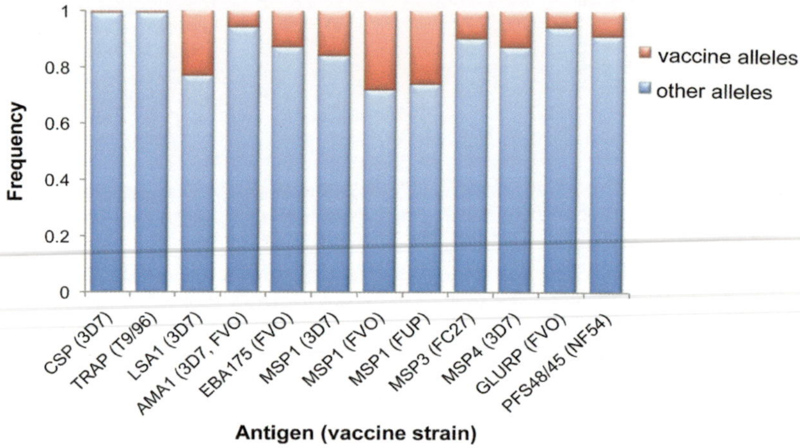

Fig. 1. Worldwide frequency of alleles represented in ten leading malaria vaccine candidates (adapted from [8]). $MSP1_{19}$ 3D7 and FVO are being developed as a combination vaccine as well as in isolation.

2. Malaria vaccines: A brief history

2.1 Early studies

The idea that a malaria vaccine might be possible was raised in the late 1800's with the observations of Robert Koch during his expedition to the Melanesian Island of Papua New Guinea (PNG). He found that while local children frequently displayed symptoms of malarial disease and harboured parasites in their blood, adults remained relatively disease and parasite-free [9]. He also noted that Malay and Chinese workers that had recently immigrated to PNG became ill with malaria more often than their counterparts who had been in residence for longer periods of time. These observations form the basis for our contemporary understanding of the epidemiology of malaria and the theory that immunity to malaria is eventually acquired in areas where people are constantly exposed to infection. In his conclusions, Dr. Koch stated that it would be possible to vaccinate against malaria toxins (and therefore the symptoms caused by infection).

Some 60 years later, the feasibility of a human malaria vaccine received a boost when Sir Ian MacGregor demonstrated that immunity was conferred by transferring hyperimmune sera (IgG) from adults to at-risk African children [10]. Soon afterward, a team at New York University (NYU) including Ruth Nussenzweig and Jerome Vanderberg showed that mice could be vaccinated against malaria with irradiated *Plasmodium bergei* sporozoites [11]. In 1973, Clyde and colleagues at the University of Maryland in collaboration with the NYU team demonstrated that infections of humans via the bite of irradiated sporozoite-positive mosquitoes protected against subsequent homologous challenge, thus providing the first real evidence that man could be vaccinated against *P. falciparum* malaria [12] and subsequently, against *P. vivax* [13]. Later work showed that this approach was also effective in protecting against heterologous strains of *P. falciparum* [14]. These studies demonstrated that a malaria vaccine could elicit sterile protective immunity, and provided the reagents and tools to identify molecules that were important immune targets, such as the circumsporozoite surface protein (CSP) [15]. Unfortunately, at the time it was impractical to vaccinate large numbers of people with irradiated sporozoites isolated from infected mosquitoes and attempts to culture sporozoites showed only limited success [16].

2.2 Subunit vaccines

The increasing availability of molecular cloning and PCR techniques in the early 1980's saw a major shift in focus to the development of synthetic "subunit" vaccines based on individual parasite proteins and peptides and the abandonment of whole-parasite approaches. Several teams around the world had identified parasite surface proteins as targets such as the sporozoite antigens: circumsporozoite surface protein (CSP) [15] and thrombospondin related antigen (TRAP, [17, 18]) ; Liver stage antigen 1 (LSA1,[19]); and the merozoite surface proteins, MSP1 [20], MSP2 [21], S-Antigen [22] and Apical Membrane Antigen 1 (AMA1, [23, 24]). Initial studies in animal models were promising but excitement began to wane as subunit vaccines showed only around half of the candidates had a protective effect in clinical trials. Of the eight malaria vaccine candidate antigens that have reached Phase II trials, only one, "RTS,S" which is based on CSP, has now been tested in Phase III clinical trials [25].

2.3 Whole parasite vaccines

The malaria parasite is a complex organism with 3000 or so known proteins [26, 27] including a few hundred that are immunogenic surface antigens [28]. This makes it a formidable target and therefore a vaccine as complex as the parasite itself may be required to immunise against malaria [29]. Evidence that sporozoite vaccinees were resistant to both homologous and heterologous challenge [14] makes whole-parasite vaccination approaches an appealing option so long as technological challenges can be overcome. New techniques for mass-producing sporozoites are reportedly in development [30] and both irradiation [31] and genetically attenuated [32, 33] parasite vaccines are being tested. Low doses of blood stage parasites have been shown to induce T-cell mediated responses targeted at cytoplasmic proteins with high levels of sequence conservation [34]. In addition, chemically- and genetically-attenuated blood-stage parasites are being developed (personal communication M. Good, Griffith University and K. Evans, Walter and Eliza Hall Institute). Consequently, whole parasite approaches have been experiencing a renaissance and have garnered much support from funding organisations [35]. As both subunit and whole parasite approaches are valid approaches [35, 36], they are being pursued in parallel. This review focuses primarily on the former approach.

2.4 Malaria vaccine subclasses

Malaria vaccines fall into three main classes based on the lifecycle stage that they target and their expected biological effects [37-39]. These include:

i. Pre-erythrocytic vaccines - based on antigens on the surface of the sporozoite or liver stage parasites or whole parasite (sporozoite approaches). These vaccines are designed to target the pre-erythrocytic stages of the parasite lifecycle and therefore inhibit infection.
ii. Blood stage vaccines - based on antigens on the surface of the blood stages such as the merozoite or intraerythrocytic stages or whole blood stage parasites. These disease-blocking vaccines are designed to control parasitaemia by preventing invasion of uninfected erythrocytes (merozoite targets) or to control disease by preventing cytoadhesion (intraerythrocyte targets), which leads to pathogenesis.
iii. Transmission blocking vaccines - based on antigens on the surface of the sexual stages, expressed either within the human host or anopheline vector. Known as transmission-blocking vaccines because they are designed to elicit antibodies within the human host that will target gametocytes (transmission forms) or to be taken up in the mosquito blood meal to target parasite proteins within the mosquito midgut.

Vaccine approaches currently being tested include individual candidates from a single lifecycle stage as well as combination vaccines formulated with targets from multiple lifecycle stages.

3. Subunit vaccine candidate antigens

The advent of recombinant DNA technology has greatly facilitated the development of subunit malaria vaccines by providing the tools with which to synthesise large amounts of parasite protein, and to disrupt gene expression for detailed functional characterisation [40-42]. Preclinical development for many candidate antigens has been successful and Phase II clinical trials have proceeded for at least eight candidate antigens, with evidence of antimalarial efficacy for MSP2 [6], CSP [43, 44], MSP3 [45] and AMA1 [46].

The release of the first full malaria genome sequence in 2002 allowed the systematic identification of novel malaria vaccine candidates amongst approximately 5300 genes. Genome wide screening for single nucleotide polymorphisms (SNPs) has been used to reveal loci under positive selection and therefore encoding proteins that may be targeted by the immune response [4, 47]. Proteomics approaches have characterised the "immunome" [48], and measured the abundance of parasite proteins on the parasite surface [49]. A pipeline of bioinformatic screens has also been used to identify surface proteins, gene knockouts and high-throughput immunological assays to identify novel surface antigens (e.g. [50]). In the last 10 years, the list of potential malaria vaccine candidates has rapidly expanded to encompass many antigens about which there is still much to be learnt. Targets that were discovered first are therefore further down the development pipeline rather than novel proteins that may ultimately be more successful.

Below, we describe the most developed malaria vaccine candidates for the two major malaria parasites, *P. falciparum* and *P. vivax* as well as some novel vaccine candidates that have recently been identified for *P. falciparum*. This is not a comprehensive listing, a complete list of preclinical, clinical and inactive or discontinued malaria vaccine projects can be found in the World Health Organisation's Malaria Vaccine Rainbow Tables [51].

3.1 *Plasmodium falciparum*

P. falciparum is responsible for most of the mortality and morbidity associated with malaria, with up to 1 million deaths and around 225 million clinical cases caused by this species [52]. It is the only major human malaria parasite for which an *in vitro* culture system is available thus making it more tractable for investigations to characterise molecular structure and function and interactions with its human and anophelene hosts. As a result, malaria research has focused on developing ways to combat this particular species with less focus on other human infecting malaria parasites. The number of well-developed *P. falciparum* vaccine candidates in advanced stages of clinical development reflects this bias and there are strong candidates for every stage of the *P. falciparum* lifecycle within the human host. Some of these are described in detail below.

3.1.1 Circumsporozoite Protein (CSP)

CSP, which is found in the outer sporozoite membrane, was shown to be a target of antibodies that prevented hepatocyte infection, thereby interrupting an obligatory stage in the parasite's lifecycle [15]. Cloning of the CSP gene (amongst other antigens) opened the doors to mass production and it was hoped, a malaria vaccine [53]. CSP contains a central (NANP) repeat region containing B-cell epitopes flanked by non-repetitive sequences containing T-cell epitopes [53-55]. In 2004, a considerable protective effect was observed with a CSP-based vaccine known as RTS,S with 49% efficacy against severe malaria for a period of 18 months in children aged 1-4 years [44]. This vaccine is composed of the central repeat and the C-terminal regions of CSP isolated from the reference strain, 3D7, combined with a Hepatitis B surface antigen (which provides protection against Hepatitis B and therefore satisfies ethical requirements). Recently published data from a phase III trial including 6000 African children has shown a 50% reduction in clinical episodes and 35% reduction in severe disease in children aged 5-18 months [25]. Therefore, RTS,S is likely to be the first licensed malaria vaccine and should be available within the next few years [56]. Most would agree though that it is an important proof of principle rather than an end to the hunt for a vaccine.

3.1.2 Thrombospondin Related Adhesion Protein (TRAP)

TRAP also known as Sporozoite Surface Protein (SSP) [18, 57] is present within the micronemes of the sporozoite and is essential for gliding motility and host cell invasion in the mosquito and human pre-erythrocyte stages [58-60]. TRAP is also expressed in the blood stages though its function in this stage is not well understood [18, 57]. TRAP is a Type I transmembrane protein consisting of multiple adhesive domains and a central repeat region flanked by unique sequence. Anti-repeat monoclonal antibodies have been shown to at least partially inhibit sporozoite invasion *in vitro* [61] and potent T-cell responses have been identified in individuals vaccinated with irradiated sporozoites [62, 63] as well as people who are naturally exposed to malaria [64]. TRAP is highly polymorphic [65] and has also been shown to be under strong diversifying selection suggesting that it is a natural immune target [66].

Mapping of inhibitory epitopes has led to the development of the multiepitope (ME)-TRAP DNA vaccine, which contains 15 TRAP T-cell epitopes. The vaccine has been delivered using a prime-boost regime involving three doses of naked DNA or DNA fused to a viral vector, to produce potent T-cell responses in both animals and humans [67]. While safety and immunogenicity trials in the UK have shown promising results [68, 69], Phase II efficacy trials conducted in semi-immune adults in The Gambia and children in Kenya provided no evidence of protective efficacy [70-73].

3.1.3 Apical Membrane Antigen 1 (AMA1)

AMA1 is an 83 kDa integral membrane protein expressed late in the asexual stages and found in the micronemes at the apical tip of merozoites [74]. Prior to schizont rupture the AMA1 prodomain is cleaved to reveal a 66 kDa protein containing three subdomains (domains I, II and III) defined by their disulfide bonds [24]. AMA1 then relocates to the parasite surface [75] where further processing during invasion leads to shedding of two fragments of 44 and 48 kDa whilst the 22kDa cytoplasmic tail remains in the membrane and is carried into the invaded erythrocyte [76, 77]. AMA1 is now known to function in formation of the tight junction through interactions with rhoptry neck proteins [78, 79]. This molecule is also expressed in sporozoites where it is involved in hepatocyte invasion [80].

Antibodies against AMA1 are found in people living in malaria endemic areas [81-83], and these have been shown to block the invasion process [84-86]. The potential of AMA1 as a malaria vaccine candidate has been demonstrated in rodent models of malaria with both strain-specific [87-89] and cross-protective [90] protection observed. High levels of polymorphism in AMA1 [8, 91, 92] due to strong balancing selection [93] has resulted in hundreds of distinct AMA1 haplotypes; this might indicate that the development of a broadly effective AMA1-based malaria vaccine will be difficult. However, little is known about the antigenic diversity of AMA1 and recent studies suggest that immunization with a small number of different alleles might give broad reactivity [94, 95]. The availability of a 3D structural model for AMA1 has greatly advanced our understanding of antibody inhibition of AMA1 function by demonstrating that several polymorphisms are found on the edge of a hydrophobic pocket within which it is thought the receptor binds [96, 97]. A cluster of polymorphisms in this region, known as the "C1L cluster" contributes to immune escape [97], but the importance of residues outside this cluster remains unclear [92].

Vaccine candidates comprising full length AMA1 originating from the 3D7 strain alone (FMP2.1, [46] and in combination with FVO (AMA1-c1, [98]), have had variable success in Phase II efficacy trials. FMP2.1 demonstrated no efficacy using the primary endpoint of a clinical malaria episode, however when the secondary endpoint of clinical infections carrying the vaccine allele was defined, a substantial efficacy of 68% above that of the control was revealed [46]. The alternative vaccine candidate, AMA1-C1, showed no allele-specific efficacy however the prevalence of the vaccine allele amongst the samples was so low that sample numbers precluded a proper assessment of any effect [98]. Additionally, the adjuvant used was alum, which is less potent.

Another approach for AMA1 that is being tested is a diversity-covering vaccine (PfAMA1 DiCo) whereby 355 published sequences were aligned and common polymorphisms (i.e. those found in >16% of sequences) were used to design three synthetic constructs, which together encompass 97% of the sequence diversity [99]. So far there have not been any clinical trials however broader parasite growth inhibitory activity was observed in animals vaccinated with the DiCo mix than those vaccinated with native AMA1 from the FVO strain [99].

3.1.4 Merozoite Surface Protein 1 (MSP1)

MSP1 is the most abundant and best studied of the *P. falciparum* merozoite surface antigens. The protein is synthesised as a 190-kDa-precursor protein that is cleaved into four fragments of 83, 30, 38, and 42 kDa [100]. These exist as a non-covalently associated complex tethered by a glycosylphosphatidylinositol (GPI) anchor at the C-terminal [101]. During erythrocyte invasion, the N-terminal fragments are shed when $MSP1_{42}$ undergoes a secondary processing event generating a further 33 kDa ($MSP1_{33}$) and 19 kDa fragment ($MSP1_{19}$) [102-104] which facilitates parasite entry into the erythrocyte [105]. The $MSP1_{19}$ fragment is retained on the surface of the invading merozoite [106].

The C-terminal end of MSP1 is a leading malaria vaccine candidate. The $MSP1_{33}$ sequence is dimorphic, with diverse alleles clustering within the two families known as K1 and Mad20 [107], however $MSP1_{19}$ is relatively conserved across the two allele families with six nonsynonymous SNPs that are commonly used to describe $MSP1_{19}$ haplotypes [108-113]. Within each of the allele-families, $MSP1_{33}$ also contains several single nucleotide polymorphisms (SNPs) and a 3 bp deletion [108, 111].

The FMP1/ASO2A vaccine, which is formulated with the 3D7 allele of $MSP1_{42}$, has been tested in Phase II trials. The vaccine initially showed promise in safety and immunogenicity trials in 40 Malian adults, with responses generated to parasite clones carrying diverse $MSP1_{42}$ alleles (FVO and Camp/FUP) [114]. Phase II efficacy trials including 400 children in Western Kenya did not protect against infection or lower parasite densities, nor did it reduce clinical episodes [115]. Though the authors stated that the vaccine was no longer a promising vaccine candidate, this was without having investigated how many vaccinees were infected with the vaccine strain. In addition, high throughput genotyping studies in Mali have demonstrated that the 3D7 allele had a prevalence of only 16% [113]. A vaccine containing both $MSP1_{42}$ 3D7 and FVO alleles fused together with conserved regions of MSP1 is currently being tested [116].

3.1.5 Merozoite Surface Protein 2 (MSP2)

MSP2, a 45-52 kDa glycoprotein is tethered to the membrane a glycosylphosphatidylinosital (GPI) anchor and is the second most abundant protein (based on copy numbers) on the merozoite surface [49]. The protein consists of highly conserved N- and C-terminal ends flanking a highly polymorphic central repeat region. MSP2 sequences fall into two distinct allelic families namely FC27 and 3D7 (IC-1) [117-120]. Within these allele-families, the central repeats vary in length, number and sequence among isolates. Allele-specific and length polymorphism in MSP2 has been used as the basis for high-resolution genotyping of *P. falciparum* isolates [121, 122].

MSP2 is a target of naturally acquired antibodies [123, 124] and antibodies are associated with protection against clinical malaria in some studies [125-128]. Longitudinal studies have suggested allele-specific antibody responses, with encountered strains not being observed in subsequent infections [129, 130], while others have shown that individuals can be re-infected with homologous strains [131]. The Combination B vaccine, which was composed of the 3D7 alleles for MSP1, MSP2 and ring-associated erythrocyte surface antigen (RESA) was tested in Phase II trials in Papua New Guinea in the early 1990's. This vaccine, which is discussed in more detail later, was shown to be efficacious, reducing parasite densities significantly with most of the activity attributed to MSP2 [6]. A combination vaccine, MSP1-C1 containing both the 3D7 and FC27 alleles has recently been tested but showed unacceptable reactogenicity due to the adjuvant used and the trial was terminated [132].

3.1.6 Merozoite Surface Protein 3

MSP3, also known as Secreted Polymorphic Antigen associated with Merozoites (SPAM) is associated with the merozoite surface. It is secreted into the parasitophorous vacuole of the mature parasite (schizont) where it undergoes proteolytic cleavage [133-135]. Upon rupture of the infected erythrocyte, some MSP3 protein remains associated with the merozoite [133]. MSP3 contains three blocks of a polymorphic heptad repeat flanked by conserved sequences [133]. While initial studies reported limited polymorphism [134, 136] analysis of several isolates has revealed that the sequence is primarily dimorphic in nature with both point mutations and repeat variations in the N-terminal half of the protein with different alleles demonstrating variable antibody binding activity [137]. Antibodies produced in mice can inhibit parasite growth *in vitro* in co-operation with monocytes [135] but are allele-specific [138]. Furthermore, antibodies to different alleles in endemic human populations are individually associated with protection against clinical episodes [138]. Sequence data from natural parasite populations has confirmed that this antigen is under strong balancing selection and therefore a natural immune target [138].

A MSP3 vaccine based on a long synthetic peptide (MSP3-LSP) covering a relatively conserved region (amino acids 181-276) from strain FC27 has been tested in Phase I trials in Switzerland and later in Burkina Faso and shown to be safe and immunogenic with a strong cytophilic response [45, 139]. Although the second trial was not designed specifically to test efficacy the number of clinical episodes was measured as a means to monitor safety. Comparison of two MSP3-LSP vaccinated groups (different adjuvants) compared to individuals that received the alternative vaccine (Hepatitis B) demonstrated that the incidence of clinical malaria was three to four-fold lower in the MSP3-LSP vaccine groups [45]. Interestingly however, the degree of protection wanes substantially during the follow up period of 60 days, suggesting that protection may be short-lived. The GMZ2 vaccine comprising a fusion protein containing conserved regions of MSP3 and Glutamate Rich Protein (GLURP) has also been confirmed as safe and immunogenic in Phase I trials [140] and Phase II trials are currently underway [51].

3.1.7 175kDa Erythrocyte Binding Antigen (EBA175)

The 175 kDa Erythrocyte Binding Antigen, EBA175, is found in the micronemes, which are located at the apical end of the merozoite [141, 142]. It is a parasite ligand that directly associates with its receptor, Glycophorin A on the surface of uninfected erythrocytes. This occurs via an interaction between sialic acids and the Glycophorin A backbone [143, 144]. The cysteine-rich binding region (RII) is a 616 amino acid region consisting of two regions – F1 and F2, which are known as Duffy binding-like (DBL) domains named so as they are homologous to *P. vivax* Duffy binding protein, DBP. These domains are found in several other adhesion ligands of *P. falciparum* including Erythrocyte Membrane Protein 1 (PfEMP1). Antibodies to EBA175-RII can be induced by immunization in animal models by recombinant EBA175 protein [143] and are acquired in humans naturally exposed to malaria [36, 145-147] and these antibodies can inhibit parasite invasion *in vitro* [142, 148]. Studies have suggested that EBA175 alleles are maintained by immune selection [149] and high levels of haplotype diversity are present, most likely as a result of recombination [8]. However, because *P. falciparum* parasites can vary the use of EBA175 to evade antibodies [150], EBA175 could not be used alone but would need to be combined with other merozoite antigens.

Vaccination of primates with the EBA175 vaccine candidate, EBA175-RII-NG, which is based on the 3D7 allele of RII, resulted in a significant decrease in parasite density after homologous challenge [151]. Clinical trials have proven the vaccines safety and shown that it produces antibody responses in vaccinated individuals. Furthermore, the serum of vaccinated individuals was shown to inhibit the binding of recombinant EBA175-RII to erythrocytes [152].

3.1.8 Pfs25 and Pfs45/48

The transmission blocking candidates Pfs25 and Pfs45/48 are found in the zygote/ookinte and gametocyte stages respectively. These antigens, which migrate as single and double bands respectively, are targets of antibodies that have been shown to block transmission of *P. falciparum* to the mosquito vector [153-156]. Pfs25 was cloned well before Pfs48/45 [157, 158] and therefore is the only candidate for which a vaccine trial has been carried out. Preclinical development studies are underway for the latter antigen. The attraction of Pfs25 as a vaccine candidate is that it is not expressed in the human host and has relatively limited polymorphism [159, 160]. It is therefore unlikely to be under the same immune pressures as other antigens, however one downside of this is that natural boosting may not occur unless long lived T-cell responses are elicited by the vaccine. Pfs48/45 gene knock out experiments demonstrate a key role in male fertility [161]. Anti-Pfs48/45 antibodies in individuals naturally exposed to malaria are associated with transmission blocking activity [162] and given that it is expressed within the human host it is likely to allow natural boosting of antibody responses. Pfs25 is relatively conserved [163] while Pfs48/45 shows high levels of diversity worldwide with evidence of diversifying selection and strong geographic structuring [8, 164, 165].

The only vaccine trial of these two antigens that has been conducted is a phase I trial of the Pfs25 vaccine candidate. However it was halted due to unexpected adverse effects [166]. Preclinical studies have demonstrated a significant increase in the immune response of animal models, and immune-sera had a significant transmission blocking effect [167]. Further clinical trials are planned [51].

3.1.9 Other *Plasmodium falciparum* vaccine candidates

There are several other malaria vaccine candidates currently under development which are based on well-known antigens, such as GLURP, which as mentioned above is being tested in combination with MSP3 [140], Liver Stage Antigen 1 (LSA1) being developed as a component of the ME-TRAP vaccine [168] and as a single component vaccine [169]; and MSP4 [170]. More recently discovered antigens demonstrate significant potential as vaccine candidates including members of the Rh family of proteins (Rh1, 2a, 2b, 4 and 5) [171, 172] and the Rh-interacting protein, RIPr [173], Serine repeat antigen 5 (SERA5, reviewed in [174]); MSP6 [175], MSP7 [176] and the pregnancy-associated malaria vaccine candidate, *var2csa* [177-179]. For some of these antigens, diversity is a significant issue that needs to be evaluated.

Combinations of antigens from different *P. falciparum* lifecycle stages have also been tested. Trials for Spf66, a synthetic combination of peptides from including CSP, MSP1 and two others of unknown origin have now been halted after it was shown to have no effect on malaria [180], NMRC-M3V-Ad-PfCA which is a combination of CSP and AMA1 and is currently in phase 2 trials in the USA [51], GMZ2 which was mentioned above (MSP3 and GLURP, [140]) and the EBA/Rh vaccine candidate, which consists of EBA175 (RIII-V) and Rh2a/b, Rh5 and RIPr binding regions [181]. This vaccine candidate is still undergoing preclinical testing and aims to target different invasion pathways used by the merozoite [172].

3.2 *Plasmodium vivax*

The increasing recognition of the importance of *Plasmodium vivax*, both as a significant cause of severe malaria and as a major obstacle to malaria control and elimination has exposed some major gaps in our knowledge of this parasite [182]. The vaccine development pipeline is lagging well behind that of *P.falciparum* and while work is progressing on vaccines targeted at the *P.vivax* Duffy-binding protein (DBP, [183]), which has long had a human genetic correlate (Duffy negative individuals have a greatly reduced risk of infection) [184], relatively little has been done on the blood-stage antigens homologous to those being intensively tested for *P.falciparum* [39]. Underlying this lack of development is an urgent need to understand more about the biology of the transmission of the parasite, the extent of its diversity at a population level, and the mechanism of acquiring immunity to it.

One major obstacle impeding *P.vivax* research is the fact that presently, *P.vivax* cannot be maintained in long-term culture or at high parasitaemias. In addition, infected individuals typically present with low parasitemia and therefore parasite material is less available than for *P. falciparum* [185]. Recombinant *P.vivax* proteins for use in immunoepidemiological studies and vaccine development therefore are often isolated from reference strains, such as Sal1 (Salvador).

Many *P. vivax* vaccine candidates currently being investigated are orthologues of *P. falciparum* vaccine candidate antigens [38, 39]. However, these two species have distinct biological features, the most obvious being the ability of *P. vivax* to form dormant liver stages, and also their variable transmission in different regions across the globe. Therefore it is difficult to base conclusions for *P.vivax*, on what is known for *P.falciparum*. Many experts believe that a malaria vaccine will need to contain a combination of both *P. falciparum* and *P. vivax* antigens to be globally effective, since many regions of the world are burdened with both species [38].

Only two *P.vivax* vaccine candidates, the circumsporozoite surface protein (CSP) and the gametocyte antigen, Pvs25, have been tested in clinical trials to date [38]. However, a host of additional *P.vivax* proteins are currently under investigation as potential vaccine candidates, including PvDBP [38], PvTRAP [186], PvMSP-1 [187], PvAMA-1 [188]; and the transmission blocking candidate, Pvs28 [38]. Additional antigens identified as potential *P.vivax* vaccine candidates include PvMSP3, PvMSP4, PvMSP5 and PvRBPs I and II [38]. PvMSP9 has also been revealed as a promising vaccine candidate in recent studies [189].

4. Variant-specific immunity

Naturally acquired immunity to malaria develops only after years of exposure to infection by Plasmodium parasites. The extensive genetic diversity that is characteristic of malaria surface antigens provides one explanation for this, especially because immune responses are variant-specific. Eventually, antibodies to all of the variants in the parasite population are acquired or reach a threshold whereby protection against clinical episodes is achieved (reviewed in [190]).

4.1 Identifying targets of human immunity

Numerous epidemiological studies have investigated the role of malarial antigens as natural targets of human immunity with conflicting estimates of their protective effect. While differences in study methodology, transmission intensity, and the rate of natural immunity acquisition [190, 191] will account for some of the discrepancies, parasite genetic diversity is likely to play a major role. This is because the prevalence of the major allelic types of specific antigens and subsequent acquisition of allele-specific immunity varies across populations.

A recent systematic review and meta-analysis investigating the protective effect of antibody responses to merozoite antigens, highlighted the issues of genetic diversity in immuno-epidemiological studies [192]. This review pooled all the published evidence for the association between anti-merozoite antibodies and the incidence of *P. falciparum* for each antigenic allele. For each allele, individual study estimates often showed large degrees of heterogeneity and comparing pooled estimates across alleles for the same antigen either showed similar (e.g. MSP1, MSP2) or very different (e.g. $MSP1_{19}$, MSP3, AMA1, GLURP) magnitudes of a protective effect.

A major contributor to the heterogeneity in protective estimates is the fact that allele-specific antibody response to the strain causing the malaria episode was not measured in these studies. If antibody-mediated protection is largely allele-specific then the true causal protective effect will be underestimated in studies that do not use allele-specific *P. falciparum* outcomes. For example, meta-analysis of studies investigating the protective effects of anti-$MSP2_{3D7}$ and $MSP2_{FC27}$ responses showed no evidence of a reduced risk of symptomatic *P. falciparum* (all strains combined) [192]. Four studies included allele-specific endpoints; two studies in PNG showed protective MSP2 responses to homologous strains [125, 128] whereas studies in South America and Africa [193, 194], show no evidence of a protective effect of pre-existing MSP2 allele-specific immunity on clinical episodes with homologous parasites.

It is clear that the importance of allele-specific immunity to malaria has been understudied in sero-epidemiological studies. There is a real need to incorporate strain-specific responses and endpoints in immuno-epidemiological studies to address whether protective responses against particular antigens are strain-transcending or strain-specific. This research is imperative so we can elucidate whether sub-unit vaccines including only one allelic type might protect against a small subset of the parasite population and thus select for parasites bearing heterologous alleles.

4.2 Vaccine trials and antigen polymorphism

Significant sequence polymorphism is present in most of the vaccine antigens that are currently in clinical trials, as well as in many of the lead candidate antigens that are in pre-clinical development. This includes *P. falciparum* antigens such as CSP (RTS,S vaccine), MSP1-42, MSP2, MSP3, AMA1, and *P. vivax* antigens, such as DBP [36]. Presently, there is only a very limited understanding of how sequence polymorphisms relate to antigenic diversity or the potential for polymorphisms to mediate vaccine escape.

Different approaches can be taken to overcome antigenic diversity present in vaccine candidates. One approach is to include multiple alleles, or variants, of an antigen such that the vaccine-induced responses cover most of the different alleles circulating in a population; referred to as multivalent vaccines. This approach has been widely used in the development of vaccines for viral and bacterial pathogens. Examples include vaccines for *Streptococcus pneumonia, Neisseria meningitidis,* and influenza. Among malaria vaccines, multivalent vaccines are in development for several antigens including MSP2 [132] and AMA1 [195] of *P. falciparum*. The level of polymorphism seen among different candidate antigens varies substantially, being high for some candidate antigens, such as AMA1, compared to others, such as EBA175 [8]. Antigens that have a lower level of diversity may be more attractive candidates for vaccine development; however, multiple factors need to be considered in prioritising the many potential antigens for development [36]. An alternative approach is to design vaccine constructs that include a conserved region of the antigen so that vaccine-induced responses would target epitopes common to all variants of the antigen. This approach is being taken for *P. falciparum* MSP3, whereby the vaccine antigen includes a conserved stretch of sequence (known as MSP3-LSP) towards the C-terminal end of MSP3 and reportedly omits the highly polymorphic epitopes [196]. Interestingly however, recent population genetic surveys have shown that T-cell epitopes within MSP3-LSP are somewhat polymorphic [138].

A well-known example of the importance of antigenic diversity in vaccine development is the phase I/IIb trial of the Combination B vaccine for *P. falciparum* malaria [6], which was mentioned earlier. The vaccine had significant efficacy in reducing parasite densities during follow-up and the anti-malarial effect of the vaccine is thought to be mediated primarily by responses to MSP2, rather than other components of the vaccine. Although MSP2 is polymorphic, nearly all sequences can be grouped into two allelic families, 3D7 and FC27. The Combination B vaccine contained only the 3D7 form of MSP2 and, consequently, infections in vaccinated individuals were over-represented by FC27 allelic types. This implies that the vaccine only had substantial efficacy against infections containing the vaccine allele, 3D7. To address this, an MSP2 vaccine containing both of the major allelic types is in development [132]. A more recent example of the challenge of antigenic diversity in malaria vaccines is AMA1. A phase II trial of a vaccine containing a single allele of *P. falciparum* AMA1 (3D7-allele) had no significant clinical efficacy when all malaria episodes were considered [46]. However, as was mentioned earlier, the vaccine demonstrated 68% efficacy against malaria episodes caused by AMA1 alleles that were similar in sequence to the vaccine allele. The development of approaches to overcome diversity in AMA1 and generate responses that give broad population coverage are ongoing.

The most advanced vaccine in development, RTS,S, is based on a region of *P. falciparum* CSP [25]. Because CSP is polymorphic, an obvious question was whether diversity in CSP may explain the partial efficacy of the RTS,S vaccine. Analyses of infecting genotypes in one phase II trial of RTS,S suggested that this was not the case as there was no evidence of selection for infections containing non-vaccine genotypes among vaccinated versus control subjects [197, 198]. These findings highlight that although antigen polymorphism needs to be considered in vaccine development, it may not be a major issue for all vaccines. Clearly, there is a lot more we need to understand about the nature and specificity of responses and the importance of sequence diversity.

There are a number of other promising antigens in pre-clinical development or early clinical trials where issues of polymorphisms have been explored. The leading *P. vivax* vaccine candidate, DBP [199] has significant polymorphism that appears to impact on the efficacy of inhibitory antibodies [200], and protective immunity shows a degree of strain-specificity [201]. The erythrocyte binding region of the *P. falciparum* vaccine candidate EBA175, also has significant polymorphism [149, 202]. Interestingly, studies suggest that these polymorphisms have little impact on the efficacy of vaccine-induced inhibitory antibodies *in vitro* [203, 204]. However, the ability of *P. falciparum* to vary the expression and use of EBA175 during invasion may be an important means of immune evasion [150], which presents different challenges in vaccine design. Another example is the PfRh invasion ligand family. One member that appears to be an important target of acquired immunity, PfRh2, has significant polymorphism in the N-terminal region [171], but studies suggest it is possible to target a C-terminal conserved stretch of the protein in vaccine design [172]. The challenge of addressing diversity in vaccine development is greatest for PfEMP1, which is expressed on the surface of infected RBCs. PfEMP1 shows extreme sequence diversity (e.g. [205, 206]) and is encoded by a family of around 60 *var* genes per genome that enables clonal antigenic variation through expression of different PfEMP1 variants [207]. A vaccine trial in non-human primates showed strain-specific protective efficacy [208] and it is not clear how this extensive antigenic diversity can be overcome. However, one specific PfEMP1 variant, known as *var2csa*, plays a key role in placental infection [209] and may be a suitable target for a vaccine that helps protect pregnant women from the complications of malaria during pregnancy. Although this single variant has a high level of polymorphism [210], recent studies suggest the extent of antigenic diversity may not be high as there appear to be many shared epitopes that are common to different variants [211, 212], and antibodies that cross-react to different variants have been induced by vaccination [213, 214] and are acquired through natural exposure [211, 215]

5. How can population genetics inform malaria vaccine development?

Population genetics is the study of allele frequency distributions and changes that occur in response to the four major forces of evolution: natural selection, genetic drift, mutation and gene flow [216]. All of the current malaria vaccine candidates are potential targets of positive balancing selection due to pressure from human immune responses. Balancing selection maintains alleles at low to medium frequencies and therefore no single allele is likely to provide broad protection [217]. Population genetic analyses can reveal insight into the extent and distribution of alleles and has been important in highlighting antigens as targets of natural immunity [218, 219].

Scores of population genetic surveys have been conducted on malaria vaccine candidates, including isolates from countries in every major malaria-endemic corner of the world. However, the data has generally not been used in the formulation of malaria candidate vaccines. Vaccine developers have included alleles isolated from well-characterised reference strains, 3D7 (and its parent NF54, origin unknown), FVO (Vietnam) or FC27 (Papua New Guinea). However, amongst the substantial sequence data available for many countries for several leading malaria vaccine antigens, these alleles are either completely absent or found at low frequencies among naturally circulating parasites (Figure 1, [8]).

A recent metapopulation genetic analysis has summarised the known diversity of twelve leading malaria vaccine candidates [8]. After compiling all available published population data on malaria vaccine candidates, either currently in vaccine trials or in preclinical development, a database of almost 5000 sequences was used to investigate the range and distribution of diversity. Only non-synonymous polymorphisms were investigated as synonymous polymorphisms do not change the protein structure and are therefore antigenically irrelevant. Table 1 summarises the results observed for the ten antigens analysed in this study, as well as other *P. falciparum* and *P. vivax* antigens that are leading malaria vaccine candidates.

The data presented in Table 1 demonstrates that the majority of current malaria vaccine candidate antigens have many distinct haplotypes and this emphasises the problem of diversity in developing a broadly effective malaria vaccine [35]. However, without knowledge of this natural diversity it will be difficult to assess vaccine trials to the full extent. In addition, for genes encoding merozoite antigens including AMA1, EBA175 and MSPs 1-4 the full breadth of diversity was present in all populations with no evidence of geographic population structure, suggesting that they are under strong immune selection. However, genes encoding the non-merozoite antigens including CSP, TRAP, LSA1 and Pfs48/45 showed variable levels of diversity, which were related to transmission levels, and there was evidence of geographic population structure [8]. The consequence of this contrasting distribution of diversity for malaria vaccine design is that a diversity-covering vaccine may be possible for merozoite antigens but for the non-merozoite antigens identifying common alleles across all populations will be difficult. Nevertheless, diversity in the non-merozoite antigens does not appear to be primarily structured by immune selection, and therefore may not be as immunologically relevant as that for the merozoite antigens.

Antigen	Expression	Domain	Continents	Countries	Total isolates sampled (range)	Total haplotypes (range)	References
Plasmodium falciparum[a]							
CSP	sporozoite	C-terminal	3	13	604 (9-143)	71 (3-20)	reviewed in [8]
TRAP	sporozoite	N-terminal	2	3	100 (8-48)	84 (8-37)	reviewed in [8]
LSA1	liver stage	N-terminal	3	4	74 (10-22)	13 (3-7)	reviewed in [8]
GLURP	sporozoite/ gametocyte	Region 0	3	3	48 (9-11)	22 (2-9)	reviewed in [8]
AMA1	merozoite	Domain I	3	11	572 (8-162)	181 (6-68)	reviewed in [8]
EBA175	merozoite	Region II	2	3	135 (30-48)	51 (15-23)	reviewed in [8]
MSP1	merozoite	MSP119	3	11	2237 (18-1368)	20 (1-15)	reviewed in [8]
MSP2	merozoite	Blocks 2 and 3	2	3	392 (n.d)	275 (n.r.)	reviewed in [8]
MSP3	merozoite	Repeat region	2	2	124 (75-86)	21 (9-12)	reviewed in [8]
MSP4	merozoite	Full length	2	4	142 (12-42)	47 (9-23)	reviewed in [8]
MSP3/6	merozoite		1	2	117(51-66)	n.r.	[218, 219]
Rh2	merozoite	Binding region	1	1	33 (15)	n.r. (13)	[171]
Rh4	merozoite	Binding region	1	1	23 (12)	9 (4)	Reiling *et al.* unpublished data
Pfs48/45	gametocyte	Full length	3	4	55 (9-15)	19 (2-8)	reviewed in [8]
Pfs28	ookinete	no population data available					
var2csa	trophozoite	DBL3	2	3	124 (15-54)	n.r.	[211]
Plasmodium vivax[b]							
CSP	pre-eryth	Central repeat	2	2	168 (31-137)	n.r. (13-25)	[220, 221]
TRAP	pre-eryth	Regions II-IV	2	2	74 (37-37)	54 (n.r.)	[222]
AMA1	merozoite	Full length[c]	2	2	96 (23-73)	n.r. (15-18)	[223] [224]
MSP1	merozoite	Full length[c]	2	7	196 (40-116)	n.r. (12-31)	[187, 225]
DBP	merozoite	Region II	2	8	675 (11-123)	n.r. (9-73)	[226]
Pvs28	ookinete	All	1	1	20	2	[227]
Pvs25	ookinete	All	1	1	30	4	[227]

[a].Total includes both natural populations and other isolates, range includes only natural populations; b. Total (range) includes only natural populations; c.Individual domains also analysed, data not shown; n.r. result not available.

Table 1. Summary of population genetic data for leading malaria vaccine candidates

5.1 Sampling diversity

An important consideration when investigating the genetic diversity of a vaccine candidate is the origin and number of samples required to obtain reliable allele frequency estimates. In early studies, only a handful of parasite isolates from diverse geographic origins were used to investigate diversity, however more recently a number of investigations on larger numbers of locally circulating field isolates which can represent natural parasite populations, have been completed (reviewed in [8], Table 1). While a geographically disparate sampling approach can provide insights into levels of polymorphism, immune selection and can allow the extent of diversity to be predicted, it cannot provide reliable information on allele frequencies. The latter approach is more appropriate if data will be used for prioritizing common alleles for vaccine development. However it is critical that large sample sizes of a minimum of 30-50 isolates be used to obtain a reliable estimate of diversity and values approaching natural allele frequencies. Once defined, natural allele frequencies can provide an indication of the minimum proportion of the parasite population that would be covered by a particular vaccine formulation. Further analysis, discussed below, can identify relationships amongst alleles and therefore the potential for cross-reactivity between distinct alleles.

5.2 Defining the extent of diversity

In population genetics, the extent of diversity at a defined locus is measured using a number of different statistics. These include statistics that are simple to estimate: e.g. the number of alleles or haplotypes and more complex statistics such as the allelic richness, which is normalised for sample size [228] and therefore is useful to compare among populations if samples sizes vary considerably. Other statistics include the nucleotide diversity (π), which is the average proportion of sites that are polymorphic within a group of sequences; the average number of differences and the expected heterozygosity, all of which can be easily calculated with the help of a myriad of population genetic software (reviewed in [229]). The most informative statistics for vaccine design includes the numbers of alleles or haplotypes that need to be considered in developing a broadly efficacious malaria vaccine. For example if we consider the data in Table 1, some antigens have larger numbers of haplotypes than others, such as CSP with 71 haplotypes while MSP3 has only 21 even though the two datasets were similar in size, showing that CSP is the more diverse antigen [8].

5.3 Defining the distribution of diversity

5.3.1 Allele and haplotype frequencies

Knowledge of the distribution of alleles and haplotypes (variants) is critical both for vaccine design and for monitoring the effects of vaccine trials. In trials for vaccine candidate antigens with allele-specific immunity, a high frequency variant has a higher likelihood of resulting in a protective effect than a low frequency variant (if the vaccine construct covers polymorphic regions). Furthermore, the identification of geographically distinct population structures is an indication that variants may be present at different frequencies. In this situation, it is possible that a vaccine based on a common allele in one population that is rare in another population, may have differential effects across the two populations. Similarly, if a vaccine is based on a variant that is found at low frequencies at a testing site, the positive effects of variant-specific immunity may be dampened by infection with parasites carrying non-vaccine alleles. The vaccine may then be interpreted as being non-protective, unless variant-specific end-points are included by genotyping post-vaccine infections. Another important consideration in this scenario is that the statistical power to measure variant-specific efficacy will be limited with only a small number of infections carrying the vaccine allele.

The importance of allele/haplotype frequencies in vaccine design has been demonstrated by a study that measured $MSP1_{19}$ diversity at a vaccine-testing site in Mali. High throughput genotyping of six common $MSP1_{19}$ polymorphisms in more than 2000 isolates showed that there were two highly prevalent haplotypes (FVO, 46% and FUP, 36%) whereas the majority of the haplotypes were relatively rare (<10%). The common haplotypes remained common over long periods of time (>44% and 34% respectively), with fluctuations that could be explained by frequency dependant selection [113]. The vaccine haplotype, 3D7, was the third most common, being found at a frequency of 16% (14-18%) throughout the study period. The authors concluded that the previous $MSP1_{19}$ vaccine trial [114] probably failed as a result of a lack of parasites harbouring 3D7 $MSP1_{19}$ haplotypes. Studies have investigated changes in vaccine antigen haplotype frequencies over time under natural conditions ([93, 230, 231]) but there have been e.g. relatively few during vaccine trials [98, 115]. More studies are needed to monitor fluctuations that occur in parasite populations over time, especially under the influence of natural immune or vaccine-mediated selection.

5.3.2 Clustering patterns

Cluster analyses have been used to identify population substructure within a given sample to understand the underlying population biology of *P. falciparum* [232]. This analysis has also been adapted to understand relationships among haplotypes of several malaria vaccine candidates [8, 91, 92, 226]. A study of 150 AMA1 sequences by Xin Zhuan Su and colleagues demonstrated that they clustered into six distinct subgroups. Some evidence was also presented that sera from rabbits immunized with AMA1 variants from one cluster tended to inhibit invasion of parasite isolates carrying sequences from the same cluster, but were less active against those from other clusters, suggesting that different clusters contain immunologically distinct sequences [91]. Later studies, including 506 AMA1 domain I sequences analysed have suggested up to 16 clusters [92]. Although the full utility of clustering patterns is yet to be confirmed, they may be used as a guide to select representative variants to cover diversity as well as to predict the effects of a vaccine trial within a defined geographic area. This is particularly important because different malaria antigens show different clustering patterns ([8], Figure 2). If clusters represent immunologically distinct subgroups, the patterns observed in Figure 2 suggest that vaccination with CSP would be significantly more effective in Africa and parts of the Americas, whereas for MSP1 the effects would be similar among many populations. Different polymorphisms have varying immunological significance [85, 97] and a better understanding of the relationship between polymorphisms and antigenic diversity will help advance the development of clustering algorithms.

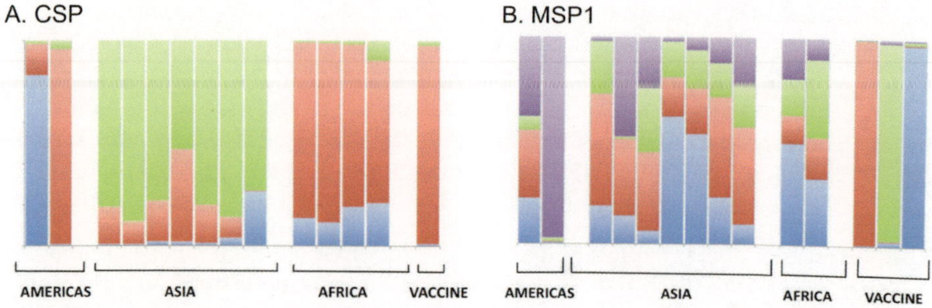

Fig. 2. Cluster analysis of sequences for (A) the pre-erythrocytic antigen, CSP and (B) the merozoite antigen, $MSP1_{19}$. Non-synonymous haplotypes were submitted to cluster analysis using STRUCTURE software [233]. Each bar represents the mean membership co-efficient for the parasite population of each country and colours represent the mean membership to each of the clusters. Vaccine alleles include CSP: 3D7; $MSP1_{19}$: 3D7, FVO or FC27. Figure adapted from [8].

5.3.3 Networks

Network analysis originated as a mathematical tool to understand social relationships and has been used to study the transmission of infectious diseases [234]. In population genetics, it has been adapted to explore relationships among sequences by linking haplotypes that are identical at a predefined proportion of polymorphic sites [8, 235]. As each haplotype (node) may have multiple connections (edges), this analysis has the potential to define not only distinct clusters or subgroups of highly related sequences but also the relationships among them. Furthermore, it can identify the location of less frequently observed admixed haplotypes in the network, which may represent novel recombinants. Barry *et al.* [8] have explored the distribution of haplotypes using network analysis and found that the network was concordant with clustering patterns for ten leading malaria vaccine antigens (Figure 3 shows the results for AMA1 as an example). In addition, they demonstrated that haplotypes

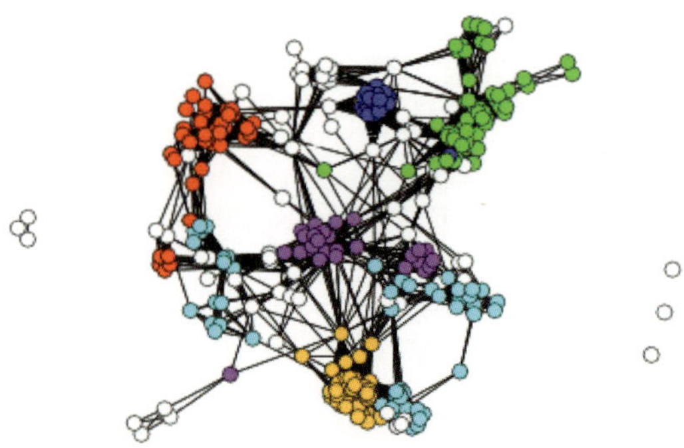

Fig. 3. Network of AMA1 (domain I) sequences. Each node (circle) represents a haplotype, shaded in colour to highlight cluster-membership or white for admixed haplotypes (as defined by the Structure analysis discussed above [233]). Nodes are tied by edges (black lines) demonstrating that they share a predefined threshold of 48 nsSNPs. Admixed haplotypes originating from isolates with unknown origin are shaded in white (unless they were vaccine haplotypes). Adapted from [8].

that were identified as "admixed" in the cluster analysis (i.e. <75% of sequences assigned into any one cluster), often formed connections between one or more lobes of the network suggesting that these represent novel recombinants resulting from exchange between sequences from the linked clusters. Such recombinants might allow evasion of naturally acquired- or vaccine-mediated immune responses if vaccine formulations were comprised only of haplotypes from distinct subgroups or clusters. Network analysis will allow shifts in the proportion of haplotypes within each cluster and admixed/recombinant haplotypes to be monitored during vaccine trials.

5.4 Immune selection

Population genetic analyses can identify signatures of balancing selection in loci that are targeted by natural immune responses and therefore allow vaccine candidates to be ranked [66, 218, 219, 236]. While data from geographically diverse isolates can be useful, the ability to identify balancing selection is strengthened by allele frequency data from natural parasite populations [237]. Comparative studies, investigating polymorphism and allele frequencies by deep population sampling of several novel vaccine candidates have been done [218, 219, 224, 237, 238]. These have demonstrated the relative levels of balancing selection and therefore whether particular candidates are stronger immune targets than others, but may also partially reflect the tolerance of a particular antigen to high levels of mutation.

Balancing selection can be measured using a variety of different statistics, however the *Hudson Kreitman Aguade ratio* (HKAr), which is determined by calculating levels of divergence between species and dividing by the amount of diversity within a species [239] has been shown to be most informative for assessing selection in any dataset, including small numbers of isolates from diverse geographic locations. However, this also relies on the availability of sequences from the most closely related species for which genome data is available, namely *Plasmodium reichenowi*. Additional *P. reichenowi* isolates have been collected by researchers and may also be used to obtain further sequence data to increase the reliability of this statistic [240]. Another statistic that has proven to be reliable for predicting balancing selection, is Tajima's D, which identifies departures from neutrality by measuring the number of polymorphic sites (S) in relation to the nucleotide diversity (π) [241]. Tajima's D requires allele frequency data and therefore can only be effectively used on population samples, with large sample sizes (>50 isolates) being the most informative [218].

5.5 Credentialing polymorphisms

It is clear that some antigens such as AMA1 and CSP have many polymorphic sites, while others such as EBA175 and MSP4 remain relatively conserved [8]. However, this is probably more a reflection of functional constraints or degree of immune exposure, than indicating their capacity to be an effective vaccine candidate. The challenge is how to determine which polymorphisms will be critical to vaccine design. Investigators have used different approaches to identify antigenically relevant polymorphisms, including three-dimensional structural modelling, immunological assays and mutational analysis [91, 97]. However, population genetic data - which may be easier to collect - can be highly informative.

When choosing which polymorphisms to consider for vaccine design it is important to define the allele frequencies for each polymorphic site. If the minor allele frequency (MAF) is <10%, at least 90% of isolates will carry the predominant allele, and therefore a vaccine candidate carrying the major allele will target the majority of the parasite population. Mapping regions of significant balancing selection (where allele frequencies will be low-medium) will identify regions that have accumulated polymorphisms as a result of being directly targeted by the immune response [236]. These analyses can help identify regions that are targets of functional immune responses. The analysis can be done by sliding window analyses of Tajima's D or measuring the HKAr for different protein domains. As balancing selection maintains balanced allele frequencies across different populations, it is also possible to use the interpopulation differentiation statistic, Wrights F_{ST} to measure differences in allele frequencies between populations. A low and insignificant Wrights F_{ST} value will demonstrate that allele frequencies are similar among populations and polymorphic regions potentially associated with immune escape [236, 242]. An additional important approach to determine key polymorphisms is by monitoring longitudinal infection dynamics in cohort studies, which may include vaccine trials [92]. If specific polymorphisms allow immune escape, then subsequent infections will carry alternative alleles to those of previous infections. Similarly, in vaccine trials, post-vaccination infections can be monitored for the presence of vaccine alleles. Antigenicity can then be determined by comparing allele frequencies in the vaccinated and control groups.

6. Conclusion: The way forward

The malaria vaccine development pipeline has suffered many setbacks and complications over the decades since the first malaria vaccine was trialed. Nevertheless, it is our opinion that with carefully planned vaccine trials and an understanding of naturally circulating parasite diversity, made possible through technological advances in next generation sequencing and dedicated bioinformatics efforts, a broadly effective subunit malaria vaccine is achievable. With respect to developing such a vaccine we put forward the following recommendations for the design and testing of the next generation of malaria vaccines:

iv. **Prioritise vaccine candidates**: Many malaria vaccine candidate antigens have reached vaccine trials simply because they were discovered first. Genome sequencing and "omic" technologies have now identified several antigens that may have greater potential to induce protective immunity to a wide variety of parasite strains than these more traditional candidates. As the pipeline to clinical trials and eventual licensing is an arduous and vastly expensive journey, a thorough review of all candidates including those recently discovered and also in development needs to be done to identify those with the greatest potential to elicit protective immunity against malaria.

v. **Prioritise vaccine alleles**: Dozens of population genetic studies have highlighted the issue of high levels of genetic diversity in candidate antigens and the low prevalence of the vaccine alleles currently being used, in natural parasite populations. Researchers now have the opportunity to mine already compiled datasets (e.g. [8]) or to rapidly sequence large numbers of field samples in vaccine testing sites to identify high frequency alleles for testing in single or multivalent vaccines. Notably, for a large number of leading malaria vaccine candidates under strong balancing selection, these alleles may be common across populations.

vi. **Allele-specific endpoints for vaccine trials:** Few malaria vaccine trials have evaluated allele frequencies either before, during, or after vaccine trials have taken place and therefore it is not possible to assess whether any allele-specific protection has been induced in individuals receiving the vaccine. Given the relatively low cost (compared to conducting a vaccine trial) and ready availability of high throughput genotyping and NextGen sequencing technologies, this step should certainly be included in future vaccine trials and could even be done in retrospect if samples are still available. However, it is important to note that in some trials where the allele used to formulate the vaccine is found at low frequencies in the testing site, sample size may be too low to evaluate any protective effects.

vii. **Parasite population monitoring:** Even after an effective vaccine(s) has been developed and rolled out, sustained and intensive surveillance efforts will be essential to monitor population allele frequencies on a regular basis. This will identify significant fluctuations that might impact on vaccine efficacy or newly emerging alleles that may allow antigenic escape. With data obtained through such a surveillance system, formulations may then be adapted n a manner analogous to the Influenza vaccine, to ensure continued protection against malaria.

A broadly effective malaria vaccine continues to be one of the most sought after strategies in the fight against malaria, however the diversity of many of the parasite antigens currently being considered as subunit vaccine candidates is an obstacle that must be overcome. Natural malaria parasite populations are complex and dynamic communities, but modern molecular and analysis technologies are providing new ways to understand them. It is therefore important that researchers consider using population genetics to inform malaria vaccine development from target discovery through to vaccine design and to assess the effects of clinical trials.

7. Acknowledgments

The authors are grateful for the support of the National Health and Medical Research Council (NHMRC) of Australia through project grants 488221 and 1003825. JB is supported by a Senior Research Fellowship; JCR by a Principal Research Fellowship; and FJIF by a Training Fellowship from the NHMRC. This work was made possible through Victorian State Government Operational Infrastructure Support and Australian Government NHMRC IRIISS.

8. References

[1] Moran, M., Guzman, J., Ropars, A, Jorgensen, M., McDonald, A., Potter, S. and Selassie, H. , *The Malaria Product Pipeline: Planning for the future*. 2007, The George Institute for International Health: Sydney.

[2] Organization, W.H., *Malaria Vaccine Rainbow Table*. 2008.

[3] Doolan, D.L., C. Dobano, and J.K. Baird, *Acquired immunity to malaria.* Clin Microbiol Rev, 2009. 22(1): p. 13-36, Table of Contents.

[4] Mu, J., et al., *Genome-wide variation and identification of vaccine targets in the Plasmodium falciparum genome.* Nat Genet, 2007. 39(1): p. 126-30.

[5] Fluck, C., et al., *Strain-specific humoral response to a polymorphic malaria vaccine.* Infect Immun, 2004. 72(11): p. 6300-5.

[6] Genton, B., et al., *A recombinant blood-stage malaria vaccine reduces Plasmodium falciparum density and exerts selective pressure on parasite populations in a phase 1-2b trial in Papua New Guinea.* J Infect Dis, 2002. 185(6): p. 820-7.

[7] Takala, S.L. and C.V. Plowe, *Genetic diversity and malaria vaccine design, testing and efficacy: preventing and overcoming 'vaccine resistant malaria'*. Parasite Immunol, 2009. 31(9): p. 560-73.

[8] Barry, A.E., et al., *Contrasting population structures of the genes encoding ten leading vaccine-candidate antigens of the human malaria parasite, Plasmodium falciparum.* PLoS One, 2009. 4(12): p. e8497.

[9] Koch, R., *Dritter Bericht uber die Thatigkeit der Malaria Expedition.* . British Medical Journal, 1900: p. 1183-1186.

[10] McGregor, I.A., *The Passive Transfer of Human Malarial Immunity.* Am J Trop Med Hyg, 1964. 13: p. SUPPL 237-9.

[11] Nussenzweig, R.S., et al., *Protective immunity produced by the injection of x-irradiated sporozoites of plasmodium berghei.* Nature, 1967. 216(111): p. 160-2.

[12] Clyde, D.F., et al., *Immunization of man against sporozite-induced falciparum malaria.* Am J Med Sci, 1973. 266(3): p. 169-77.

[13] Clyde, D.F., et al., *Specificity of protection of man immunized against sporozoite-induced falciparum malaria.* Am J Med Sci, 1973. 266(6): p. 398-403.

[14] Hoffman, S.L., et al., *Protection of humans against malaria by immunization with radiation-attenuated Plasmodium falciparum sporozoites.* J Infect Dis, 2002. 185(8): p. 1155-64.

[15] Yoshida, N., et al., *Hybridoma produces protective antibodies directed against the sporozoite stage of malaria parasite.* Science, 1980. 207(4426): p. 71-3.

[16] Vanderberg, J.P., M.M. Weiss, and S.R. Mack, *In vitro cultivation of the sporogonic stages of Plasmodium: a review.* Bull World Health Organ, 1977. 55(2-3): p. 377-92.

[17] Robson, K.J., et al., *A highly conserved amino-acid sequence in thrombospondin, properdin and in proteins from sporozoites and blood stages of a human malaria parasite.* Nature, 1988. 335(6185): p. 79-82.

[18] Rogers, W.O., et al., *Characterization of Plasmodium falciparum sporozoite surface protein 2.* Proc Natl Acad Sci U S A, 1992. 89(19): p. 9176-80.

[19] Guerin-Marchand, C., et al., *A liver-stage-specific antigen of Plasmodium falciparum characterized by gene cloning.* Nature, 1987. 329(6135): p. 164-7.

[20] Holder, A.A., et al., *A malaria merozoite surface protein (MSP1)-structure, processing and function.* Mem Inst Oswaldo Cruz, 1992. 87 Suppl 3: p. 37-42.

[21] Smythe, J.A., et al., *Identification of two integral membrane proteins of Plasmodium falciparum.* Proc Natl Acad Sci U S A, 1988. 85(14): p. 5195-9.

[22] Coppel, R.L., et al., *Isolate-specific S-antigen of Plasmodium falciparum contains a repeated sequence of eleven amino acids.* Nature, 1983. 306(5945): p. 751-6.

[23] Deans, J.A., et al., *Vaccination trials in rhesus monkeys with a minor, invariant, Plasmodium knowlesi 66 kD merozoite antigen.* Parasite Immunol, 1988. 10(5): p. 535-52.

[24] Hodder, A.N., et al., *The disulfide bond structure of Plasmodium apical membrane antigen-1.* J Biol Chem, 1996. 271(46): p. 29446-52.

[25] Agnandji, S.T., et al., *First results of phase 3 trial of RTS,S/AS01 malaria vaccine in African children.* N Engl J Med, 2011. 365(20): p. 1863-75.

[26] Florens, L., et al., *A proteomic view of the Plasmodium falciparum life cycle.* Nature, 2002. 419(6906): p. 520-6.

[27] Gardner, M.J., et al., *Genome sequence of the human malaria parasite Plasmodium falciparum.* Nature, 2002. 419(6906): p. 498-511.

[28] Doolan, D.L., et al., *Profiling humoral immune responses to P. falciparum infection with protein microarrays.* Proteomics, 2008. 8(22): p. 4680-94.

[29] Doolan, D.L., et al., *Utilization of genomic sequence information to develop malaria vaccines.* J Exp Biol, 2003. 206(Pt 21): p. 3789-802.

[30] Butler, D., *Mosquito production mooted as fast track to malaria vaccine.* Nature, 2003. 425(6957): p. 437.

[31] Epstein, J.E., et al., *Live attenuated malaria vaccine designed to protect through hepatic CD8 T cell immunity.* Science, 2011. 334(6055): p. 475-80.

[32] van Dijk, M.R., et al., *Genetically attenuated, P36p-deficient malarial sporozoites induce protective immunity and apoptosis of infected liver cells.* Proc Natl Acad Sci U S A, 2005. 102(34): p. 12194-9.

[33] Butler, N.S., et al., *Superior antimalarial immunity after vaccination with late liver stage-arresting genetically attenuated parasites.* Cell Host Microbe, 2011. 9(6): p. 451-62.

[34] Woodberry, T., et al., *Human T cell recognition of the blood stage antigen Plasmodium hypoxanthine guanine xanthine phosphoribosyl transferase (HGXPRT) in acute malaria.* Malar J, 2009. 8: p. 122.

[35] Good, M.F., *A whole parasite vaccine to control the blood stages of Plasmodium: the case for lateral thinking.* Trends Parasitol, 2011. 27(8): p. 335-40.

[36] Richards, J.S. and J.G. Beeson, *The future for blood-stage vaccines against malaria.* Immunol Cell Biol, 2009. 87(5): p. 377-90.

[37] Moorthy, V.S., M.F. Good, and A.V. Hill, *Malaria vaccine developments.* Lancet, 2004. 363(9403): p. 150-6.

[38] Arevalo-Herrera, M., C. Chitnis, and S. Herrera, *Current status of Plasmodium vivax vaccine.* Hum Vaccin, 2010. 6(1): p. 124-32.

[39] Galinski, M.R. and J.W. Barnwell, *Plasmodium vivax: who cares?* Malar J, 2008. 7 Suppl 1: p. S9.

[40] Crabb, B.S. and A.F. Cowman, *Characterization of promoters and stable transfection by homologous and nonhomologous recombination in Plasmodium falciparum.* Proc Natl Acad Sci U S A, 1996. 93(14): p. 7289-94.

[41] Wu, Y., L.A. Kirkman, and T.E. Wellems, *Transformation of Plasmodium falciparum malaria parasites by homologous integration of plasmids that confer resistance to pyrimethamine.* Proc Natl Acad Sci U S A, 1996. 93(3): p. 1130-4.

[42] Wu, Y., et al., *Transfection of Plasmodium falciparum within human red blood cells.* Proc Natl Acad Sci U S A, 1995. 92(4): p. 973-7.

[43] Alonso, P.L., et al., *Duration of protection with RTS,S/AS02A malaria vaccine in prevention of Plasmodium falciparum disease in Mozambican children: single-blind extended follow-up of a randomised controlled trial.* Lancet, 2005. 366(9502): p. 2012-8.

[44] Alonso, P.L., et al., *Efficacy of the RTS,S/AS02A vaccine against Plasmodium falciparum infection and disease in young African children: randomised controlled trial.* Lancet, 2004. 364(9443): p. 1411-20.

[45] Sirima, S.B., S. Cousens, and P. Druilhe, *Protection against malaria by MSP3 candidate vaccine.* N Engl J Med, 2011. 365(11): p. 1062-4.

[46] Thera, M.A., et al., *A field trial to assess a blood-stage malaria vaccine.* N Engl J Med, 2011. 365(11): p. 1004-13.

[47] Volkman, S.K., et al., *A genome-wide map of diversity in Plasmodium falciparum.* Nat Genet, 2007. 39(1): p. 113-9.

[48] Doolan, D.L., *Plasmodium immunomics.* Int J Parasitol, 2010.

[49] Sanders, P.R., et al., *Distinct protein classes including novel merozoite surface antigens in Raft-like membranes of Plasmodium falciparum.* J Biol Chem, 2005. 280(48): p. 40169-76.

[50] Arumugam, T.U., et al., *Discovery of GAMA, a Plasmodium falciparum merozoite micronemal protein, as a novel blood-stage vaccine candidate antigen.* Infect Immun, 2011. 79(11): p. 4523-32.

[51] Organisation, W.H. *Malaria Vaccine Rainbow Tables.* . 2010 December 2010; Available from: http://www.who.int/vaccine_research/links/Rainbow/en/index.html.

[52] Snow, R.W., et al., *The global distribution of clinical episodes of Plasmodium falciparum malaria.* Nature, 2005. 434(7030): p. 214-7.

[53] Enea, V., et al., *DNA cloning of Plasmodium falciparum circumsporozoite gene: amino acid sequence of repetitive epitope.* Science, 1984. 225(4662): p. 628-30.

[54] Dame, J.B., et al., *Structure of the gene encoding the immunodominant surface antigen on the sporozoite of the human malaria parasite Plasmodium falciparum.* Science, 1984. 225(4662): p. 593-9.

[55] Good, M.F., et al., *Human T-cell recognition of the circumsporozoite protein of Plasmodium falciparum: immunodominant T-cell domains map to the polymorphic regions of the molecule.* Proc Natl Acad Sci U S A, 1988. 85(4): p. 1199-203.

[56] *First Results of Phase 3 Trial of RTS,S/AS01 Malaria Vaccine in African Children.* N Engl J Med, 2011.

[57] Cowan, G., et al., *Expression of thrombospondin-related anonymous protein in Plasmodium falciparum sporozoites.* Lancet, 1992. 339(8806): p. 1412-3.

[58] Ghosh, A.K., et al., *Malaria parasite invasion of the mosquito salivary gland requires interaction between the Plasmodium TRAP and the Anopheles saglin proteins.* PLoS Pathog, 2009. 5(1): p. e1000265.

[59] Sultan, A.A., et al., *TRAP is necessary for gliding motility and infectivity of plasmodium sporozoites.* Cell, 1997. 90(3): p. 511-22.

[60] Kappe, S., et al., *Conservation of a gliding motility and cell invasion machinery in Apicomplexan parasites.* J Cell Biol, 1999. 147(5): p. 937-44.

[61] Charoenvit, Y., et al., *Development of two monoclonal antibodies against Plasmodium falciparum sporozoite surface protein 2 and mapping of B-cell epitopes.* Infect Immun, 1997. 65(8): p. 3430-7.

[62] Wizel, B., et al., *Irradiated sporozoite vaccine induces HLA-B8-restricted cytotoxic T lymphocyte responses against two overlapping epitopes of the Plasmodium falciparum sporozoite surface protein 2.* J Exp Med, 1995. 182(5): p. 1435-45.

[63] Wizel, B., et al., *HLA-A2-restricted cytotoxic T lymphocyte responses to multiple Plasmodium falciparum sporozoite surface protein 2 epitopes in sporozoite-immunized volunteers.* J Immunol, 1995. 155(2): p. 766-75.

[64] Aidoo, M., et al., *Identification of conserved antigenic components for a cytotoxic T lymphocyte-inducing vaccine against malaria.* Lancet, 1995. 345(8956): p. 1003-7.

[65] Robson, K.J., et al., *Natural polymorphism in the thrombospondin-related adhesive protein of Plasmodium falciparum.* Am J Trop Med Hyg, 1998. 58(1): p. 81-9.

[66] Weedall, G.D., et al., *Differential evidence of natural selection on two leading sporozoite stage malaria vaccine candidate antigens.* Int J Parasitol, 2007. 37(1): p. 77-85.

[67] Gilbert, S.C., et al., *Synergistic DNA-MVA prime-boost vaccination regimes for malaria and tuberculosis.* Vaccine, 2006. 24(21): p. 4554-61.

[68] McConkey, S.J., et al., *Enhanced T-cell immunogenicity of plasmid DNA vaccines boosted by recombinant modified vaccinia virus Ankara in humans.* Nat Med, 2003. 9(6): p. 729-35.

[69] Bejon, P., et al., *Calculation of liver-to-blood inocula, parasite growth rates, and preerythrocytic vaccine efficacy, from serial quantitative polymerase chain reaction studies of volunteers challenged with malaria sporozoites.* J Infect Dis, 2005. 191(4): p. 619-26.

[70] Bejon, P., et al., *A phase 2b randomised trial of the candidate malaria vaccines FP9 ME-TRAP and MVA ME-TRAP among children in Kenya.* PLoS Clin Trials, 2006. 1(6): p. e29.

[71] Bejon, P., et al., *Extended follow-up following a phase 2b randomized trial of the candidate malaria vaccines FP9 ME-TRAP and MVA ME-TRAP among children in Kenya.* PLoS One, 2007. 2(8): p. e707.

[72] Moorthy, V.S., et al., *A randomised, double-blind, controlled vaccine efficacy trial of DNA/MVA ME-TRAP against malaria infection in Gambian adults.* PLoS Med, 2004. 1(2): p. e33.

[73] Moorthy, V.S., et al., *Phase 1 evaluation of 3 highly immunogenic prime-boost regimens, including a 12-month reboosting vaccination, for malaria vaccination in Gambian men.* J Infect Dis, 2004. 189(12): p. 2213-9.

[74] Peterson, M.G., et al., *Integral membrane protein located in the apical complex of Plasmodium falciparum.* Mol Cell Biol, 1989. 9(7): p. 3151-4.

[75] Narum, D.L. and A.W. Thomas, *Differential localization of full-length and processed forms of PF83/AMA-1 an apical membrane antigen of Plasmodium falciparum merozoites.* Mol Biochem Parasitol, 1994. 67(1): p. 59-68.

[76] Howell, S.A., et al., *Proteolytic processing and primary structure of Plasmodium falciparum apical membrane antigen-1.* J Biol Chem, 2001. 276(33): p. 31311-20.

[77] Howell, S.A., et al., *A single malaria merozoite serine protease mediates shedding of multiple surface proteins by juxtamembrane cleavage.* J Biol Chem, 2003. 278(26): p. 23890-8.

[78] Collins, C.R., et al., *An inhibitory antibody blocks interactions between components of the malarial invasion machinery.* PLoS Pathog, 2009. 5(1): p. e1000273.

[79] Besteiro, S., et al., *Export of a Toxoplasma gondii rhoptry neck protein complex at the host cell membrane to form the moving junction during invasion.* PLoS Pathog, 2009. 5(2): p. e1000309.

[80] Silvie, O., et al., *Malaria sporozoite: migrating for a living.* Trends Mol Med, 2004. 10(3): p. 97-100; discussion 100-1.

[81] Johnson, A.H., et al., *Human leukocyte antigen class II alleles influence levels of antibodies to the Plasmodium falciparum asexual-stage apical membrane antigen 1 but not to merozoite surface antigen 2 and merozoite surface protein 1.* Infect Immun, 2004. 72(5): p. 2762-71.

[82] Thomas, A.W., et al., *Aspects of immunity for the AMA-1 family of molecules in humans and non-human primates malarias.* Mem Inst Oswaldo Cruz, 1994. 89 Suppl 2: p. 67-70.

[83] Cortes, A., et al., *Allele specificity of naturally acquired antibody responses against Plasmodium falciparum apical membrane antigen 1.* Infect Immun, 2005. 73(1): p. 422-30.

[84] Hodder, A.N., P.E. Crewther, and R.F. Anders, *Specificity of the protective antibody response to apical membrane antigen 1.* Infect Immun, 2001. 69(5): p. 3286-94.

[85] Kennedy, M.C., et al., *In vitro studies with recombinant Plasmodium falciparum apical membrane antigen 1 (AMA1): production and activity of an AMA1 vaccine and generation of a multiallelic response.* Infect Immun, 2002. 70(12): p. 6948-60.

[86] Kocken, C.H., et al., *High-level expression of the malaria blood-stage vaccine candidate Plasmodium falciparum apical membrane antigen 1 and induction of antibodies that inhibit erythrocyte invasion.* Infect Immun, 2002. 70(8): p. 4471-6.

[87] Yoshida, S., et al., *Plasmodium berghei circumvents immune responses induced by merozoite surface protein 1- and apical membrane antigen 1-based vaccines.* PLoS One, 2010. 5(10): p. e13727.

[88] Miura, K., et al., *In immunization with Plasmodium falciparum apical membrane antigen 1, the specificity of antibodies depends on the species immunized.* Infect Immun, 2007. 75(12): p. 5827-36.

[89] Narum, D.L., et al., *Passive immunization with a multicomponent vaccine against conserved domains of apical membrane antigen 1 and 235-kilodalton rhoptry proteins protects mice against Plasmodium yoelii blood-stage challenge infection.* Infect Immun, 2006. 74(10): p. 5529-36.

[90] Barclay, V.C., et al., *Mixed allele malaria vaccines: host protection and within-host selection.* Vaccine, 2008. 26(48): p. 6099-107.

[91] Duan, J., et al., *Population structure of the genes encoding the polymorphic Plasmodium falciparum apical membrane antigen 1: implications for vaccine design.* Proc Natl Acad Sci U S A, 2008. 105(22): p. 7857-62.

[92] Takala, S.L., et al., *Extreme polymorphism in a vaccine antigen and risk of clinical malaria: implications for vaccine development.* Sci Transl Med, 2009. 1(2): p. 2ra5.

[93] Cortes, A., et al., *Geographical structure of diversity and differences between symptomatic and asymptomatic infections for Plasmodium falciparum vaccine candidate AMA1.* Infect Immun, 2003. 71(3): p. 1416-26.

[94] Kusi, K.A., et al., *Generation of humoral immune responses to multi-allele PfAMA1 vaccines; effect of adjuvant and number of component alleles on the breadth of response.* PLoS One, 2010. 5(11): p. e15391.

[95] Kusi, K.A., et al., *Humoral immune response to mixed PfAMA1 alleles; multivalent PfAMA1 vaccines induce broad specificity.* PLoS One, 2009. 4(12): p. e8110.

[96] Dutta, S., et al., *Alanine mutagenesis of the primary antigenic escape residue cluster, c1, of apical membrane antigen 1.* Infect Immun, 2010. 78(2): p. 661-71.

[97] Dutta, S., et al., *Structural basis of antigenic escape of a malaria vaccine candidate.* Proc Natl Acad Sci U S A, 2007. 104(30): p. 12488-93.

[98] Ouattara, A., et al., *Lack of allele-specific efficacy of a bivalent AMA1 malaria vaccine.* Malar J, 2010. 9: p. 175.

[99] Remarque, E.J., et al., *A diversity-covering approach to immunization with Plasmodium falciparum apical membrane antigen 1 induces broader allelic recognition and growth inhibition responses in rabbits.* Infect Immun, 2008. 76(6): p. 2660-70.

[100] McBride, J.S. and H.G. Heidrich, *Fragments of the polymorphic Mr 185,000 glycoprotein from the surface of isolated Plasmodium falciparum merozoites form an antigenic complex.* Mol Biochem Parasitol, 1987. 23(1): p. 71-84.

[101] Gerold, P., et al., *Structural analysis of the glycosyl-phosphatidylinositol membrane anchor of the merozoite surface proteins-1 and -2 of Plasmodium falciparum.* Mol Biochem Parasitol, 1996. 75(2): p. 131-43.

[102] Barale, J.C., et al., *Plasmodium falciparum subtilisin-like protease 2, a merozoite candidate for the merozoite surface protein 1-42 maturase.* Proc Natl Acad Sci U S A, 1999. 96(11): p. 6445-50.

[103] Hackett, F., et al., *PfSUB-2: a second subtilisin-like protein in Plasmodium falciparum merozoites.* Mol Biochem Parasitol, 1999. 103(2): p. 183-95.

[104] Harris, P.K., et al., *Molecular identification of a malaria merozoite surface sheddase.* PLoS Pathog, 2005. 1(3): p. 241-51.

[105] Blackman, M.J., et al., *Antibodies inhibit the protease-mediated processing of a malaria merozoite surface protein.* J Exp Med, 1994. 180(1): p. 389-93.

[106] Blackman, M.J., et al., *A single fragment of a malaria merozoite surface protein remains on the parasite during red cell invasion and is the target of invasion-inhibiting antibodies.* J Exp Med, 1990. 172(1): p. 379-82.

[107] Tanabe, K., et al., *Allelic dimorphism in a surface antigen gene of the malaria parasite Plasmodium falciparum.* J Mol Biol, 1987. 195(2): p. 273-87.

[108] Miller, L.H., et al., *Analysis of sequence diversity in the Plasmodium falciparum merozoite surface protein-1 (MSP-1).* Mol Biochem Parasitol, 1993. 59(1): p. 1-14.

[109] Da Silveira, L.A., et al., *Sequence diversity and linkage disequilibrium within the merozoite surface protein-1 (Msp-1) locus of Plasmodium falciparum: a longitudinal study in Brazil.* J Eukaryot Microbiol, 2001. 48(4): p. 433-9.

[110] Ferreira, M.U., et al., *Sequence diversity and evolution of the malaria vaccine candidate merozoite surface protein-1 (MSP-1) of Plasmodium falciparum.* Gene, 2003. 304: p. 65-75.

[111] Qari, S.H., et al., *Predicted and observed alleles of Plasmodium falciparum merozoite surface protein-1 (MSP-1), a potential malaria vaccine antigen.* Mol Biochem Parasitol, 1998. 92(2): p. 241-52.

[112] Sakihama, N., et al., *Allelic recombination and linkage disequilibrium within Msp-1 of Plasmodium falciparum, the malignant human malaria parasite.* Gene, 1999. 230(1): p. 47-54.

[113] Takala, S.L., et al., *Dynamics of polymorphism in a malaria vaccine antigen at a vaccine-testing site in Mali.* PLoS Med, 2007. 4(3): p. e93.

[114] Thera, M.A., et al., *Safety and allele-specific immunogenicity of a malaria vaccine in Malian adults: results of a phase I randomized trial.* PLoS Clin Trials, 2006. 1(7): p. e34.

[115] Ogutu, B.R., et al., *Blood stage malaria vaccine eliciting high antigen-specific antibody concentrations confers no protection to young children in Western Kenya.* PLoS One, 2009. 4(3): p. e4708.

[116] Goodman, A.L., et al., *New candidate vaccines against blood-stage Plasmodium falciparum malaria: prime-boost immunization regimens incorporating human and simian adenoviral vectors and poxviral vectors expressing an optimized antigen based on merozoite surface protein 1.* Infect Immun, 2010. 78(11): p. 4601-12.

[117] Fenton, B., et al., *Structural and antigenic polymorphism of the 35- to 48-kilodalton merozoite surface antigen (MSA-2) of the malaria parasite Plasmodium falciparum.* Mol Cell Biol, 1991. 11(2): p. 963-71.

[118] Smythe, J.A., et al., *Structural diversity in the Plasmodium falciparum merozoite surface antigen 2.* Proc Natl Acad Sci U S A, 1991. 88(5): p. 1751-5.

[119] Smythe, J.A., et al., *Structural diversity in the 45-kilodalton merozoite surface antigen of Plasmodium falciparum.* Mol Biochem Parasitol, 1990. 39(2): p. 227-34.

[120] Snewin, V.A., et al., *Polymorphism of the alleles of the merozoite surface antigens MSA1 and MSA2 in Plasmodium falciparum wild isolates from Colombia.* Mol Biochem Parasitol, 1991. 49(2): p. 265-75.

[121] Falk, N., et al., *Comparison of PCR-RFLP and Genescan-based genotyping for analyzing infection dynamics of Plasmodium falciparum.* Am J Trop Med Hyg, 2006. 74(6): p. 944-50.

[122] Schoepflin, S., et al., *Comparison of Plasmodium falciparum allelic frequency distribution in different endemic settings by high-resolution genotyping.* Malar J, 2009. 8: p. 250.

[123] Ranford-Cartwright, L.C., et al., *Differential antibody recognition of FC27-like Plasmodium falciparum merozoite surface protein MSP2 antigens which lack 12 amino acid repeats.* Parasite Immunol, 1996. 18(8): p. 411-20.

[124] Taylor, R.R., et al., *Human antibody response to Plasmodium falciparum merozoite surface protein 2 is serogroup specific and predominantly of the immunoglobulin G3 subclass.* Infect Immun, 1995. 63(11): p. 4382-8.

[125] Stanisic, D.I., et al., *Immunoglobulin G subclass-specific responses against Plasmodium falciparum merozoite antigens are associated with control of parasitemia and protection from symptomatic illness.* Infect Immun, 2009. 77(3): p. 1165-74.

[126] Taylor, R.R., et al., *IgG3 antibodies to Plasmodium falciparum merozoite surface protein 2 (MSP2): increasing prevalence with age and association with clinical immunity to malaria.* Am J Trop Med Hyg, 1998. 58(4): p. 406-13.

[127] Metzger, W.G., et al., *Serum IgG3 to the Plasmodium falciparum merozoite surface protein 2 is strongly associated with a reduced prospective risk of malaria.* Parasite Immunol, 2003. 25(6): p. 307-12.

[128] al-Yaman, F., et al., *Assessment of the role of the humoral response to Plasmodium falciparum MSP2 compared to RESA and SPf66 in protecting Papua New Guinean children from clinical malaria.* Parasite Immunol, 1995. 17(9): p. 493-501.

[129] Bruce, M.C., et al., *Genetic diversity and dynamics of plasmodium falciparum and P. vivax populations in multiply infected children with asymptomatic malaria infections in Papua New Guinea.* Parasitology, 2000. 121 (Pt 3): p. 257-72.

[130] Franks, S., et al., *Frequent and persistent, asymptomatic Plasmodium falciparum infections in African infants, characterized by multilocus genotyping.* J Infect Dis, 2001. 183(5): p. 796-804.

[131] Weisman, S., et al., *Antibody responses to infections with strains of Plasmodium falciparum expressing diverse forms of merozoite surface protein 2.* Infect Immun, 2001. 69(2): p. 959-67.

[132] McCarthy, J.S., et al., *A pilot randomised trial of induced blood-stage Plasmodium falciparum infections in healthy volunteers for testing efficacy of new antimalarial drugs.* PLoS One, 2011. 6(8): p. e21914.

[133] McColl, D.J., et al., *Molecular variation in a novel polymorphic antigen associated with Plasmodium falciparum merozoites.* Mol Biochem Parasitol, 1994. 68(1): p. 53-67.

[134] McColl, D.J. and R.F. Anders, *Conservation of structural motifs and antigenic diversity in the Plasmodium falciparum merozoite surface protein-3 (MSP-3).* Mol Biochem Parasitol, 1997. 90(1): p. 21-31.

[135] Oeuvray, C., et al., *Merozoite surface protein-3: a malaria protein inducing antibodies that promote Plasmodium falciparum killing by cooperation with blood monocytes.* Blood, 1994. 84(5): p. 1594-602.

[136] Huber, W., et al., *Limited sequence polymorphism in the Plasmodium falciparum merozoite surface protein 3.* Mol Biochem Parasitol, 1997. 87(2): p. 231-4.
[137] Okenu, D.M., A.W. Thomas, and D.J. Conway, *Allelic lineages of the merozoite surface protein 3 gene in Plasmodium reichenowi and Plasmodium falciparum.* Mol Biochem Parasitol, 2000. 109(2): p. 185-8.
[138] Polley, S.D., et al., *Plasmodium falciparum merozoite surface protein 3 is a target of allele-specific immunity and alleles are maintained by natural selection.* J Infect Dis, 2007. 195(2): p. 279-87.
[139] Audran, R., et al., *Phase I malaria vaccine trial with a long synthetic peptide derived from the merozoite surface protein 3 antigen.* Infect Immun, 2005. 73(12): p. 8017-26.
[140] Mordmuller, B., et al., *Safety and immunogenicity of the malaria vaccine candidate GMZ2 in malaria-exposed, adult individuals from Lambarene, Gabon.* Vaccine, 2010. 28(41): p. 6698-703.
[141] Camus, D. and T.J. Hadley, *A Plasmodium falciparum antigen that binds to host erythrocytes and merozoites.* Science, 1985. 230(4725): p. 553-6.
[142] Sim, B.K., et al., *Primary structure of the 175K Plasmodium falciparum erythrocyte binding antigen and identification of a peptide which elicits antibodies that inhibit malaria merozoite invasion.* J Cell Biol, 1990. 111(5 Pt 1): p. 1877-84.
[143] Sim, B.K., et al., *Receptor and ligand domains for invasion of erythrocytes by Plasmodium falciparum.* Science, 1994. 264(5167): p. 1941-4.
[144] Tolia, N.H., et al., *Structural basis for the EBA-175 erythrocyte invasion pathway of the malaria parasite Plasmodium falciparum.* Cell, 2005. 122(2): p. 183-93.
[145] Okenu, D.M., et al., *Analysis of human antibodies to erythrocyte binding antigen 175 of Plasmodium falciparum.* Infect Immun, 2000. 68(10): p. 5559-66.
[146] Okoyeh, J.N., C.R. Pillai, and C.E. Chitnis, *Plasmodium falciparum field isolates commonly use erythrocyte invasion pathways that are independent of sialic acid residues of glycophorin A.* Infect Immun, 1999. 67(11): p. 5784-91.
[147] Richards, J.S., et al., *Association between naturally acquired antibodies to erythrocyte-binding antigens of Plasmodium falciparum and protection from malaria and high-density parasitemia.* Clin Infect Dis, 2010. 51(8): p. e50-60.
[148] Narum, D.L., et al., *Antibodies against the Plasmodium falciparum receptor binding domain of EBA-175 block invasion pathways that do not involve sialic acids.* Infect Immun, 2000. 68(4): p. 1964-6.
[149] Baum, J., A.W. Thomas, and D.J. Conway, *Evidence for diversifying selection on erythrocyte-binding antigens of Plasmodium falciparum and P. vivax.* Genetics, 2003. 163(4): p. 1327-36.
[150] Persson, K.E., et al., *Variation in use of erythrocyte invasion pathways by Plasmodium falciparum mediates evasion of human inhibitory antibodies.* J Clin Invest, 2008. 118(1): p. 342-51.
[151] Jones, T.R., et al., *Protection of Aotus monkeys by Plasmodium falciparum EBA-175 region II DNA prime-protein boost immunization regimen.* J Infect Dis, 2001. 183(2): p. 303-312.
[152] El Sahly, H.M., et al., *Safety and immunogenicity of a recombinant nonglycosylated erythrocyte binding antigen 175 Region II malaria vaccine in healthy adults living in an area where malaria is not endemic.* Clin Vaccine Immunol, 2010. 17(10): p. 1552-9.
[153] Rener, J., et al., *Target antigens of transmission-blocking immunity on gametes of plasmodium falciparum.* J Exp Med, 1983. 158(3): p. 976-81.

[154] Vermeulen, A.N., et al., *Sequential expression of antigens on sexual stages of Plasmodium falciparum accessible to transmission-blocking antibodies in the mosquito.* J Exp Med, 1985. 162(5): p. 1460-76.

[155] Quakyi, I.A., et al., *The 230-kDa gamete surface protein of Plasmodium falciparum is also a target for transmission-blocking antibodies.* J Immunol, 1987. 139(12): p. 4213-7.

[156] Barr, P.J., et al., *Recombinant Pfs25 protein of Plasmodium falciparum elicits malaria transmission-blocking immunity in experimental animals.* J Exp Med, 1991. 174(5): p. 1203-8.

[157] Kocken, C.H., et al., *Cloning and expression of the gene coding for the transmission blocking target antigen Pfs48/45 of Plasmodium falciparum.* Mol Biochem Parasitol, 1993. 61(1): p. 59-68.

[158] Kaslow, D.C., et al., *Comparison of the primary structure of the 25 kDa ookinete surface antigens of Plasmodium falciparum and Plasmodium gallinaceum reveal six conserved regions.* Mol Biochem Parasitol, 1989. 33(3): p. 283-7.

[159] Shi, Y.P., et al., *Single amino acid variation in the ookinete vaccine antigen from field isolates of Plasmodium falciparum.* Mol Biochem Parasitol, 1992. 50(1): p. 179-80.

[160] Kaslow, D.C., et al., *A vaccine candidate from the sexual stage of human malaria that contains EGF-like domains.* Nature, 1988. 333(6168): p. 74-6.

[161] van Dijk, M.R., et al., *A central role for P48/45 in malaria parasite male gamete fertility.* Cell, 2001. 104(1): p. 153-64.

[162] Roeffen, W., et al., *Association between anti-Pfs48/45 reactivity and P. falciparum transmission-blocking activity in sera from Cameroon.* Parasite Immunol, 1996. 18(2): p. 103-9.

[163] Duffy, P.E. and D.C. Kaslow, *A novel malaria protein, Pfs28, and Pfs25 are genetically linked and synergistic as falciparum malaria transmission-blocking vaccines.* Infect Immun, 1997. 65(3): p. 1109-13.

[164] Anthony, T.G., et al., *Evidence of non-neutral polymorphism in Plasmodium falciparum gamete surface protein genes Pfs47 and Pfs48/45.* Mol Biochem Parasitol, 2007. 156(2): p. 117-23.

[165] Conway, D.J., et al., *Extreme geographical fixation of variation in the Plasmodium falciparum gamete surface protein gene Pfs48/45 compared with microsatellite loci.* Mol Biochem Parasitol, 2001. 115(2): p. 145-56.

[166] Wu, Y., et al., *Phase 1 trial of malaria transmission blocking vaccine candidates Pfs25 and Pvs25 formulated with montanide ISA 51.* PLoS One, 2008. 3(7): p. e2636.

[167] Kubler-Kielb, J., et al., *Long-lasting and transmission-blocking activity of antibodies to Plasmodium falciparum elicited in mice by protein conjugates of Pfs25.* Proc Natl Acad Sci U S A, 2007. 104(1): p. 293-8.

[168] Reyes-Sandoval, A., et al., *Prime-boost immunization with adenoviral and modified vaccinia virus Ankara vectors enhances the durability and polyfunctionality of protective malaria CD8+ T-cell responses.* Infect Immun, 2010. 78(1): p. 145-53.

[169] Hillier, C.J., et al., *Process development and analysis of liver-stage antigen 1, a preerythrocyte-stage protein-based vaccine for Plasmodium falciparum.* Infect Immun, 2005. 73(4): p. 2109-15.

[170] Goschnick, M.W., et al., *Merozoite surface protein 4/5 provides protection against lethal challenge with a heterologous malaria parasite strain.* Infect Immun, 2004. 72(10): p. 5840-9.

[171] Reiling, L., et al., *Evidence that the erythrocyte invasion ligand PfRh2 is a target of protective immunity against Plasmodium falciparum malaria.* J Immunol, 2010. 185(10): p. 6157-67.
[172] Lopaticki, S., et al., *Reticulocyte and erythrocyte binding-like proteins function cooperatively in invasion of human erythrocytes by malaria parasites.* Infect Immun, 2011. 79(3): p. 1107-17.
[173] Chen, L., et al., *An EGF-like protein forms a complex with PfRh5 and is required for invasion of human erythrocytes by Plasmodium falciparum.* PLoS Pathog, 2011. 7(9): p. e1002199.
[174] Palacpac, N.M., et al., *Plasmodium falciparum serine repeat antigen 5 (SE36) as a malaria vaccine candidate.* Vaccine, 2011. 29(35): p. 5837-45.
[175] Demanga, C.G., et al., *Toward the rational design of a malaria vaccine construct using the MSP3 family as an example: contribution of antigenicity studies in humans.* Infect Immun, 2010. 78(1): p. 486-94.
[176] Pachebat, J.A., et al., *Extensive proteolytic processing of the malaria parasite merozoite surface protein 7 during biosynthesis and parasite release from erythrocytes.* Mol Biochem Parasitol, 2007. 151(1): p. 59-69.
[177] Barfod, L., et al., *Baculovirus-expressed constructs induce immunoglobulin G that recognizes VAR2CSA on Plasmodium falciparum-infected erythrocytes.* Infect Immun, 2006. 74(7): p. 4357-60.
[178] Salanti, A., et al., *Several domains from VAR2CSA can induce Plasmodium falciparum adhesion-blocking antibodies.* Malar J, 2010. 9: p. 11.
[179] Srivastava, A., et al., *Full-length extracellular region of the var2CSA variant of PfEMP1 is required for specific, high-affinity binding to CSA.* Proc Natl Acad Sci U S A, 2010. 107(11): p. 4884-9.
[180] Snounou, G. and L. Renia, *The vaccine is dead--long live the vaccine.* Trends Parasitol, 2007. 23(4): p. 129-32.
[181] Tham, W.H., Healer, J.,Cowman, A.F., *Erythrocyte and reticulocyte binding-like proteins of Plasmodium falciparum.* Trends in Parasitology, 2011. In press.
[182] Mueller, I., et al., *Key gaps in the knowledge of Plasmodium vivax, a neglected human malaria parasite.* Lancet Infect Dis, 2009. 9(9): p. 555-66.
[183] Chitnis, C.E. and A. Sharma, *Targeting the Plasmodium vivax Duffy-binding protein.* Trends Parasitol, 2008. 24(1): p. 29-34.
[184] Miller, L.H., et al., *The resistance factor to Plasmodium vivax in blacks. The Duffy-blood-group genotype, FyFy.* N Engl J Med, 1976. 295(6): p. 302-4.
[185] Gentil, F., et al., *A recombinant vaccine based on domain II of Plasmodium vivax Apical Membrane Antigen 1 induces high antibody titres in mice.* Vaccine, 2010. 28(38): p. 6183-90.
[186] Castellanos, A., et al., *Plasmodium vivax thrombospondin related adhesion protein: immunogenicity and protective efficacy in rodents and Aotus monkeys.* Mem Inst Oswaldo Cruz, 2007. 102(3): p. 411-6.
[187] Putaporntip, C., et al., *Mosaic organization and heterogeneity in frequency of allelic recombination of the Plasmodium vivax merozoite surface protein-1 locus.* Proc Natl Acad Sci U S A, 2002. 99(25): p. 16348-53.
[188] Cheng, Q. and A. Saul, *Sequence analysis of the apical membrane antigen I (AMA-1) of Plasmodium vivax.* Mol Biochem Parasitol, 1994. 65(1): p. 183-7.

[189] Lima-Junior, J.C., et al., *Promiscuous T-cell epitopes of Plasmodium merozoite surface protein 9 (PvMSP9) induces IFN-gamma and IL-4 responses in individuals naturally exposed to malaria in the Brazilian Amazon.* Vaccine, 2010. 28(18): p. 3185-91.

[190] Marsh, K. and S. Kinyanjui, *Immune effector mechanisms in malaria.* Parasite Immunol, 2006. 28(1-2): p. 51-60.

[191] Gupta, S., et al., *Immunity to non-cerebral severe malaria is acquired after one or two infections.* Nat Med, 1999. 5(3): p. 340-3.

[192] Fowkes, F.J., et al., *The relationship between anti-merozoite antibodies and incidence of Plasmodium falciparum malaria: A systematic review and meta-analysis.* PLoS Med, 2010. 7(1): p. e1000218.

[193] Scopel, K.K., et al., *Variant-specific antibodies to merozoite surface protein 2 and clinical expression of Plasmodium falciparum malaria in rural Amazonians.* Am J Trop Med Hyg, 2007. 76(6): p. 1084-91.

[194] Osier, F.H., et al., *Allele-specific antibodies to Plasmodium falciparum merozoite surface protein-2 and protection against clinical malaria.* Parasite Immunol, 2010. 32(3): p. 193-201.

[195] Kusi, K.A., et al., *Safety and immunogenicity of multi-antigen AMA1-based vaccines formulated with CoVaccine HT and Montanide ISA 51 in rhesus macaques.* Malar J, 2011. 10: p. 182.

[196] Druilhe, P., et al., *A malaria vaccine that elicits in humans antibodies able to kill Plasmodium falciparum.* PLoS Med, 2005. 2(11): p. e344.

[197] Waitumbi, J.N., et al., *Impact of RTS,S/AS02(A) and RTS,S/AS01(B) on genotypes of P. falciparum in adults participating in a malaria vaccine clinical trial.* PLoS One, 2009. 4(11): p. e7849.

[198] Enosse, S., et al., *RTS,S/AS02A malaria vaccine does not induce parasite CSP T cell epitope selection and reduces multiplicity of infection.* PLoS Clin Trials, 2006. 1(1): p. e5.

[199] Beeson, J.G. and B.S. Crabb, *Towards a vaccine against Plasmodium vivax malaria.* PLoS Med, 2007. 4(12): p. e350.

[200] VanBuskirk, K.M., et al., *Antigenic drift in the ligand domain of Plasmodium vivax duffy binding protein confers resistance to inhibitory antibodies.* J Infect Dis, 2004. 190(9): p. 1556-62.

[201] Cole-Tobian, J.L., et al., *Strain-specific duffy binding protein antibodies correlate with protection against infection with homologous compared to heterologous plasmodium vivax strains in Papua New Guinean children.* Infect Immun, 2009. 77(9): p. 4009-17.

[202] Verra, F., et al., *Contrasting signatures of selection on the Plasmodium falciparum erythrocyte binding antigen gene family.* Mol Biochem Parasitol, 2006. 149(2): p. 182-90.

[203] Mamillapalli, A., et al., *Polymorphism and epitope sharing between the alleles of merozoite surface protein-1 of Plasmodium falciparum among Indian isolates.* Malar J, 2007. 6: p. 95.

[204] Jiang, L., et al., *Evidence for erythrocyte-binding antigen 175 as a component of a ligand-blocking blood-stage malaria vaccine.* Proc Natl Acad Sci U S A, 2011. 108(18): p. 7553-8.

[205] Barry, A.E., et al., *Population genomics of the immune evasion (var) genes of Plasmodium falciparum.* PLoS Pathog, 2007. 3(3): p. e34.

[206] Chen, D.S., et al., *A molecular epidemiological study of var gene diversity to characterize the reservoir of Plasmodium falciparum in humans in Africa.* PLoS One, 2011. 6(2): p. e16629.

[207] Smith, J.D., et al., *Switches in expression of Plasmodium falciparum var genes correlate with changes in antigenic and cytoadherent phenotypes of infected erythrocytes.* Cell, 1995. 82(1): p. 101-10.

[208] Baruch, D.I., et al., *Immunization of Aotus monkeys with a functional domain of the Plasmodium falciparum variant antigen induces protection against a lethal parasite line.* Proc Natl Acad Sci U S A, 2002. 99(6): p. 3860-5.

[209] Salanti, A., et al., *Evidence for the involvement of VAR2CSA in pregnancy-associated malaria.* J Exp Med, 2004. 200(9): p. 1197-203.

[210] Trimnell, A.R., et al., *Global genetic diversity and evolution of var genes associated with placental and severe childhood malaria.* Mol Biochem Parasitol, 2006.

[211] Hommel, M., et al., *Evaluation of the antigenic diversity of placenta-binding Plasmodium falciparum variants and the antibody repertoire among pregnant women.* Infect Immun, 2010. 78(5): p. 1963-78.

[212] Bockhorst, J., et al., *Structural polymorphism and diversifying selection on the pregnancy malaria vaccine candidate VAR2CSA.* Mol Biochem Parasitol, 2007. 155(2): p. 103-12.

[213] Avril, M., et al., *Antibodies to a full-length VAR2CSA immunogen are broadly strain-transcendent but do not cross-inhibit different placental-type parasite isolates.* PLoS One, 2011. 6(2): p. e16622.

[214] Bigey, P., et al., *The NTS-DBL2X region of VAR2CSA induces cross-reactive antibodies that inhibit adhesion of several plasmodium falciparum isolates to chondroitin sulfate A.* J Infect Dis, 2011. 204(7): p. 1125-33.

[215] Beeson, J.G., et al., *Antigenic differences and conservation among placental Plasmodium falciparum-infected erythrocytes and acquisition of variant-specific and cross-reactive antibodies.* J Infect Dis, 2006. 193(5): p. 721-30.

[216] Hartl, D.L., Clark, A.G. , *Principles of Population Genetics.* 3 ed. 1997, Sunderland, Maryland: Sinauer Associates.

[217] Conway, D.J., *Natural selection on polymorphic malaria antigens and the search for a vaccine.* Parasitol Today, 1997. 13(1): p. 26-9.

[218] Tetteh, K.K., et al., *Prospective identification of malaria parasite genes under balancing selection.* PLoS One, 2009. 4(5): p. e5568.

[219] Ochola, L.I., et al., *Allele frequency-based and polymorphism-versus-divergence indices of balancing selection in a new filtered set of polymorphic genes in Plasmodium falciparum.* Mol Biol Evol, 2010. 27(10): p. 2344-51.

[220] Guerra, C.A., et al., *The international limits and population at risk of Plasmodium vivax transmission in 2009.* PLoS Negl Trop Dis, 2010. 4(8): p. e774.

[221] Zakeri, S., et al., *Circumsporozoite protein gene diversity among temperate and tropical Plasmodium vivax isolates from Iran.* Trop Med Int Health, 2006. 11(5): p. 729-37.

[222] Putaporntip, C., et al., *Diversity in the thrombospondin-related adhesive protein gene (TRAP) of Plasmodium vivax.* Gene, 2001. 268(1-2): p. 97-104.

[223] Ord, R.L., A. Tami, and C.J. Sutherland, *ama1 genes of sympatric Plasmodium vivax and P. falciparum from Venezuela differ significantly in genetic diversity and recombination frequency.* PLoS One, 2008. 3(10): p. e3366.

[224] Gunasekera, A.M., et al., *Genetic diversity and selection at the Plasmodium vivax apical membrane antigen-1 (PvAMA-1) locus in a Sri Lankan population.* Mol Biol Evol, 2007. 24(4): p. 939-47.

[225] Moon, S.U., et al., *High frequency of genetic diversity of Plasmodium vivax field isolates in Myanmar.* Acta Trop, 2009. 109(1): p. 30-6.

[226] Nobrega de Sousa, T., L.H. Carvalho, and C.F. Alves de Brito, *Worldwide genetic variability of the Duffy binding protein: insights into Plasmodium vivax vaccine development.* PLoS One, 2011. 6(8): p. e22944.

[227] Zakeri, S., S. Razavi, and N.D. Djadid, *Genetic diversity of transmission blocking vaccine candidate (Pvs25 and Pvs28) antigen in Plasmodium vivax clinical isolates from Iran.* Acta Trop, 2009. 109(3): p. 176-80.

[228] Hurlbert, S.H., *The non-concept of species diversity: a critique and alternative parameters.* . Ecology, 1971. 52(577-586).

[229] Excoffier, L. and G. Heckel, *Computer programs for population genetics data analysis: a survival guide.* Nat Rev Genet, 2006. 7(10): p. 745-58.

[230] Jalloh, A., et al., *Sequence variation in the T-cell epitopes of the Plasmodium falciparum circumsporozoite protein among field isolates is temporally stable: a 5-year longitudinal study in southern Vietnam.* J Clin Microbiol, 2006. 44(4): p. 1229-35.

[231] Tanabe, K., N. Sakihama, and A. Kaneko, *Stable SNPs in malaria antigen genes in isolated populations.* Science, 2004. 303(5657): p. 493.

[232] Mu, J., et al., *Recombination Hotspots and Population Structure in Plasmodium falciparum.* PLoS Biol, 2005. 3(10): p. e335.

[233] Pritchard, J.K., M. Stephens, and P. Donnelly, *Inference of population structure using multilocus genotype data.* 2000. 155(2): p. 945.

[234] Friedman, S.R. and S. Aral, *Social networks, risk-potential networks, health, and disease.* J Urban Health, 2001. 78(3): p. 411-8.

[235] Bull, P.C., et al., *Plasmodium falciparum antigenic variation. Mapping mosaic var gene sequences onto a network of shared, highly polymorphic sequence blocks.* Mol Microbiol, 2008. 68(6): p. 1519-34.

[236] Conway, D.J., et al., *A principal target of human immunity to malaria identified by molecular population genetic and immunological analyses.* Nat Med, 2000. 6(6): p. 689-92.

[237] Weedall, G.D. and D.J. Conway, *Detecting signatures of balancing selection to identify targets of anti-parasite immunity.* Trends Parasitol, 2010. 26(7): p. 363-9.

[238] Cui, L., et al., *The genetic diversity of Plasmodium vivax populations.* Trends Parasitol, 2003. 19(5): p. 220-6.

[239] Innan, H., *Modified Hudson-Kreitman-Aguade test and two-dimensional evaluation of neutrality tests.* Genetics, 2006. 173(3): p. 1725-33.

[240] Prugnolle, F., et al., *African great apes are natural hosts of multiple related malaria species, including Plasmodium falciparum.* Proc Natl Acad Sci U S A, 2010. 107(4): p. 1458-63.

[241] Tajima, F., *Statistical method for testing the neutral mutation hypothesis by DNA polymorphism.* Genetics, 1989. 123(3): p. 585-95.

[242] Polley, S.D., W. Chokejindachai, and D.J. Conway, *Allele frequency-based analyses robustly map sequence sites under balancing selection in a malaria vaccine candidate antigen.* Genetics, 2003. 165(2): p. 555-61.

12

The Impact of Immune Responses on the Asexual Erythrocytic Stages of *Plasmodium* and the Implication for Vaccine Development

Elke S. Bergmann-Leitner, Elizabeth H. Duncan and Evelina Angov
Department of Molecular Parasitology, Division of Malaria Vaccine Development, Walter Reed Army Institute of Research, USA

1. Introduction

Natural immunity against malaria is acquired after repeated infections for an extended period of time resulting in a state of immunological non-responsiveness against the malaria parasite. This state ultimately prevents the onset of severe disease such as cerebral malaria thereby reducing the risk of death from malaria. Individuals with acquired natural immunity to malaria still harbor parasites (albeit in low densities) in the blood, and therefore natural immunity against malaria is not sterile. For this reason, natural immunity to malaria cannot be compared to immunity achieved against other diseases where the immune response neutralizes and eliminates the pathogen. The second hallmark of natural immunity to malaria is that protection wanes once a "protected" individual leaves the malaria-endemic area indicating that protection depends on continued antigen exposure. Immunity to malaria is stage- and species-specific and distinct immune mechanisms confer protection against the different developmental stages of the parasite. In the case of blood stage infection, passive transfer experiments with purified human immunoglobulins derived from immune individuals living in malaria-endemic areas have demonstrated that antibodies can mediate protection (Cohen et al., 1961; Butcher et al., 1970; Bouharoun-Tayoun et al., 1990). Mechanistic studies revealed that the effect of blood stage-specific antibodies on the asexual erythrocytic parasite depends on their antigen-specificity; antibodies can bind to merozoites, opsonize and target them towards phagocytic cells of the host (Groux and Gysin, 1990), or prevent invasion of new erythrocytes (Perkins, 1991). Once infected, antibodies against asexual blood stage antigens such as Pf332 or MSP-1 inhibit the intra-erythrocytic development of *Plasmodium falciparum* (Ahlborg et al., 1996; Siddique et al., 1998; Bergmann-Leitner et al., 2009). Antibodies directed to antigens expressed by sexual erythrocytic stages (gametocytes) have been shown to prevent transmission of malaria by blocking either the infection of the mosquito or the development in the mosquito (Lavazec and Bourqouin, 2008). As will be outlined in this chapter, it becomes increasingly clear that a blood stage vaccine may never be able to induce sterile protection, but can prevent mortality. Why bother developing blood stage vaccines? Extensive studies characterizing the leading pre-erythrocytic vaccine RTS,S have shown approximately 40% sterile protection of vaccinated US individuals (Kester et al., 2007). Protection in the field is restricted to reduced mortality and morbidity and requires vaccination of young children that have continued exposure to the parasite. Under these circumstances, partial protection (when defined as time to first clinical episode) was approx 30% (Sacarlal et al., 2009). The limited efficacy of pre-erythrocytic vaccines appears to be the result of the fact that even a few sporozoites which escape the vaccine-induced immune response are still capable of establishing full blown blood stage infection. Combining a pre-erythrocytic vaccine such as RTS,S with a blood stage vaccine would assure that individuals, who did not develop sterile immunity (sterile immunity has never been achieved in field trials) would have a reduced risk of dying as a result of the added blood stage component.

This chapter will highlight the major readout methods that are currently used to gauge the efficacy of blood stage vaccines. In the absence of 'protection' models, the study of blood stage vaccines requires the development of *in vitro* assays that predict vaccine efficacy. In the absence of a definitive correlate of protection, the predictive value of these assays still awaits validation. Various target antigens for vaccine development will be highlighted with a special focus on the Merozoite Surface Protein (MSP)-1. Lastly, we will discuss modes of action of immune effector mechanisms against blood stage parasites and provide a preview of next-generation malaria vaccines.

2. Methodological tools to study anti-parasite activities mediated by *Plasmodium*-specific antibodies

The ability to culture blood stage parasites of *P. falciparum* has greatly assisted in our understanding of events associated with maturation of the intra-erythrocytic parasite (Trager and Jensen, 1976; Haynes and Moch, 2002; Haynes et al., 2002). This is underscored by the lack of knowledge for other *Plasmodium* species that have not been successfully established in culture. Once the liver schizonts have reached maturity, the hepatocyte membrane dissolves and the merosome, *i.e.*, the parasitophorous vacuole which resembles a bag containing infectious merozoites, is released from the liver destined for the lung capillaries where infection of erythrocytes occurs (Baer et al., 2007). The erythrocytic life cycle of *P. falciparum* blood stage parasites ranges from 38-48 hrs. During the first 24 hrs the parasite has a ring-like morphology (ring stage parasite) which subsequently develops into a trophozoite that is clearly distinguishable by the increasing amount of DNA and cytoplasm. Further maturation of the parasite into the schizont stage is marked by DNA segmentation resulting in individual nuclei. Additionally, schizonts have increasing amounts of digested hemoglobin (*aka*, malaria pigment or hemozoin). The schizonts rupture after first dissolving the parasitophorous vacuole and then the erythrocyte membrane, thus releasing 16-32 infectious merozoites per new infected erythrocyte (Cowman and Crabb, 2006). This event typically occurs in post capillary venules where the flow rate of the blood is low thereby favoring the rapid invasion of erythrocytes. Free merozoites have a relatively short lifespan and thus it is thought that the invasion event occurs quickly (within 5 minutes). This poses a significant challenge for effector antibodies which have to engage the parasite during this brief period of vulnerability and to block the interactions between host cells and merozoites. Successful active or passive immunotherapy requires providing an ample supply of antigen-specific, high-affinity antibodies capable of blocking a 'tsunami' of parasites every 38-48 hours. Whether this will be achievable to prevent morbidity or whether blood stage vaccine-induced antibodies will only be able to prevent severe disease and mortality is currently the focus of erythrocytic vaccines. Ideally, *in vitro* methods and/or preclinical models would assist in the down-selection of vaccine candidates. However, currently there is no preclinical model that adequately simulates human malaria. In contrast, there are several *in vitro* methods that have been used for analyzing functional antibodies against blood stage parasites *in vitro*. The following methods have been employed extensively in the evaluation of blood stage vaccines and we outline the advantages and drawbacks of the various methods as well as their predictive value.

2.1 Functional assays capturing the biological activity of blood stage, parasite-specific antibodies

Various methods have been developed that allow the measurement of the biological functionality displayed by either the antibodies themselves (growth inhibition assays (GIA) and invasion inhibition assays (IIA)) or antibodies in collaboration with immune cells expressing Fc-receptors (receptors that naturally bind certain immunoglobulin isotypes in order to eliminate antigens bound by antibodies). Antibodies bind their specific pathogen and form "immune complexes". Depending on the class and isotype of the antibody in the immune complex, this interaction leads to different outcomes: (1) the immune complex activates the complement system, *i.e.* complement fixation (which ultimately results in the lysis of the attached pathogen) or (2) the immune complex binds to Fc-receptors, *i.e.* opsonization (mediating uptake of the bound pathogen by the immune cells) or (3) antibody binds to the antigen and inactivates (neutralizes) the pathogen and thus prevents infection. The functional analysis of anti-blood stage antibodies, especially when obtained from individuals in endemic areas, is complicated by the presence of toxic factors or lipids in sera or plasma (such as anti-malarial drugs and anti-coagulants, or oxidized lipids due to long or inadequate sample storage). Eliminating nonspecific toxicities requires purification of the antibodies from serum or plasma using either bulk enrichment techniques (such as precipitation with ammonium sulfate and caprylic acid) or immunoglobulin purification methods (*e.g.*, the use of Protein A, G , L-columns). It should be noted that most anti-malarial drugs can be removed by simply dialyzing the samples (Sy et al., 1990; Persson et al., 2006) which allows the testing of samples where only small volumes are available as is often the case for pediatric specimen. When comparing various methods in regards to yield, purity, integrity and retention of functional activity of recovered antibodies, we found that some methods lead to the selective enrichment of certain isotypes or in some cases fairly unstable immunoglobulin preparations (Bergmann-Leitner et al., 2008b). Also, not all purification methods perform equally well when purifying immunoglobulins from different species. The choice of purification method greatly influences the results obtained in the functional assay and can lead to significant artifacts.

2.1.1 Microscopic analysis

Microscopic evaluation of blood smears stained with Giemsa is the classic method for detecting parasitized erythrocytes (pRBC) and remains the gold standard in clinical trials. It is also used for studying the effect of antibodies on the morphology of the intra-erythrocytic parasite. To detect parasitemia in the blood, thick film-smears are prepared and 100 microscopic fields are screened for the presence of parasites at a 1000x magnification. For quantitation, 200 leukocytes and all pRBC in the respective fields of a thin film-smear are counted. If nine or less pRBC per 200 leukocytes are detected the quantitation is extended to 500 leukocytes. The equipment is readily available in all clinical labs and is fairly cheap. However, since the analysis is done by humans, it is essential that it is performed in a double-blinded fashion to avoid introduction of bias and subjectivity. Moreover, the microscopists have to be highly trained and experienced in slide reading in order to reliably identify malaria parasites in thick and thin film blood smears. The expertise of microscopists has long been recognized as the key issue for evaluating vaccine and malarial drug trials as quantifying parasitemia of malaria infected individuals commonly defines a study's primary endpoint. Furthermore, manual analysis, *i.e.* individual slide reading, is also rather slow and therefore not suitable for high-throughput screening. The microscopic analysis permits the quantification of parasitemia, but cannot objectively characterize changes in morphology which would indicate developmental growth inhibition or retardation.

2.1.2 Flow cytometric analysis

Flow cytometry is an ideal methodology for the automated and objective analysis of large numbers of cells. It provides information about the number of positively stained cells as well as the intensity of staining (Shapiro, 2004). Staining of mature human erythrocytes with DNA dyes allows for the detection of *Plasmodium* infection as these host cells are devoid of DNA unless parasites are present. This analysis reveals both the percentage parasitemia in the culture (% DNA containing cells) as well as the intracellular DNA content which is indicative of the parasite's maturation stages within the infected cells. Various DNA dyes have been reported to be useful for the detection and quantification of pRBC (reviewed in (Grimberg, 2011)). We have compared several DNA dyes side-by-side (*i.e.*, Syto-16, SybrGreen and Hydroethidine) in order to determine their usefulness in measuring invasion and growth inhibition of anti-blood stage antibodies. Using standard DNA binding dyes such as Syto-16 (Brand et al., 2003) and SybrGreen allows only the quantification of pRBC in culture and does not assess the viability of the intra-erythrocytic parasite (Green et al., 1981; Pang et al., 1999; Tebo et al., 2001; Haynes and Moch, 2002). If invasion occurs but the parasite fails to thrive, then the infected cell is detectable. Thus this approach measures only invasion inhibition since antibodies that block invasion result in either low or no parasitemia. In order to assess actual developmental growth inhibition, a different strategy has to be employed:

(1) Measurement of the DNA content of the pRBC as a correlate of the maturation stage of the parasite (Figure 1). A prerequisite for this approach is the tight synchronization of the parasites - either through repeated Percoll/Sorbitol purification or growth in temperature-cycling incubators - prior to setting up the experiment as the analysis requires setting strict cut-off values (see Fig. 1) for the different maturation stages of the parasite (ring/trophozoite/schizont). Such cut-off values have to be established for every parasite clone and isolate and have to be revised whenever culture conditions (new batch of serum/ culture media) change. Failure to control for these changes and the different growth kinetics of isolates and clones results in inaccurate estimates of parasite growth and yields uninterpretable results.

(2) Use of viability DNA stains such as hydroethidine (HE) (van der Heyde et al., 1995). HE-staining depends on the intracellular conversion of HE into ethidium by parasitic NADPH oxidase and has been described in various protozoan systems including malaria to be a reliable metabolic indicator of parasite viability (Wyatt et al., 1991; van der Heyde et al., 1995). The host erythrocytes' enzymatic activity is not sufficient to convert the dye and, therefore, host cells do not introduce artifacts into this analysis.

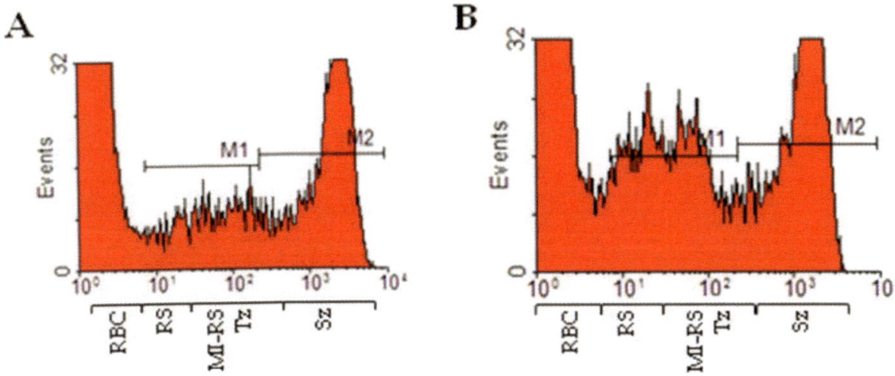

Fig. 1. DNA content of blood cultures infected with *P. falciparum* in the presence of control (malaria-naïve, not growth inhibitory) serum (Panel A) or immune serum (Panel B) determined by flow cytometric analysis. X-axis = Mean fluorescence intensity of Syto-16 DNA staining, Y-axis = arbitrary unit for cell number. Brackets under X-axis indicate the DNA content of uninfected erythrocytes (RBC), ring stage parasites (RS), multiply infected ring stage parasites (MI-RS) and trophozoites (Tz) and schizont stage parasites (Sz). Marker M1 captures young pRBC and M2 mature pRBC and the changes of the proportion have been used to calculate growth inhibition. Panel A serves as reference for healthy, un-impaired parasite growth. Panel B indicates growth retardation as there is a higher prevalence of ring and trophozoite stage parasites compared to the control serum. The difference between the area under the curve for M1 of the test culture and the control culture is used to report the percentage of growth inhibition.

2.1.3 Measurement of invasion inhibition by using transgenic parasites

In an attempt to identify the contribution of MSP-1 mediated invasion inhibition, O'Donnell *et al.* (O'Donnell et al., 2001) developed a *P. falciparum* D10 clone (MAD 20 allele) transgenic in the MSP-1p19 portion where the wildtype sequence was replaced by the p19 of *P. chabaudi*. Testing the inhibitory activity of antibodies against the parental D10 compared to the transgenic parasites identifies the contribution of *P.falciparum* MSP-1 mediated parasite inhibition. Other transgenic parasites have been developed that express the green fluorescence protein to facilitate the detection of the parasites within erythrocytes (O'Donnell et al., 2000). This approach eliminates the need for intracellular DNA staining of pRBCs. Using these parasites requires maintaining an additional parasite strain in the laboratory, which adds cost and labor, but it greatly facilitates the analysis because no additional manipulation of the cultures, *i.e.*, DNA staining, is required to perform the analysis. The analysis would yield similar results as staining with a general DNA dye such as SybrGreen, which allows accurate detection of invasion inhibition while the quantitation of growth inhibition is challenging as outlined above.

2.1.4 Measurement of the metabolic activity of the intra-erythrocytic parasite

An alternative to quantifying either parasitized cells or the DNA content of infected erythrocytes is the measurement of enzymatic activity. The following approaches have been previously described: (1) the quantification of ^{3}H-hypoxanthine incorporation into newly synthesized DNA (Bungener and Nielsen, 1968; Rahman, 1997), (2) the conversion of hydroethidine to ethidium (Wyatt et al., 1991; van der Heyde et al., 1995), and (3) detection/measurement of the parasite-derived lactate dehydrogenase (pLDH) (Makler and Hinrichs, 1993; Prudhomme and Sherman, 1999). Measuring the metabolic activity allows for the detection of parasitized erythrocytes that are viable and metabolically active thus enabling the quantitation of growth inhibition. It should be pointed out that multiple LDH-substrates have been described in the literature for *Plasmodium ssp*. There are, however, qualitative differences between these substrates that will affect the sensitivity and the signal-to-noise ratio. The protocol developed at NIAID/NIH (Kennedy et al., 2002) has demonstrated robustness, reproducibility and specificity (Corran PH, manuscript in preparation). This basic protocol was optimized in our laboratory to accommodate small sample volumes (< 50 μl) and high throughput screening utilizing 384 well plates and assay volumes of ≤ 20 μl (Bergmann-Leitner et al., 2008a).

2.2 The quest for the most sensitive method for identifying anti-parasite activity of anti-malarial antibodies

We have compared four methods in an attempt to identify the most sensitive method capable of measuring an array of functional activities displayed by immune antibodies, namely: (1) GIEMSA-staining of blood smears (with visual detection); (2) flow cytometric analysis using either a standard DNA binding dye (Syto-16) or (3) hydroethidine; and (4) pLDH detection using a substrate specific for the parasitic enzyme LDH (Bergmann-Leitner et al., 2006). The model system to evaluate anti-parasite activities was based on the use of immune sera specific for either AMA-1 (Kennedy et al., 2002) or MSP-1p42 (Angov et al., 2003; Darko et al., 2005) and previously established *P. falciparum* parasite clones (namely 3D7 and FVO). While staining with Giemsa revealed antibody-induced morphological changes in parasite development after exposure to immune serum, directly correlating these changes with parasite viability and thus efficacy of the antibodies is limited due to the subjective nature of the readout method. The DNA dye Syto16 readily permeates membranes of both viable and non-viable cells and thus cannot be used to determine the parasites' viability since any erythrocyte with DNA content will equally be identified as an "infected cell", thus under-estimating the inhibition. Growth inhibition (viability), however, can be determined by either flow cytometric analysis of parasites whose DNA was stained with HE or by measuring the enzymatic activity of pLDH. The conclusion from this comparative study was that the mode of action of antibodies directed against malaria blood stage antigens depends on not only the target antigen but also on the parasite strain. In cases where antibodies primarily mediated invasion inhibition, such as anti-AMA-1 specific antibodies (Triglia et al., 2000; Healer et al., 2004), all four methods yielded similar results.

However, antibodies directed against MSP-1p42 preferentially inhibited invasion or inhibited either parasite growth and development, depending on the parasite test strain. MSP-1 specific antibodies acted on the FVO parasite clone mainly by inhibiting invasion. In contrast, the same antibodies mediated invasion- and growth inhibition in the case of 3D7 parasites (the exact mechanisms involved in this anti-parasite activity will be discussed in section 5). This study demonstrated that readout methods, which can distinguish between invasion inhibition and growth inhibition of the intra-erythrocytic parasite must be employed in order to comprehensively define the antibodies' mechanism of action.

In an effort to increase the sensitivity of the readout methods used to assess the anti-parasite activity through DNA dyes and flow cytometric analysis, multi-cycle experiments have been evaluated (Haynes et al., 2002; Persson et al., 2006), (Bergmann-Leitner, unpublished observations). To this end, cultures were not limited to the length of a single life cycle (40-48 hours duration), but allowed to continue for at least another cycle (72-96 hours duration). Several caveats are associated with this experimental setup: (1) The starting parasitemia of the culture has to be adjusted for each isolate/clone to assure that the parasites will not overgrow after the completion of the first cycle. This would result in the depletion of nutrients and the exhausted culture conditions would result in an overestimation of growth inhibition. One remedy has been to feed the cultures once or repeatedly. This can, however, pose yet another challenge as the exchange of media dilutes the antibodies and without knowing at which stage they will take effect, this manipulation could reduce their biological activity. Replenishing the antibodies when changing the media may lead to an overestimation of the biological effect in cases where the antibodies have already bound to the surface of the pRBC or entered the parasitophorous vacuole. Therefore, adding more antibody artificially increases the total antibody concentration; (2) Outgasing of cultures (*i.e.*, change in the ratio of CO_2 and O_2 in the atmosphere due to exposure to regular air) during the feeding process, can result in reduced invasion or slowed growth; (3) Interrupting invasion events when feeding occurs very closely to the time of schizont rupture. Estimating a safe time frame may be challenging because antibodies may slow the growth of the parasite, but not inhibit it and the growth inhibitory effect would be amplified; and (4) Controlling for proper starting parasitemia and modifying feeding times still leads to reduced multiplication rates in static cultures. Using suspension cultures for larger culture vessels such as 24-well plates and culture flasks yielded similar multiplication rates of the parasites during the second cycle compared to the first cycle (when feeding was also performed). It should be noted, however, that we have been unable to replicate the beneficial effect of suspension cultures when scaling down the assay format to 96 well and 48 well plates (Bergmann-Leitner, unpublished observation).

2.3 Functional assays to evaluate antibody dependent cellular cytotoxicity (ADCC)

Early studies have shown that antibodies *per se* may not be sufficient to block the blood stage parasites (Bouharoun-Tayoun et al., 1990; Ouevray et al., 1994) and a cellular component is involved in the antibody-mediated anti-parasitic effect. Compared to classic antibody-dependent cellular cytotoxicity (ADCC), the postulated antibody-dependent cellular inhibition (ADCI) is mediated only by blood monocytes (not macrophages, polymorphonuclear neutrophils (PMN), lymphocytes, platelets) and primarily by cytophilic immunoglobulin classes (particularly IgG3) that target merozoite surface antigens

(Bouharoun-Tayoun et al., 1995; Tebo et al., 2001). The activation of monocytes through FcγRII triggers the release of soluble TNF-α that in turn blocks the development of adjacent intra-erythrocytic parasites (Bouharoun-Tayoun et al., 1995). Furthermore, a role of FcγRI in contributing to clinical malaria has been suggested based on the functional properties of recombinant human antibodies derived from immune Gambian adults (McIntosh et al., 2007). These antibodies were tested in mice transgenic for human Fc-receptors challenged with transgenic rodent malaria parasites (expressing *Pf*MSP-1p19) in an effort to evaluate the role of antibodies in protection. Another study demonstrated that the activation of monocytic cells requires two distinct Fcγ receptors (FcγRII and FcγRIII) simultaneously engaged by a least two cytophilic IgG molecules, which are part of the same immune complexes (Jafarshad et al., 2007). Finally, the concept of the contribution of Fc receptors in natural immunity is supported by epidemiological studies (Shi et al., 2001; Israelsson et al., 2008; Leoratti et al., 2008).

We conclude from these studies that ADCI as an anti-parasite defense mechanism depends on the target antigen, a concept with significant implications for vaccine development (revisited below in section 4). Experiments measuring the ADCI activity of anti-blood stage antibodies are set up in principle as described for growth/invasion inhibition assays (above): parasite cultures are established at a defined percentage of parasitemia in the presence or absence of immune antibodies and – in addition - in the presence of monocytic cells. Readout methods used are the same as for the standard "growth inhibition" assays as described earlier (our lab prefers the pLDH assay for this purpose). Note that the source and quality of the monocytic cells will greatly influence the results obtained in these experiments: (1) freshly isolated PBMC (plastic adherence *vs.* CD14 MACS separated cells *vs.* monocytic tumor cell lines); (2) resting *vs.* cytokine activated cells; or (3) inter-donor variations. When optimizing the ADCI protocol, it is important that the *in vitro* conditions including the cell types of phagocytes used simulate the *in vivo* setting as closely as possible in order to reproduce the conditions in the malaria infected host. Using cancer cells such as the monocytic tumor cell line THP-1 may not adequately mimic the effector population found in the patient. This is underscored by recent findings that infection and acute malaria can drastically change the phenotype of monocytic subpopulations (Chimma et al., 2009). This includes changes in chemokine receptors as well as functional properties. This was evidenced as monocytic cells derived from patients during an acute malaria infection were superior over the monocytes derived from healthy donor individuals. However, other studies have described significant impairments of monocyte functions due to malaria infection, such as their ability to phagocytize (Leitner and Krzych, 1997). This underscores that there is more to monocytic cells than just the expression of Fc-receptors and that these observations warrant the characterization of effector cells used for *in vitro* assays in an effort to minimize *in vitro* artifacts.

To this end, we tested various methods for generating activated monocytic cells *in vitro* and found that the purification of monocytes with magnetic bead labeled anti-CD14 monoclonal antibody resulted in higher and more reproducible ADCI-activities as compared to cells that were isolated by plastic adherence. Moreover, pre-activating the isolated cells overnight with 300 U/ml IFN-γ reduced the inter-assay variability. Pre-activation also decreased the variability observed between different blood donors consistent with the concept that the stimulation "normalizes" the activation state of the cells (data not published).

What role does the parasite isolate or clone play when measuring ADCI activity? Using a sample from an individual from a malaria-endemic area (Lyon et al., 1997) we were able to detect a differential contribution of ADCI in the growth-inhibition of two *P. falciparum* clones: various amounts of serum in the assay in the presence or absence of monocytes were tested against the 3D7 and FVO parasite clones (Figure 2). The main difference in the clones is the fact that they represent the two distinct MSP-1 alleles (the MAD20 and the Wellcome K1 allele, respectively) and they have also been described as invading either through sialic acid independent (3D7) or dependent (FVO) pathways. The inhibitory activity of serum against 3D7 parasites was not increased by the presence of monocytes while the inhibition of FVO parasites could be amplified by adding monocytes (data not published). This synergistic effect of antibodies and monocytes became apparent when limiting the amount of serum in the assay. More studies are needed to determine the underlying mechanism for this differential effect as this may be a matter of antibody fine specificity (discussed in section 5).

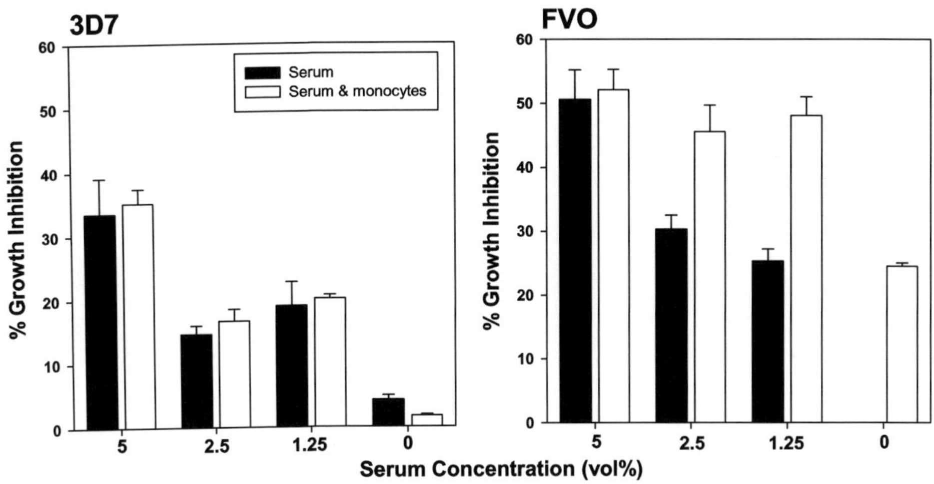

Fig. 2. Effect of inhibitory antibodies and antibody-dependent cellular inhibition on growth of 3D7 (left Panel) and FVO (right Panel) parasite clones. X-axis indicates percentage of human malaria-immune serum in the culture; y-axis shows the % growth inhibition measured by quantifying pLDH. White bars = growth inhibition induced by serum only, black bars = growth inhibition induced by serum and $CD14^{+}$ IFN-γ activated monocytes. Data expressed as mean % growth inhibition, error bars indicate SD.

3. Anti-parasite activities in sera from individuals living in malaria-endemic areas

Protection against malaria mediated by antibodies recognizing the erythrocytic parasite or the parasitized erythrocyte is mediated by several distinct mechanisms: (1) Binding of the antibody to the surface of merozoites can interfere with the invasion of new erythrocytes and opsonize the merozoite, which results in complement activation and/or phagocytosis; (2) Binding to the merozoite may not suffice to block invasion, but antibodies carried into the infected RBC by the merozoite can result in growth inhibition; (3) Binding to pRBC can prevent sequestration, thus exposing the pRBC to conditions that are unfavorable for development, which may lead to increased clearance of pRBC by the spleen; and (4) Binding to pRBC can interfere with rosetting, a prerequisite for invasion. Studying the invasion of erythrocytes by merozoites has resulted in the identification of various invasion pathways, which the parasite can utilize. These pathways can be categorized broadly into: (1) sialic acid dependent and (2) sialic acid independent pathways. Field studies of the anti-parasite activity in sera from individuals with acquired natural immunity have shown that one of the earliest mechanisms to block blood stage parasites is to develop antibodies that interfere with the sialic acid dependent invasion (Baum et al., 2003; Nery et al., 2006; Persson et al., 2008). Antibodies obtained from sera of young African children are more likely to block sialic acid dependent pathways while the ability to block sialic acid independent pathways is acquired after years of exposure to the parasite and with age. Antibodies capable of inhibiting rosetting can mediate protection, which reduces the risk of cerebral malaria (Vigan-Womas et al., 2010). Nevertheless, the actual role of antibodies in protecting against disease in the field remains controversial. While they may reduce the parasite load of individuals living in endemic areas, they do not mediate sterile protection or total suppression of parasites in the blood (Genton et al., 2002). Recently, an apical merozoite antigen (AMA)-1 based vaccine that induces high antibody titers, and high GIA responses *in vitro* in human vaccinees (Ellis et al., 2009) was evaluated for its protective effect in a blood challenge. To this end, the vaccinees were immunized and then challenged with blood infected with the 3D7 parasite clone. While the vaccine was able to reduce the multiplication rate *in vivo*, it was unable to mediate complete elimination of the parasites after a blood challenge (Duncan et al., 2011). This may indicate that either a single antigen such as AMA-1 or blood-stage antigens in general may be able to alleviate the morbidity associated with disease (as seen in the case of natural immunity), but may not be able to induce complete protection against disease.

Longitudinal studies in hyper-endemic malaria transmission areas have revealed factors related to the development (or lack thereof) of malaria-specific antibodies. Due to overlapping malaria infections in high transmission areas, where infections can occur frequently or even daily, it is difficult to study immune responses elicited by and maintained after a discrete infection. Studies in high transmission areas have a limited ability to consider age because participants suffer many unrelated infections during their first 5 years of life, including viral, bacterial and other parasitic diseases. One example is nematode infections, which are quite common in malaria-endemic areas and predispose the host to Th2-type immune responses. Exposure to malaria is an important potential confounder in immune-epidemiological studies. Therefore, the inadequate measurement and adjustment for differences in exposure may lead to the underestimation of the strength of associations between immunological variables and malaria incidence (Kinyanjui et al., 2009). The strongest evidence that antibodies are important mediators of naturally acquired immunity is from passive transfer experiments of antibody from immune adults used to treat children with severe *P. falciparum* malaria (Cohen et al., 1961; McGregor and Carrington, 1963; Bouharoun-Tayoun et al., 1990). IgG and IgM antibodies present in sera of malaria-exposed individuals recognize and bind directly to trophozoites or schizonts. Neutralization and agglutination of merozoites and pRBC by these antibodies are reported as possible protective mechanisms during *Plasmodium* infection (Cohen and Butcher, 1971).

IgM antibodies are characterized by lower affinity for antigen compared to their IgG counterparts because little or no somatic hypermutation and clonal selection has occurred. IgM antibodies form pentamers to compensate for the lower affinity, which results in a higher overall avidity due to increased number of binding sites. Evidence for a protective role of IgM against malaria infection (Wahlgren et al., 1986; Boudin et al., 1993) or against severe malaria (Brasseur et al., 1990) has been reported.

Evidence from field studies in Ghana (Dodoo et al., 2000), Senegal (Oeuvray et al., 2000) and East Asia (Soe et al., 2004) suggest that cytophilic antibodies are associated with a lower risk for subsequent clinical malaria episodes. These isotypes are also associated with the antibody-dependent cellular inhibition as discussed above. The importance of immunoglobulin isotypes in addition to the antigen specificity of the humoral response is underscored by studies that report an association between the levels of noncytophilic antibodies and clinical malaria incidence. IgG4 antibodies are preferentially induced after repeated exposure (Aalberse et al., 1983a; Aalberse et al., 1983b) and this isotype is associated with enhanced risk of infection and with a high risk of clinical malaria episodes (Aucan et al., 2000).

The attitude towards the use of measuring growth inhibition as an immune correlate has changed over the past five years. Invasion or growth inhibitory (GIA) activity was considered a reliable predictor of vaccine efficacy and the results from these assays were used to down-select potential vaccine candidates. Initially, GIA activity was determined by using purified immunoglobulins from preclinical or clinical trials at high concentrations and from these studies, strong inhibition was frequently observed. However, the same vaccines that generated very "high" GIA activities in rabbits and other preclinical models failed to induce protection in naïve US individuals (Spring et al., 2009; Duncan et al., 2011). In residents from malaria-endemic areas, GIA activity is, however, a common factor associated with protection against clinical disease (Dent et al., 2008). In this study, malaria-infected participants were drug-cured and followed up until their next malaria infection. Participants whose sera exhibited higher growth inhibition prior to drug cure were protected for significantly longer periods of time than those participants whose antibodies mediated only low GIA activities. Moreover, an age-dependent effect was observed in that GIA activity inversely correlated with the age of study participants. Another confounding factor is the historical exposure of study participants as vaccine efficacy differs dramatically between individuals with no prior malaria history *vs.* residents from malaria-endemic areas. For example, an AMA-1 vaccine tested in US naïve study participants resulted in relatively high GIA activities, but the same vaccine failed to induce either GIA activity or protection as defined by time to the next malaria episode when given to individuals in Mali (Miura et al., 2011).

Review of the scientific literature on blood stage malaria vaccines reveals no straightforward strategy for evaluating a successful blood stage vaccine. A variety of reasons may be responsible for the contradictory outcomes.

- Differences in the transmission rates (intensity and stability) and the short lifespan of malaria specific antibodies can skew the measurements and conclusions. Therefore, directly comparing study results from different geographic regions that are not matched by transmission rates and seasons should be avoided. Transmission rates may have an impact on the clinical outcome of malaria episodes as well as on the induction of natural immunity.

- Differences in the kinetics of induction of natural immunity (mainly caused by high transmission rates) may influence the immune factors mediating protection.
- Differences in the definitions of clinical malaria and study endpoints. In some settings, are the individuals with no signs of malaria truly protected or simply not exposed to the parasite?
- The quality of plate antigens used for the ELISA: Proteins used for *in vitro* analyses may be of inferior quality due to misfolding or truncation. Recombinant proteins may not represent the native antigen structure. Moreover, for the analysis of MSP-1 specific immune responses induced by natural exposure to the parasite, most investigators have focused on the MSP-1p19 fragment rather than the MSP-1p42 protein, which is initially presented on the merozoite surface.
- Mismatching of recombinant antigens and parasite phenotype: In many studies, the parasite variant prevalent in the study area is not matched with the recombinant protein used for the *in vitro* analysis (*e.g.*, plate antigen for ELISA assay).
- Differences in the age of study participants: concentrations of malaria-specific antibodies are age dependent and, therefore, only comparisons of study participants with similar ages are valid.
- Lack of information about study participants' conditions such as the use of bed nets, use of anti-malarial drugs or folk-medicine, co-infection with other parasites, bacteria and viruses.
- Incompatibility in study design: in some cases study participants are pre-treated with anti-malarial drugs to clear parasites from the circulation prior to immunization while in other studies vaccines are administered while study participants have – in some cases significant numbers of- parasites in the blood. Therefore, it is inappropriate to compare vaccine potency and efficacy between such studies.

4. Identification of antigens that are targeted by immune responses in immune individuals

The merozoite consists of the merozoite surface coat, the micronemes, the rhoptries, apicoplast and a nucleus. From each of these components several antigens have been isolated and their immunological potential and biological function has been evaluated.

4.1 Merozoite surface coat antigens

Several antigens expressed on the merozoite surface coat have been evaluated as vaccine candidates. Highlighted in this section are the most frequently targeted of those antigens:

- MSP-1: the properties and functions of this antigen will be discussed in detail in Section 5 since this antigen represents a major blood stage vaccine candidate (Ockenhouse et al., 2006; Ogutu et al., 2009).
- MSP-2: immunization with the recombinant protein MSP-2 protects non-human primates and has yielded allele-specific reduced parasite density in field studies (Genton et al., 2002). Much of the development of MSP-2 as a vaccine in the field has been hampered by the fact that MSP-2 is an unstructured protein that tends to form amyloid fibrils in solution (Genton et al., 2003). Therefore, quality control of manufactured vaccines is difficult without a known structure or conformation-dependent antibodies.

- MSP-3: this protein is non-covalently attached to the surface of the merozoite. This is different from MSP-1 and MSP-2, which are GPI-anchored proteins. Disruption of the MSP-3 gene is not lethal while genetic knockouts of MSP-1 and MSP-2 are. Similar to MSP-1, allelic dimorphism has been reported. MSP-3 specific antibodies found in sera from malaria-endemic areas are associated with protective immunity (Soe et al., 2004). MSP-3 based vaccines have been designed as long peptides representing the conserved C-terminus of the antigen (Druilhe et al., 2005; Sirima et al., 2007). Anti-parasite activity of MSP-3 specific antibodies was not evident unless monocytic cells were used in the assay (ADCI).
- Glutamate-rich protein (GLURP): this antigen is not only expressed on the merozoite surface, but also on the liver stage parasite making it an attractive potential target for a multi-stage vaccine. The N-terminal region of the antigen is quite conserved and thus synthetic peptides representing the N-terminal non-repeat region have been tested in the clinic. Antibodies induced by these GLURP-peptides were able to inhibit parasite growth in the presence of monocytes indicating that - similar to MSP-3 - anti-GLURP antibodies act through ADCI (Hermsen et al., 2007). Several clinical studies have been conducted with GLURP alone (Hermsen et al., 2007) or in combination with MSP-3 (Esen et al., 2009; Belard et al., 2011).

4.2 Antigens within merozoite organelles

Antigens found in the apical organelles of the merozoites such as the apical membrane antigen (AMA)-1 or the erythrocyte binding antigen (EBA-175 RII) have long been studied due to their immunogenicity or biological function. While the exact function of AMA-1 is unknown, EBA-175 has been better characterized. EBA-175 is found in the micronemes of the merozoite and is secreted by merozoites in order to bind to erythrocytes that are ready for invasion. This binding facilitates the attachment of merozoites to the coated erythrocytes in a strain-specific manner (Camus and Hadley, 1985). EBA-175 is a member of a family of binding proteins such as EBA-140, EBA-181, MAEBL; all of these antigens share a receptor binding domain (Region (R)-II). The analysis of sera from malaria-endemic areas for the presence of EBA-175 specific antibodies revealed some association with protection in children that have higher antibody titers (reviewed in (Fowkes et al., 2010)). Recently, an EBA-175 based vaccine yielded some clinical efficacy (El Sahly et al., 2010).

AMA-1 is a highly polymorphic antigen generated in the rhoptries of the merozoites and it appears on the parasite's surface just before invasion occurs. AMA-1 is highly immunogenic and anti-AMA-1 antibody responses are found in sera from individuals living in malaria-endemic areas. Another promising feature of this antigen is the fact that AMA-1 is expressed on sporozoites and thus the antigen could act as a pre-erythrocytic as well as an erythrocytic vaccine. Analysis of AMA-1 specific antibodies in growth inhibition assays provided even more promise as the antibody activity is typically very high compared to other blood stage antigens. A clinical study in which volunteers were challenged by mosquito bite revealed that vaccination with AMA-1 was unable to provide sterile protection and only yielded a limited delay in the development of parasitemia in vaccinees compared to challenge control subjects (Spring et al., 2009). Characterization of the AMA-1 gene sequence revealed a fatal characteristic of this antigen which will likely preclude its use as a malaria vaccine in the field: well over 150 allelic variants of the antigen have been reported (Takala et al., 2009) and humoral responses against AMA-1 indicate that immunity is allele-specific and therefore, an AMA-based vaccine would primarily provide strain-specific protection at best. Efforts are underway to develop AMA-1 vaccines that induce allele-cross-reactive responses to overcome this limitation (Remarque et al., 2008; Dutta et al., 2010). However, the success of any AMA-1 based malaria vaccines is also impeded by the fact that sera from malaria-endemic areas appear to contain antibodies capable of blocking the activity of AMA-1 specific antibodies (Miura et al., 2008).

4.3 Antigens expressed on the surface of infected erythrocytes

The access of antibodies to merozoite antigens is limited as merozoites quickly invade new erythrocytes. Antibodies have the ability to gain entry to into infected erythrocytes (Bergmann-Leitner et al., 2009), but cannot mediate ADCI and would act independently of phagocytic cells as described above. Therefore, efforts are underway to identify antigens on pRBC which are theoretically always accessible for binding by specific antibodies. The surface localization of the antigens indicates that they are crucial for sequestration of the pRBC in the placenta or post-capillary venules. This warrants their exploration as potential vaccine targets. The variant surface antigens (VSA) (reviewed in (Hviid, 2010)) have been shown to mediate sequestration of the parasite and immune responses towards these antigens confer protection in a strain-specific manner. One of the members, the *P. falciparum* erythrocyte membrane protein (*Pf*EMP)-1, has been reported to be encoded by the *var* gene family and displays varying immunogenicity depending on the variant that is generated (Bull et al., 2005). One of these variants, *var2csa* is expressed by parasites that sequester in the placenta leading to severe malaria attacks in primagravid women often resulting in miscarriage and/or death of the mother (reviewed in (Beeson and Duffy, 2005)). This has led to efforts to develop vaccines that will be administered prior to or early in pregnancy (Avril et al., 2009).

4.4 Multi-antigen responses: Reducing the risk for clinical infection or reducing parasite density

The analysis of naturally acquired antibodies induced by the malaria parasite in an attempt to identify their antigen-specificity is challenging. Studies have frequently focused on a few select antigens, thus ignoring this complexity and the possibility of synergy in the response to multiple antigens. The complexity of these humoral responses was demonstrated using microarray assays in which 18 recombinant antigen fragments spanning various regions and alleles of four leading vaccine candidates (namely, MSP-1, MSP-2, MSP-3 and AMA-1) were tested (Gray et al., 2007). The results clearly demonstrate complex combinations of specific antibodies leading to an association with some form of protection. Reactivity to individual antigens did not correlate with protection, but combinations of antibodies to AMA-1 and allelic variants of MSP-2 were prevalent in individuals protected against clinical malaria.

A field study in Senegal in which factors such as reappearance of parasites, asymptomatic carriage of parasites, time to first clinical episode, and incidence of clinical episodes were considered led to the observation that antibodies to NANP, MSP-1p19, *Pf*EMP-3, *Pf*EB200 were associated with a lower risk for severe disease (Perraut et al., 2003). Another comprehensive study conducted in Senegal (305 children followed over 1 year) showed that different mechanisms mediate protection: higher levels of IgG1 specific for GLURP and IgG3 for MSP-2 in children correlate with resistance to malaria and high-level parasitemia compared to malaria-susceptible children (Courtin et al., 2009). Higher anti-MSP-1 IgG1 levels were associated with protection against high-density parasitemia. The study also evaluated the *in vitro* anti-parasite activity of the sera from these children and reported an age-dependent decline in the *in vitro* GIA activity of the sera. The GIA activity was dependent on anti-MSP-1, anti-AMA-1 and anti-MSP-2 specific antibody titers.

A recent comprehensive meta-analysis of 33 clinical studies investigated the relationship between anti-merozoite antibodies and the incidence rate of malaria (Fowkes et al., 2010). The closest association between antibody titers and reduced risk was observed with IgG specific for the C-terminus of MSP-3 and MSP-1 (MSP-1p19). In contrast, antibodies directed to the N-terminus of MSP-1 and the presence of antibodies to MSP-2 was not significantly associated with protection. The analysis also revealed a positive association between reduced risk for infection and antibody titers against AMA-1 and GLURP-R0.

5. MSP-1 and its role in immunity and infection

Our laboratory has focused on the major merozoite surface protein -1 (MSP-1). This antigen was identified in immune complexes from merozoite lysates (gp195), which provided the rationale for developing vaccines against it (Lyon et al., 1997). MSP-1 is first produced as a 195kD precursor that undergoes two successive proteolytic cleavage events (Blackman et al., 1994). The second processing event occurs immediately before invasion, resulting in the cleavage of the p42 molecule into a p33 and a p19 fragment. The p19 fragment remains attached to the merozoite surface through a GPI anchor (Gerold et al., 1996) and is comprised of two epidermal growth factor (EGF)-like domains (Morgan et al., 1999), which may have a role in the invading complex. Serological studies have provided significant evidence suggesting that immune responses directed against the C-terminus of MSP-1 (MSP-1p19 and MSP-1p42) are associated with immunity in preclinical models (Long et al., 1994; Egan et al., 1999; Darko et al., 2005; Parkkinen et al., 2006). Moreover, protective immunity as defined by lower mortality and morbidity of individuals residing in endemic areas was also associated with MSP-1p19 (Egan et al., 1999; John et al., 2004).

5.1 The role of MSP-1 in natural immunity

Various biological factors influencing the function of MSP-1 specific antibodies have been reported in individuals with natural immunity:

(1) The role of MSP-1 specific antibody titers, isotype and the association with protection and/or reduction in morbidity:

A meta-analysis of 33 clinical studies revealed that the presence of MSP-1p19 specific antibodies is associated with a lower incidence rate of malaria (Fowkes et al., 2010). Moreover, high levels of anti-PfMSP-1p19 immunoglobulin G were associated with reduced malaria in an age-adjusted multivariate analysis (Perraut et al., 2005). In contrast, other reports failed to show any associations between MSP-1p19 (MSP-1) Abs and clinical outcome (Dodoo et al., 1999; Nebie et al., 2008). At this point we can only speculate about the cause of this discrepancy. As outlined above, the differences in the methodology and/or choice of plate antigen may be responsible for some of these issues. It is, however, interesting to note that full length MSP-1p42 was only used in one study as the plate antigen and this study reported a reduced risk of malaria (Al-Yaman et al., 1996).

(2) The role of antibody isotype and functional activity against the parasite:

Longitudinal studies have demonstrated an association between the IgM and IgG responses to MSP-1p19 and the degree of clinical disease and anemia in infants and pregnant women (Branch et al., 1998). Similarly, high antibody levels of MSP-1 specific IgG1 were associated with reduced morbidity (Riley et al., 1992; Al-Yaman et al., 1996) with protection against high-level parasitemia (Fowkes et al., 2010) and clinical disease (Egan et al., 1996; Cavanagh et al., 2004; Soe et al., 2004).

(3) The role of fine specificity of antibodies and association with protection:

IgG derived from sera obtained from Kenyan residents were tested for their impact on parasite viability and growth. The results demonstrated that the invasion inhibitory antibodies were specific for the C-terminal MSP-1p19 (John et al., 2004). Overall, there was a lack of association of total IgG or IgG subclass Abs to MSP-1p19 measured by ELISA with either invasion-inhibitory activity or protection against infection. In contrast, a study analyzing sera from children in West Africa (Sierra Leone and Gambia) demonstrated a strong association between antibody titers to the C-terminus of MSP-1 (MSP-1p19) and protection against clinical malaria and high level parasitemia (Egan et al., 1996). Thus, the fine specificity (*i.e.*, epitope specificity) of the MSP-1 specific antibodies appears to be important and testing only for antibody titers to the total molecule or a fragment may result in the loss of an association with a clinical response (Corran et al., 2004; Okech et al., 2004). The C-terminus of the MSP-1 is comprised of two EGF-like domains and depending on which of the domains the antibodies recognize results in either growth inhibition or no functional activity against the parasite (Chappel et al., 1994; Darko et al., 2005).

5.2 Efficacy of MSP-1 based vaccines in naïve and malaria-exposed individuals

Several clinical trials have been conducted testing either MSP-1p42 or MSP-1p19 as vaccine candidates. The objective of using the larger subunit, MSP-1p42, was to ensure that potential helper epitopes, which can induce antibodies are present in the immunogen. Moreover, the N-terminus p33 portion of the molecule contains most of the known T cell epitopes. The nature of the C-terminus, *i.e.*, due to several disulfide bridges associated with the EGF-like domains, renders the structure rigid and thus resistant to processing by antigen presenting cells, and therefore does not contain any dominant T cell epitopes. Thus, using the full length p42 fragment, which is expressed on pRBC starting at the trophozoite stage, would allow antibodies to bind to the parasites even inside the pRBC thereby potentially preventing the rupture of schizonts. This fact motivated two institutions (National Institute of Health (NIH) and Walter Reed Army Institute of Research (WRAIR)) to proceed with two independent MSP-1p42 based vaccines. At the NIH, a mixture of MSP-1p42 (FVO) and MSP-1p42 (3D7) was adjuvanted with Alhydrogel together with or without the addition of CpG7909 (Ellis et al., 2010) while the WRAIR vaccine consisted of single-allele vaccines, MSP-1p42 (3D7) (Ockenhouse et al., 2006) or MSP-1p42 (FVO) (Spring et al., manuscript in preparation), adjuvanted with GSK's adjuvant system, $AS02_A$ or $AS01_B$, respectively. Both were tested in US naïve individuals. All studies reported good immunogenicity and - in the case of the single allele vaccine - moderate growth inhibitory activity was induced. The MSP-1p42 vaccines generated at WRAIR underwent further clinical evaluation in Phase Ib studies conducted in Kenya (Stoute et al., 2007) and Mali (Thera et al., 2006), where adults were immunized with the MSP-1p42 (3D7) adjuvanted in $AS02_A$. In Kenya, although pre-existing MSP-1p42 antibody titers in the participants were high, they could be boosted by the vaccine. In addition, Phase Ib (Withers et al., 2006) and Phase IIb (Ogutu et al., 2009) studies were conducted in Kenyan children (1-4 years old) using the same vaccine formulation. Results from this study indicated that younger children mounted stronger vaccine responses in terms of the magnitude of the antibody response. Sera from the Phase IIb study displayed strong growth inhibitory activity against the heterologous FVO parasites indicating that the predominant strain circulating at the time of natural exposure was different from the vaccine strain 3D7 (Angov et al., manuscript in preparation). Growth inhibitory activity to the 3D7 parasites was only observed in a small proportion of the study population with no significant difference between the rabies control group (Rabipur) and the malaria vaccine group. Some 3D7 specific GIA activity was reversible by antigen add-back confirming that some of the activity in the sera was due to MSP-1 specific antibodies. The major conclusion from this trial was that although the vaccine was safe and immunogenic, in the context of the heterologous exposure, the vaccine did not induce sufficiently cross-reactive responses. Future studies should include MSP-1p42 allele(s) that are better matched to the dominant circulating parasites. Another important consideration is to clear parasitemia in the study participants prior to and during the course of the vaccination. The presence of parasites during vaccination could lead to competitive immune responses thus curtailing the vaccine's potential.

Some vaccine approaches have focused on the MSP-1p19 fragment rather than the full-length MSP-1p42 since this region of the molecule contains the highly conserved functionally important B cell dominant epitopes. In one particular construct, helper T cell epitopes from tetanus toxoid were used to generate a chimeric P30P2-MSP-1p19 protein (Keitel et al., 1999). Others approached the lack of T cell help by generating a chimeric AMA-1/MSP-1p19 vaccine, which was tested in a Phase Ia trial (Malkin et al., 2008). This vaccine induced antibodies to both antigens; however the antibodies reacted primarily to the recombinant antigens by ELISA, less well by immunofluorescence assay (IFA) on whole parasites, and showed no activity in growth inhibition assays.

Therefore, with regards to further characterizing of MSP-1-based vaccine approaches, there is a need for reliable readout preclinical methods to enable prediction of protection and to facilitate the down-selection of vaccine candidates. One such attempt was the development of a transgenic rodent malaria parasite (*P. berghei*) expressing the *P. falciparum* MSP-1p19 transgene (De Koning-Ward et al., 2003). These parasites may be useful in the down-selection of vaccine candidates by either immunization strategies in the murine model (which does not necessarily address immunogenicity in humans) or passive transfer strategies to characterize the immune potential of antibodies induced in vaccinated individuals. Moreover, a recent report suggests that some anti-MSP-1 specific antibodies may mediate ADCI. Due to the incomplete compatibility between human Abs and murine Fc receptors, current mouse models are unable to use this pathway and may lead to false negative results. There are some experimental alternatives such as transgenic mice that express one of the human Fc receptors (CD32 or CD64) or humanized mice. Humanization refers to irradiated mice that have been reconstituted with human leukocytes (Badell et al., 2000; Pleass et al., 2003) or hematopoietic stem cells which leads to the production of an array of human blood cells in the mice.

5.3 Biological effect of MSP-1 specific antibodies on parasite growth and function

Characterizing immune responses induced by MSP-1 vaccines revealed that several factors impact the immunogenicity and functional activity of the induced antibodies (vaccine platforms will be discussed in detail in Section 6): (1) the expression system used for the production of the recombinant protein (*i.e., E. coli*, baculovirus, or yeast) (Arnot et al., 2008; Reed et al., 2009), (2) the amino-acid sequence used for vaccine development (*i.e.* full length gp195, MSP-1p42 or MSP-1p19) (Stowers et al., 2001; Woehlbier et al., 2006) and (3) the vaccine platform used to deliver the MSP vaccine (*i.e*, recombinant protein, recombinant viral vectors or DNA vaccines).

Our laboratory has intensively studied the anti-parasite effects induced by MSP-1p42 specific antibodies. Early observations indicated that MSP-1 specific antibodies impacted the various parasite strains differently depending on their classification as MAD20 or Wellcome/K1-like. These two alleles differ markedly in their p33 fragments while only by four amino acids (E-TSR *vs.* Q-KNG, respectively) in the p19 portion of the molecule. To this end, MSP-1 specific antibodies were able to significantly delay the intra-erythrocytic development of the 3D7, but not the FVO parasite clone (Bergmann-Leitner et al. 2009). In the case of FVO parasites, anti-MSP-1p42 antibodies prevented schizont rupturing by stalling or arresting intra-erythrocytic parasite development likely through direct interactions with intra-erythrocytic parasites within the parasitophorous vacuole, which is putatively connected to the surface of the pRBC by the parasitophorous duct. This duct gives antibodies, but not larger immune components access to the parasite inside the vacuole (Bergmann-Leitner et al., 2009). In contrast, the same antisera tested on the 3D7 parasite clone were unable to interfere with the release of the merozoites. These antibodies were still able to agglutinate merozoites and interfere with invasion. We expanded our analysis to the parasite clone CAMP/FUP that has a p33 and a p19 EGF-like domain 1 identical to the sequence of the 3D7 parasite clone, and an EGF-like domain 2 identical to the FVO parasite clone. We observed the same response pattern as reported for the FVO parasite indicating that antibodies within the EGF-like domain might be responsible for stalling the rupture of the schizonts. In contrast, no significant growth inhibition was observed following successful invasion indicating that EGF-like domain 1 specific antibodies may be mediating this particular biological effect. To test this working hypothesis, the activity of affinity purified antibodies specific to the entire p19 or each of the EGF-like domains were compared to the source material (antibodies induced by immunization with the MSP-1p42 vaccine representing either the FVO or the 3D7 allele). We concluded that only antibodies that bound to regions within the p42 or to the p19 subunit, but not the EGF-like domain 1 or 2 subunits, displayed growth inhibitory activities. This was surprising given previous observations suggesting that responses directed to the p19 were associated with reduced parasite density or clinical disease (see above). However, the proper folding of the recombinant fragments used, which represent the two EGF-like domains has not yet been confirmed. This result may indicate that protective epitopes may depend on proper tertiary structure of the molecule. In support of this theory, it has been reported that inhibitory anti-MSP-1 specific antibodies map to epitopes formed through the "properly" folded p19 subunit and not to its sub-domains (McBride and Heidrich, 1987; Uthaipibull et al., 2001).

One biological function known to be displayed by some MSP-1 specific antibodies is the inhibition of the secondary processing of the MSP-1 molecule into the p33 and the p19 portion (Blackman et al., 1994). This activity was found in sera from individuals with acquired natural immunity (Patino et al., 1997). In this assay, merozoites are prepared from synchronized blood stage cultures and their ability to process MSP-1p42 into p33 and p19 in the presence or absence of immune antibodies is evaluated. This method is qualitative at best and due to its nature not designed for high-throughput testing. Thus, very few laboratories use the technique for the evaluation of functional activity in immune sera.

6. Future direction

The current body of literature clearly supports the development of a blood stage vaccine. Although such a vaccine would not prevent infection, it can reduce morbidity and mortality associated with malaria infection and therefore such a vaccine would save the lives of many residents of malaria-endemic areas. The experience and knowledge gained from these studies should be used to rationally design new vaccine formulations and future clinical trials. Factors that need to be considered for their success are:

(1) *Vaccine platform.* Most erythrocytic vaccines tested so far are based on recombinant, soluble proteins. When using recombinant proteins it is paramount to assure proper, thus native-like, protein folding. Sera from malaria-endemic areas are a useful tool to establish the degree of cross-reactivity between the recombinant vaccine and the "native" antigen. Alternative vaccine platforms to those primarily described here, soluble proteins plus adjuvant, are particle-based approaches. When using this approach it is important to assure proper orientation of the protein on the particle. Some proteins that are inherently unstructured such as MSP-2 could benefit from particle formation because the particle provides a stabilizing scaffold. Moreover, the distance between the epitopes and the density may be crucial in order to induce proper immune responses. Such particle presentation could be achieved by using either recombinantly expressed antigen on whole-killed bacteria or viruses. For example, mouse studies using recombinant adenovirus encoding MSP-1 demonstrated "protection" (defined by the authors as delayed and lower parasitemia) (Draper et al., 2009).

(2) *Development of preclinical and clinical models that better predict human anti-malarial responses.* When using preclinical animal models, the parasite growth kinetic is frequently different between those *Plasmodium* species that are suitable for the respective animal model and *P. falciparum* thus failing to simulate the clinical situation. Testing vaccine candidates in animals can be challenging when testing *P. falciparum* antigens: except for one confirmed antigen, *Pf*CelTOS, (Bergmann-Leitner et al., 2010), malaria antigens are relatively species-specific, *i.e.,* immunization with *P. falciparum* antigens does not confer protection against a heterologous *Plasmodium* species. Thus, investigators often make their decisions based solely on immunogenicity in the animal model (cellular and/or humoral responses notionally thought to be important). Alternatively, investigators have searched for orthologs of the *P. falciparum* antigen in the respective *Plasmodium* species relevant for their preclinical model to conduct immunization and challenge studies. A caveat of this approach is that the ortholog may have a different function than the *P. falciparum* antigen in human malaria or there simply may not be a valid ortholog (*e.g. P. falciparum* LSA-1 does not have an ortholog in

rodent *Plasmodia*). Another important consideration for the establishment of relevant models of human malaria is the immunization and challenge routes. Challenge routes should take into consideration the natural inoculation route. Our work with pre-erythrocytic antigens has shown that vaccine efficacy can vary significantly if the challenge route is changed (intravenous *vs.* mosquito bite) and thus the efficacy of a vaccine could be over- or underestimated if an artificial challenge method is used (Leitner et al., 2010) which may bypass vaccine-induced effector mechanisms (Vanderberg et al., 2007). For erythrocytic antigens this has been an issue as well because - until recently - it was ethically inconceivable to challenge human volunteers with malaria-infected blood due to the risk of transmitting life threatening blood borne diseases. However, extensive testing of the blood source used for the challenge has allowed a limited challenge study with the understanding that significant improvements are needed before blood challenges can be performed routinely similar to the mosquito bite challenges (Moorthy et al., 2009). A final issue to consider is that blood stage challenge in humans may not fully predict the situation where an individual receives a blood stage vaccine followed by mosquito bite challenge, as the vaccine-induced immune responses may be edited (*i.e.*, altered) by the sporozoite and the liver-stage infection.

(3) Improving surrogate readout assays to down-select vaccine candidates. At this time, different assays are being used as surrogate markers for down-selecting vaccine candidates. Without an immune correlate of protection, the predictive value of these readout methods remains questionable. Therefore, identifying immune correlates for the various target antigens is necessary to 'validate' the readout methods and allow their use for rational down-selection of vaccine candidates

7. Acknowledgments

This work was supported by the U.S. Agency for International Development under project number 936-3118, award number GHA-T-00-08-00007-01, and by the United States Army Medical Research and Materiel Command.

8. Disclaimer

The authors' views are private and are not to be construed as official policy of the Department of Defense or the U.S. Army or the Centers for Disease Control.

9. References

Aalberse, R.C., Dieges, P.H., Knul-Bretlova, V., et al., 1983a. IgG4 as a blocking antibody. Clin Rev Allergy 1, 289-302.

Aalberse, R.C., van der Gaag, R. & van Leeuwen, J., 1983b. Serological aspect of IgG4 antibodies. I. Prolonged immunization results in an IgG4-restricted response. J Immunol 130, 722-726.

Ahlborg, N., Igbal, J., Bjork, L., et al., 1996. *Plasmodium falciparum*: differential parasite growth inhibition mediated by antibodies to the antigens Pf332 and Pf155/RESA. Exp Parasitol 82, 155-163.

Al-Yaman, F., Genton, B., Kramer, K.J., et al., 1996. Assessment of the role of naturally acquired antibody levels to *Plasmodium falciparum* merozoite surface protein-1 in protecting Papua New Guinean children from malaria morbidity. Am J Trop Med Hyg 54, 443-448.

Angov, E., Aufiero, B.M., Turgeon, A.M., et al., 2003. Development and pre-clinical analysis of a *Plasmodium falciparum* Merozoite Surface Protein-1(42) malaria vaccine. Mol Biochem Parasitol 128, 195-204.

Arnot, D.E., Cavanagh, D.R., Remarque, E.J., et al., 2008. Comparative testing of six antigen-based malaria vaccine candidates directed toward merozoite-stage *Plasmodium falciparum*. Clin. Vaccine Immunol 15, 1345-1355.

Aucan, C., Traore, Y., Tall, F., et al., 2000. High immunoglobulin G2 (IgG2) and low IgG4 levels are associated with human resistance to *Plasmodium falciparum* malaria. Infect Immun 68, 1252-1258.

Avril, M., Hathaway, M.J., Carrwright, M.M., et al., 2009. Optimizing expression of the pregnancy malaria vaccine candidate,VAR2CSA in *Pichia pastoris*. Mal J 8, e143.

Badell, E., Oeuvray, C., Moreno, A., et al., 2000. Human malaria in immunocompromised mice: an *in vivo* model to study defense mechanisms against *Plasmodium falciparum*. J Exp Med 192, 1653-1660.

Baer, K., Klotz, C., Kappe, S.H., et al., 2007. Release of hepatic *Plasmodium yoelii* merozoites in the pulmonary microvasculature. PLoS Pathog 3, e171.

Baum, J., Pinder, M. & Conway, D.J., 2003. Erythrocyte invasion phenotypes of *Plasmodium falciparum* in The Gambia. Infect Immun 71, 1856-1863.

Beeson, J.G. & Duffy, P.E., 2005. The immunology and pathogenesis of malaria during pregnancy. Curr Top Microbiol Immunol 297, 187-227.

Belard, S., Issifou, S., Hounkpatin, A.B., et al., 2011. A randomized controlled phase Ib trial of the malaria vaccine candidate GMZ2 in African children. PLoS ONE 6, e22525.

Bergmann-Leitner, E.S., Duncan, E.H., Mullen, G.E., et al., 2006. Critical evaluation of different methods for measuring the functional activity of antibodies against malaria blood stage antigens. Am J Trop Med Hyg 75, 437-442.

Bergmann-Leitner, E.S., Duncan, E.H., Burge, J.R., et al., 2008a. Miniaturization of a high-throughput pLDH-based *Plasmodium falciparum* growth inhibition assay for small volume samples from preclinical and clinical vaccine trials. Am J Trop Med Hyg 78, 468-471.

Bergmann-Leitner, E.S., Mease, R.M., Duncan, E.H., et al., 2008b. Evaluation of immunoglobulin purification methods and their impact on quality and yield of antigen-specific antibodies. Malar J 7, 129.

Bergmann-Leitner, E.S., Duncan, E.H. & Angov, E., 2009. MSP-1p42-specific antibodies affect growth and development of intra-erythrocytic parasites of *Plasmodium falciparum*. Malar J 8, 183.

Bergmann-Leitner, E.S., Mease, R.M., De La Vega, P., et al., 2010. Immunization with pre-erythrocytic antigen CelTOS from *Plasmodium falciparum* elicits cross-species protection against heterologous challenge with *Plasmodium berghei*. PLoS ONE 5, e12294.

Blackman, M.J., Scott-Finnigan, T.J., Shai, S., et al., 1994. Antibodies inhibit the protease-mediated processing of a malaria merozoite surface protein. J Exp Med 180, 389-393.

Boudin, C., Chumpitazi, B., Dziegiel, M.H., et al., 1993. Possible role of specific immunoglobulin M antibodies to *Plasmodium falciparum* antigens in immunoprotection of humans living in a hyperendemic area, Burkina Faso. J Clin Microbiol 31, 636-641.

Bouharoun-Tayoun, H., Attanath, P., Sabchareon, A., et al., 1990. Antibodies that protect humans against *Plasmodium falciparum* blood stages do not on their own inhibit parasite growth and invasion in vitro, but act in cooperation with monocytes. J Exp Med 172, 1633-1641.

Bouharoun-Tayoun, H., Oeuvray, C., Lunel, F., et al., 1995. Mechanisms underlying the monocyte-mediated antibody-dependent killing of *Plasmodium falciparum* asexual blood stages. J Exp Med 182, 409-418.

Branch, O.H., Udhayakumar, V., Hightower, A.W., et al., 1998. A longitudinal investigation of IgG and IgM antibody responses to the merozoite surface protein-1 19-kiloDalton domain of *Plasmodium falciparum* in pregnant women and infants: associations with febrile illness, parasitemia, and anemia. Am J Trop Med Hyg 58, 211-219.

Brand, V., Sandu, C.D., Duranton, C., et al., 2003. Dependence of *Plasmodium falciparum in vitro* growth on the cation permeability of the human host erythrocyte. Cell Physiol Biochem 13, 347-356.

Brasseur, P., Ballet, J.J. & Druilhe, P., 1990. Impairment of *Plasmodium falciparum*-specific antibodies in severe malaria. J Clin Microbiol 28, 265-268.

Bull, P.C., Berriman, M., Kyes, S., et al., 2005. *Plasmodium falciparum* variant surface antigen expression patterns during malaria. PLoS Pathog 1, e26.

Bungener, W. & Nielsen, G., 1968. Nucleic acid metabolism in experimental malaria. 2. Incorporation of adenosine and hypoxanthine into the nucleic acids of malaria parasites (*Plasmodium berghei* and *Plasmodium vinckei*). Z Tropenmed Parasitol 19, 185-197.

Butcher, G.A., Cohen, S. & Garnham, P.C., 1970. Passive immunity in *Plasmodium knowlesi* malaria. Trans R Soc Trop Med Hyg 64, 850-856.

Camus, D. & Hadley, T.J., 1985. A *Plasmodium falciparum* antigen that binds to host erythrocytes and merozoites. Science 230, 553-556.

Cavanagh, D.R., Dodoo, D., Hviid, L., et al., 2004. Antibodies to the N-terminal block 2 of *Plasmodium falciparum* merozoite surface protein 1 are associated with protection against clinical malaria. Infect Immun 72, 6492-6502.

Chappel, J.A., Egan, A.F., Riley, E.M., et al., 1994. Naturally acquired human antibodies which recognize the first epidermal growth factor-like module on the *Plasmodium falciparum* merozoite surface protein 1 do not inhibit parasite growth in vitro. Infect Immun 62, 4488-4494.

Chimma, P., Rouissilhon, C., Sratongno, P., et al., 2009. A distinct peripheral blood monocyte phenotype is associated with parasite inhibitory activity in acute uncomplicated *Plasmodium falciparum* malaria. PLoS Pathog 5, e1000631.

Cohen, J. & Butcher, G.A., 1971. Serum antibody in acquired malarial immunity. Trans R Soc Trop Med Hyg 65, 125-135.

Cohen, S., McGregor, I.A. & Carrington, S., 1961. Gamma-globulin and acquired immunity to human malaria. Nature 192, 733-737.

Corran, P.H., O'Donnel, R.A., Todd, J., et al., 2004. The fine specificity, but not the invasion inhibitory activity of the 19-kilodalton merozoite surface protein 1-specific antibodies is associated with resistance to malarial parasitemia in a cross-sectional survey in The Gambia. Infect Immun 72, 6185-6189.

Courtin, D., Oesterholt, M., Huismans, H., et al., 2009. The quantity and quality of African children's IgG responses to merozoite surface antigens reflect protection against *Plasmodium falciparum* malaria. PLoS ONE 4, e7590.

Cowman, A.F. & Crabb, B.S., 2006. Invasion of red blood cells by malaria parasites. Cell 124, 755-768.

Darko, C.A., Angov, E., Collins, W.E., et al., 2005. The clinical-grade 42-kilodalton fragment of merozoite surface protein 1 of *Plasmodium falciparum* strain FVO expressed in *Escherichia coli* protects *Aotus nancymai* against challenge with homologous erythrocytic-stage parasites. Infect Immun 73, 287-297.

De Koning-Ward, T.F., O'Donnel, R.A., Drew, D.R., et al., 2003. A new rodent model to assess blood stage immunity to the *Plasmodium falciparum* antigen merozoite surface protein 1_{19} reveals a protective role for invasion inhibitory antibodies. J Exp Med 198, 869-875.

Dent, A.E., Bergmann-Leitner, E.S., Wilson, D.W., et al., 2008. Antibody-mediated growth inhibition of *Plasmodium falciparum*: relationship to age and protection from parasitemia in Kenyan children and adults. PLoS ONE 3, e3557.

Dodoo, D., Theander, T.G., Kurtzhals, J.A., et al., 1999. Levels of antibody to conserved parts of *Plasmodium falciparum* merozoite surface protein 1 in Ghanaian children are not associated with protection from clinical malaria. Infect Immun 67, 2131-2137.

Dodoo, D., Theisen, M., Kurtzhals, J.A., et al., 2000. Naturally acquired antibodies to the glutamate-rich protein are associated with protection against *Plasmodium falciparum* malaria. J Infect Dis 181, 1202-1205.

Draper, S.J., Goodman, A.L., Biswas, S., et al., 2009. Recombinant viral vaccines expressing merozoite surface protein-1 induce antibody- and T cell-mediated multistage protection against malaria. Cell Host Microbe 5, 95-105.

Druilhe, P., Spertini, F., Soesoe, D., et al., 2005. A malaria vaccine that elicits in humans antibodies able to kill *Plasmodium falciparum*. PLoS Med 2, e344.

Duncan, C.J.A., Sheehy, S.H., Ewer, K.J., et al., 2011. Impact on malaria parasite multiplication rates in infected volunteers of the protein-in-adjuvant vaccine AMA1-C1/Alhydrogel+CPG 7909. PLoS ONE 6, e22271.

Dutta, S., Dlugosz, L.S., Clayton, J.W., et al., 2010. Alanine mutagenesis of the primary antigenic escape residue cluster, c1, of apical membrane antigen 1. Infect Immun 78, e 661-671.

Egan, A.F., Morris, J., Barnish, G., et al., 1996. Clinical immunity to *Plasmodium falciparum* malaria is associated with serum antibodies to the 19kDa C-terminal fragment of the merozoite surface antigen, PfMSP-1. J Infect Dis 173, 765-769.

Egan, A.F., Burghaus, P., Druilhe, P., et al., 1999. Human antibodies to the 19kDa C-terminal fragment of *Plasmodium falciparum* merozoite surface protein 1 inhibit parasite growth *in vitro*. Parasite Immunol 21, 133-139.

El Sahly, H.M., Patel, S.M., Atmar, R.L., et al., 2010. Safety and immunogenicity of a recombinant nonglycosylated erythrocyte binding antigen 175 region II malaria vaccine in healthy adults living in an area where malaria is not endemic. Clin Vaccin Immunol 17, 1552-15559.

Ellis, R.D., Mullen, G.E., Pierce, M., et al., 2009. A Phase 1 study of the blood-stage malaria vaccine candidate AMA-C1/Alhydrogel with CPG 7909, using two different formulations and dosing intervals. Vaccine 27, 4104-4109.

Ellis, R.D., Martin, L.B., Shaffer, D., et al., 2010. Phase 1 trial of the *Plasmodium falciparum* blood stage vaccine MSP1(42)-C1/Alhydrogel with and without CPG7909 in malaria naive adults. PLoS ONE 5, e8787.

Esen, M., Kremsner, P.G., Schleucher, R., et al., 2009. Safety and immunogenicity of MGZ2 - a MSP3-GLURP fusion protein malaria vaccine candidate. Vaccine 27, 6862-6868.

Fowkes, F.J.I., Richards, J.S., Simpson, J.A., et al., 2010. The relationship between anti-merozoite antibodies and incidence of *Plasmodium falciparum* malaria: a systematic review and meta-analysis. PLoS Med 7, e1000218.

Genton, B., Betuela, I., Felger, I., et al., 2002. A recombinant blood-stage malaria vaccine reduces *Plasmodium* density and exerts selective pressure on parasite populations in a phase 1-2b trial in Papua New Guinea. J Infect Dis 185, 820-827.

Genton, B., Al-Yaman, F., Betuela, I., et al., 2003. Safety and immunogenicity of a three-component blood-stage malaria vaccine (MSP1, MSP2, RESA) against *Plasmodium falciparum* in Papua New Guinean children. Vaccine 22, 30-41.

Gerold, P., Schofield, L., Blackman, M.J., et al., 1996. Structural analysis of the glycosyl-phosphatidylinositol membrane anchor of the merozoite surface proteins-1 and -2 of *Plasmodium falciparum*. Mol. Biochem. Parasitol 75, 131-143.

Gray, J.C., Corran, P.H., Mangia, E., et al., 2007. Profiling th antibody immune response against blood stage malaria vaccine candidates. Clin Chem 53, 1244-1253.

Green, T.J., Morhardt, M., Brackett, R.G., et al., 1981. Serum inhibition of merozoite dispersal from *Plasmodium falciparum* schizonts: indicator of immune status. Infect Immun 31, 1203-1208.

Grimberg, B.T., 2011. Methodology and application of flow cytometry for investigation of human malaria parasites. J Immunol Meth 367, 1-16.

Groux, H. & Gysin, J., 1990. Opsonization as an effector mechanism in human protection against asexual blood stages of *Plasmodium falciparum*: functional role of IgG subclasses. Res Immunol 141, 529-542.

Haynes, J.D. & Moch, J.K., 2002. Automated synchronization of *Plasmodium falciparum* parasites by culture in a temperature-cycling incubator. Methods Mol Med 72, 489-497.

Haynes, J.D., Moch, J.K. & Smoot, D.S., 2002. Erythrocytic malaria growth or invasion inhibition assays with emphasis on suspension culture GIA. Methods Mol Med 72, 535-554.

Healer, J., Murphy, V., Hodder, A.N., et al., 2004. Allelic polymorphisms in apical membrane antigen-1 are responsible for evasion of antibody-mediated inhibition in *Plasmodium falciparum*. Mol Microbiol 52, 159-168.

Hermsen, C.C., Verhage, D.F., Telgt, D.S., et al., 2007. Glutamate-rich protein (GLURP) induces antibodies that inhibit in vitro growth of *Plasmodium falciparum* in a phase 1 malaria vaccine trial. Vaccine 25, 2930-3940.

Hviid, L., 2010. The role of *Plasmodium falciparum* variant surface antigens in protective immunity and vaccine development. Hum Vaccin 6, 84-89.

Israelsson, E., Vafa, M., Maiga, B., et al., 2008. Differences in Fc gamma receptor IIa genotypes and IgG subclass pattern of anti-malarial antibodies between sympatric ethnic groups in Mali. Malar J e 15.

Jafarshad, A., Dziegiel, M.H., Lundquist, R., et al., 2007. A novel antibody-dependent cellular cytotoxicity mechanism involved in defense against malaria requires costimulation of monocytes FcgammaRII and FcgammaRIII. J Immunol 178, 3099-3106.

John, C.C., O'Donnell, R.A., Sumba, P.O., et al., 2004. Evidence that invasion-inhibitory antibodies specific for the 19-kDa fragment of the merozoite surface protein-1 (MSP-1_{19}) can play a protective role against Blood-stage *Plasmodium falciparum* infection in individuals in a malaria endemic area of Africa. J Immunol 173, 666-672.

Keitel, W.A., Kester, K.E., Atmar, R.L., et al., 1999. Phase I trial of two recombinant vaccines containing the 19kd carboxy terminal fragment of *Plasmodium falciparum* merozoite surface protein 1 (MSP-1(19)) and T helper epitopes of tetanus toxoid. Vaccine 18, 531-539.

Kennedy, M.C., Wang, J., Zhang, Y., et al., 2002. In vitro studies with recombinant *Plasmodium falciparum* apical membrane antigen 1 (AMA1): production and activity of an AMA1 vaccine and generation of a multiallelic response. Infect Immun 70, 6948-6960.

Kester, K.E., McKinney, D., Tornieporth, N., et al., 2007. A phase I/IIa safety, immunogenicity, and efficacy bridging randomized study of a two-dose regimen of liquid and lyophilized formulations of the candidate malaria vaccine RTS,S/ASO2A in malaria-naive adults. Vaccine 25, 5359-5366.

Kinyanjui, S.M., Bejon, P., Osier, F.H., et al., 2009. What you see is not what you get: implications of the brevity of antibody responses to malaria antigens and transmission heterogeneity in longitudinal studies of malaria immunity. Malar J 8, e242.

Lavazec, C. & Bourqouin, C., 2008. Mosquito-based transmission blocking vaccinees for interrupting *Plasmodium* development. Microbes Infect 10, 845-849.

Leitner, W.W. & Krzych, U., 1997. *Plasmodium falciparum* malaria blood stage parasites preferentially inhibit macrophages with high phagocytic activity. Parasite Immunol 19, 103-110.

Leitner, W.W., Bergmann-Leitner, E.S. & Angov, E., 2010. Comparison of *Plasmodium berghei* challenge models for the evaluation of pre-erythrocytic malaria vaccines and their effect on perceived vaccine efficacy. Malar J 9, 145.

Leoratti, F.M., Durlacher, R.R., Lacerda, M.V., et al., 2008. Pattern of humoral immune response to *Plasmodium falciparum* blood stages in individuals presenting different clinical expressions of malaria. Malar J 7, e186.

Long, C.A., Daly, T.M., Kima, P., et al., 1994. Immunity to erythrocytes stages of malarial parasites. Am J Trop Med Hyg 50, 27-32.

Lyon, J.A., Carter, J.M., Thomas, A.W., et al., 1997. Merozoite surface protein-1 epitopes recognized by antibodies that inhibit *Plasmodium falciparum* merozoite dispersal. Mol Biochem Parasitol 90, 223-234.

Makler, M.T. & Hinrichs, D.J., 1993. Measurement of the lactate dehydrogenase activity of *Plasmodium falciparum* as an assessment of parasitemia. Am J Trop Med Hyg 48, 205-210.

Malkin, E., Hu, J., Li, Z., et al., 2008. A phase 1 trial of PfCP2.9: an AMA1/MSP1 chimeric recombinant protein vaccine for *Plasmodium falciparum* malaria. Vaccine 26, 6864-6873.

McBride, J.S. & Heidrich, H.G., 1987. Fragments of the polymorphic Mr 185,000 glycoprotein from the surface of isolated *Plasmodium falciparum* merozoites form an antigenic complex. Mol Biochem Parasitol 23, 71-84.

McGregor, I. & Carrington, S., 1963. Treatment of East African *P. falciparum* malaria with West African human-globulin. Trans R Soc Trop Med Hyg 57, 170-175.

McIntosh, R.S., Shi, J., Jennings, R.M., et al., 2007. The importance of human Fc gamma RI in mediating protection to malaria. PLoS Pathog 3, e72.

Miura, K., Zhou, H., Moretz, S.E., et al., 2008. Comparison of biological activity of human anti-apical membrane antigen-1 antibodies induced by natural infection and vaccination. J Immunol 181, 8776-8783.

Miura, K., Zhou, H., Diouf, A., et al., 2011. Immunological responses against *Plasmodium falciparum* Apical Membrane Antigen 1 vaccines vary depending on the population immunized. Vaccine 29, 2255-2261.

Moorthy, V.S., Diggs, C., Ferro, S., et al., 2009. Report of a consultation on the optimization of clinical challenge trials for evaluation of candidate blood stage malaria vaccines. 18-19 March 2009. Bethesda, MD, USA. Vaccine 27, 5719-5725.

Morgan, W.D., Birdsall, B., Frenkiel, T.A., et al., 1999. Solution structure of an EGF module pair from the *Plasmodium falciparum* merozoite surface protein 1. J Mol Biol 289, 113-122.

Nebie, I., Diarra, A., Ouedraogo, A., et al., 2008. Humoral responses to *Plasmodium falciparum* blood-stage antigens and association with incidence of clinical malaria in children living in an area of seasonal malaria transmission in Burkina Faso, West Africa. Infect Immun 76, 759-766.

Nery, S., Deans, A.M., Mosobo, M., et al., 2006. Expression of *Plasmodium falciparum* genes involved in erythrocyte invasion varies among isolates cultured directly from patients. Mol Biochem Parasitol 149, 208-215.

O'Donnell, R.A., Saul, A., Cowman, A.F., et al., 2000. Functional conservation of the malaria vaccine antigen MSP-1_{19} across distantly related *Plasmodium* species. Nat Med 6, 91-95.

O'Donnell, R.A., Koning-Ward, T.F.d., Burt, R.A., et al., 2001. Antibodies against Merozoite Surface Protein (MSP)-1_{19} are the major component of the invasion-inhibitory response in individuals immune to malaria. J Exp Med 193, 1403-1412.

Ockenhouse, C., Angov, E., Kester, K.E., et al., 2006. Phase I safety and immunogenicity trial of FMP1/ASO2A, a *Plasmodium falciparum* MSP-1 asexual blood stage vaccine. Vaccine 24, 3009-3017.

Oeuvray, C., Theisen, M., Rogier, C., et al., 2000. Cytophilic immunoglobulin responses to *Plasmodium falciparum* glutamate-rich protein are correlated with protection against clinical malaria Dielmo, Senegal. Infect Immun 68, 2617-2620.

Ogutu, B.R., Apollo, O.J., McKinney, D., et al., 2009. Blood stage malaria vaccine eliciting high antigen-specific antibody concentrations confers no protection to young children in Western Kenya. PLoS ONE 4, e4708.

Okech, B.A., Corran, P.H., Todd, J., et al., 2004. Fine specificity of serum antibodies to *Plasmodium falciparum* merozoite surface protein, PfMSP-1(19), predicts protection from malaria infection and high-density parasitemia. Infect Immun 72, 1557-1567.

Ouevray, C., Bouharoun-Tayoun, H., Grass-Masse, H., et al., 1994. A novel merozoite surface antigen of *Plasmodium falciparum* (MSP-3) identified by cellular-antibody cooperative mechanism antigenicity and biological activity of antibodies. Mem. Inst. Oswaldo Cruz 89, 77-80.

Pang, X.-L., Mitamura, T. & Horii, T., 1999. Antibodies reactive with the N-terminal domain of *Plasmodium falciparum* serine repeat antigen inhibit cell proliferation by agglutinating merozoites and schizonts. Infect Immun 67, 1821-1827.

Parkkinen, J., Rahola, A., von Bonsdorff, L., et al., 2006. A modified caprylic acid method for manufacturing immunoglobulin G from human plasma with high yield and efficient virus clearance. Vox Sang 90, 97-104.

Patino, G.A., Holder, A.A., McBride, J.S., et al., 1997. Antibodies that inhibit malaria merozoite surface protein-1 processing and erythrocyte invasion are blocked by naturally acquired human antibodies. J Exp Med 186, 1689-1699.

Perkins, M., 1991. Approaches to study merozoite invasion of erythrocytes. Res Immunol 141, 662-665.

Perraut, R., Marrama, L., Diouf, B., et al., 2003. Distinct surrogate markers for protection against *Plasmodium falciparum* infection and clinical malaria identified in a Senegalese community after radical drug cure. J Infect Dis 188, 1940-1950.

Perraut, R., Marrama, L., Diouf, B., et al., 2005. Antibodies to the conserved C-terminal domain of the *Plasmodium falciparum* merozoite surface protein 1 and to the merozoite extract and their relationship with *in vitro* inhibitory antibodies and protection against clinical malaria in a Senegalese village. J Infect Dis 191, 264-271.

Persson, K.E., Lee, C.T., Marsh, K., et al., 2006. Development and optimization of high-throughput methods to measure *Plasmodium falciparum*-specific growth inhibitory antibodies. J Clin Microbiol 44, 1665-1673.

Persson, K.E., McCallum, F.J., Reiling, L., et al., 2008. Variation in use of erythrocyte invasion pathways by *Plasmodium falciparum* mediates evasion of human inhibitory antibodies. J Clin Invest 118, 342-351.

Pleass, R.J., Ogun, S.A., McGuiness, D.H., et al., 2003. Novel antimalarial antibodies highlight the importance of the antibody Fc region in mediating protection. Blood 102, 4424-4430.

Prudhomme, J.G. & Sherman, I.W., 1999. A high capacity in vitro assay for measuring the cytoadherence of *Plasmodium falciparum*-infected erythrocytes. J Immunol Meth 229, 169-176.

Rahman, N.N., 1997. Evaluation of the sensitivity in vitro of *Plasmodium falciparum* and *in vivo* of *Plasmodium chabaudi* Malaria to various drugs and their combinations. Med J malaysia 52, 390-398.

Reed, Z.H., Kieny, M.P., Engers, H., et al., 2009. Comparison of immunogenicity of five MSP1-based malaria vaccine candidate antigens in rabbits. Vaccine 27, 1651-1660.

Remarque, E.J., Faber, B.W., Kocken, C.H., et al., 2008. A diversity-covering approach to immunization with *Plasmodium falciparum* apical membrane antigen 1 induces broader allelic recognition and growth inhibition responses in rabbits. Infect Immun 76, 2660-2670.

Riley, E.M., Allen, S.J., Wheeler, J.G., et al., 1992. Naturally acquired cellular and humoral immune responses to the major merozoite surface antigen (PfMSP1) of *Plasmodium falciparum* are associated with reduced malaria morbidity. Parasite Immunol 14, 321-337.

Sacarlal, J., Aide, P., Aponte, J.J., et al., 2009. Long-term safety and efficacy of the RTS,S/ASO2A malaria vaccine in Mozambican children. J Infect Dis 200, 329-336

Shapiro, H.M., 2004. The evolution of cytometers. Cytometry A 58, 13-20.

Shi, Y.P., Nahlen, B.L., Kariuki, H.C., et al., 2001. Fcgamma receptor IIa (CD32) polymorphism is associated with protection in infants against high-density *Plasmodium falciparum* infection. VII. Asembo Bay Cohort Project. J Infect Dis 184, 107-111.

Siddique, A.B., Ahlborg, N., Wahlin Flyg, B., et al., 1998. Antibodies to sequences in a non-repeat region of *Plasmodium falciparum* antigen Pf155/RESA inhibit either cytoadherence or parasite growth in vitro. Parasitology 117 (Pt 3), 209-216.

Sirima, S.B., Nebie, I., Ouedraogo, A., et al., 2007. Safety and immunogenicity of the *Plasmodium falciparum* merozoite surface protein-3 long synthetic peptide (MSP3-LSP) malaria vaccine in healthy, semi-immune adult males in Burkina Faso, West Africa. Vaccine 25, 2723-2732.

Soe, S., Theisen, M., Rouissilhon, C., et al., 2004. Association between protection against clinical malaria and antibodies to merozoite surface antigens in an area of hyperendemicity in Myanmar: complementarity between responses to merozoite surface protein 3 and the 220-kilodalton glutamate-rich protein. Infect Immun 72, 247-252.

Spring, M.D., Cummings, J.F., Ockenhouse, C.F., et al., 2009. Phase 1/2a study of the malaria vaccine candidate apical membrane antigen-1 (AMA-1) administered in adjuvant system AS01B or AS02A. PLoS ONE 4, e5254.

Stoute, J.A., Gombe, J., Withers, M.R., et al., 2007. Phase 1 randomized double-blind safety and immunogenicity trial of *Plamodium falciparum* malaria merozoite surface protein FMP1 vaccine, adjuvanted with ASO2A in adults in western Kenya. Vaccine 25, 176-184.

Stowers, A.W., Cioce, V., Shimp, R.L., et al., 2001. Efficacy of two alternate vaccines based on *Plasmodium falciparum* merozoite surface protein 1 in an *Aotus* challenge trial. Infect Immun 69, 1536-1546.

Sy, N.E., Oberst, R.B., Macalagay, P.S., et al., 1990. *In vitro* growth inhibition of *Plasmodium falciparum* by sera from different regions of the Phillipines. Am J Trop Med Hyg 43, 243-247.

Takala, S.L., Coulibaly, B., Mahamadou, A.T., et al., 2009. Extreme polymorphism in a vaccine antigen and risk of clinical malaria: implications for vaccine development. Sci Transl Med 1, 2ra5.

Tebo, A.E., Kremsner, P.G. & Luty, A.J., 2001. *Plasmodium falciparum:* a major role for IgG3 in antibody-dependent monocyte-mediated cellular inhibition of parasite growth *in vitro*. Exp Parasitol 98, 20-28.

Thera, M.A., Doumbo, O.K., Coulibaly, B., et al., 2006. Safety and allele-specific immunogenicity of a malaria vaccine in Malian adults: results of a phase I randomized trial. Plos Clin Trials 1, e34.

Trager, W. & Jensen, J.B., 1976. Human malaria parasites in continuous culture. Science 193, 673-675.

Triglia, T., Healer, J., Caruana, S.R., et al., 2000. Apical membrane antigen 1 plays a central role in erythrocyte invasion by *Plasmodium* species. Mol Microbiol 38, 706-718.

Uthaipibull, C., Aufiero, B., Syed, S.E., et al., 2001. Inhibitory and blocking monoclonal antibody epitopes on merozoite surface protein 1 of the malaria parasite *Plasmodium falciparum*. J Mol Biol 307, 1381-1394.

van der Heyde, H.C., Elloso, M.M., vande Waa, J., et al., 1995. Use of hydroethidine and flow cytometry to assess the effects of leukocytes on the malarial parasite *Plasmodium falciparum*. Clin Diagn Lab Immunol 2, 417-425.

Vanderberg, J., Mueller, A.K., Heiss, K., et al., 2007. Assessment of antibody protection against malaria sporozoites must be done by mosquito injection of sporozoites. Am J Pathol 171, 1405-1406.

Vigan-Womas, I., Lokossou, A., Guillotte, M., et al., 2010. The humoral response to *Plasmodium falciparum* VarO rosetting variant and its association with protection against malaria in Beninese children. Malar J 9, e 267.

Wahlgren, M., Bjorkman, A., Perlmann, H., et al., 1986. Anti-*Plasmodium falciparum* antibodies acquired by residents in a holoendemic area of Liberia during development of clinical immunity. Am J Trop Med Hyg 35, 22-29.

Withers, M.R., McKinney, D., Ogutu, B.R., et al., 2006. Safety and reactogenicity of an MSP-1 malaria vaccine candidate: a randomized phase Ib dose-escalation trial in Kenyan children. PLoS Clin Trials 1, e32.

Woehlbier, U., Epp, C., Kauth, C.W., et al., 2006. Analysis of antibodies directed against merozoite surface protein 1 of the human malaria parasite *Plasmodium falciparum*. Infect Immun 74, 1313-1322.

Wyatt, C.R., Goff, W. & Davis, W.C., 1991. A flow cytometric method for assessing viability of intraerythrocytic hemoparasites. J Immunol Meth 140, 117-122.

Part 6

Genomics of Malaria

13

In Silico Resources for Malaria Drug Discovery

Pieter B. Burger and Fourie Joubert
University of Pretoria
South Africa

1. Introduction

Drugs currently in use against the malaria parasite have been derived from known natural compounds, or discovered serendipitously. The completion of the *Plasmodium falciparum* genome project at the turn of the century (Gardner *et al.*, 2002) raised great hopes for the identification of a wealth of targets against which to design new and novel drugs. However, it soon became apparent that the challenges associated with the annotation of the malaria proteome was creating a significant hurdle to be overcome already in the early stages. In addition, the complexity introduced by the multitude of factors that need consideration in selecting suitable drug targets made it difficult to perform the selection of target proteins in a high-throughput automated fashion. The need for the development of effective *in silico* approaches required to successfully address these problems were identified and addressed by the malaria community.

This chapter focuses on *in silico* resources that are available to support researchers working in the area of malaria drug discovery. It aims to facilitate the researcher's entry into early phase drug discovery by lowering the initial barrier to data mining sometimes perceived as a daunting task due to information overload. While *in silico* experimentation is not intended to replace detailed experimental work, it may be extremely useful in decreasing the size of the protein and chemical space to be investigated *in vitro*, and may help guide the experimentalist's decision making during the selection process. These resources are intended to assist the researcher in rationally selecting a relatively small number of targets out of the whole for further detailed investigation. The *in silico* resources discussed here vary from primary data repositories, to advanced data mining systems, and provide information on a variety of different levels in discovery research.

Genome databases are often the first point of access. Whereas they always contain the primary data generated during the genome project, they usually contain significant amounts of annotations regarding gene structures and gene products including nucleotide and protein sequences. The annotation detail may vary, as is the case with the malaria genomes. *Plasmodium falciparum* has been annotated extensively, but the level of annotation for the other Plasmodia may range widely. The genome database for malaria parasites additionally provides extensive information on gene variation, protein features, expression and a wide variety of other molecular properties and is a rich resource from which to embark on further study. Each entry also provides many external links for exploration.

The more specialized databases are typically derived from the data present in the genome database, and provide focussed information on specific aspects related to the molecules available. There are several resources containing information around metabolic pathways of the malaria parasites, assisting researchers in understanding the pathways present in the organisms, and the role of specific proteins or compounds in the organisms' metabolic activity, which is especially useful in deciding on aspects of the parasite metabolism that may be selected for interference. Protein-protein interaction resources highlight interacting proteins, but additionally allow the researcher to begin understanding the interaction and regulatory network that the parasite requires for growth and survival, together with possible ways to manipulate this homeostasis. Gene expression resources provide insights into the regulatory mechanisms of gene expression, especially in terms of changes in expression profiles over the different stages of the parasite. Functional prediction resources attempt to expand the annotation of novel and unassigned proteins produced by the parasites, particularly by attempting to use methods that may be independent from the protein sequence of the molecule using eg. guilt-by-association approaches. Protein structure databases provide the researcher with experimentally-determined structures or models to help understand molecular mechanisms, and for further use in comparative undertakings and molecular modeling projects. Literature resources focus on articles published on the many aspects of malaria and its molecules, and may attempt to automatically extract value-added information from the text. Drug discovery resources attempt to integrate many of the aspects already mentioned here into a single system, where researchers may perform the selection and scoring of possible drug targets and lead compounds in an automated or semi-automated fashion.

A summary of the resource discussed in this Chapter is presented in Table 1.

Name	**URL**
PlasmoDB	http://www.plasmodb.org
Malaria Parasite Metabolic Pathways	http://sites.huji.ac.il/malaria
PlasmoCyc	http://plasmocyc.stanford.edu
KEGG	http://www.genome.jp/kegg
PlasmoMap	http://www.cbil.upenn.edu/plasmoMAP
IDC Strain Comparison Database	http://malaria.ucsf.edu
PlasmoDraft	http://www.atgc-montpellier.fr/PlasmoDraft
Protein Structure Database	http://www.pdb.org
TDI Kernel	http://tropicaldisease.org/kernel
ModBase	http://modbase.compbio.ucsf.edu
Malaria Literature Database	http://carrier.gnf.org/publications/Py
ChEMBL	http://www.ebi.ac.uk/chembldb
TDR Targets	http://tdrtargets.org
Discovery	http://discovery.bi.up.ac.za

Table 1. A summary of resources discussed in this chapter

2. Malaria genome databases

2.1 PlasmoDB

URL: http://www.plasmodb.org

PlasmoDB (Aurrecoechea *et al.*, 2009) is the primary resource for malaria genome information, and is part of the larger EuPathDB project (Aurrecoechea *et al.*, 2010) which is focussed on eukaryotic pathogens. The PlasmoDB resource contains genome data for *P. falciparum*, *P. vivax*, *P. yoelii*, *P. berghei*, *P. chabaudi* and *P. knowlesi*. PlasmoDB is regarded as the primary distribution point for malaria sequence data, and while genome and proteome data are available for download, an advanced data mining system is provided for complex queries in gene, protein and related features. The most basic mechanism to access the PlasmoDB site is by searching using either a known accession number or a keyword. The more useful approach is to perform a text-based query, where series of species and data fields may be selected for searching. This will provide the user with a list of entries matching the search criteria. When an entry is selected, a page for the molecule is displayed, containing the genomic context, together with annotation, protein, expression and sequence information.

Each of these categories has a rich subset of information, which may be selected for display, including single nucleotide polymorphisms, sequence aligment vs. the other malaria species, links to annotation information in other databases, orthologs and paralogs, ontology information, metabolism information, physical-chemical information, structural information, immunological information, microarray and proteomics results (Figure 1). Some of the additional data is generated by the PlasmoDB group, while other data is linked to 3rd-party sites and research groups.

While a simple text search may be useful in straight-forward cases, the powerful query engine underlying the resource provides the user with the capability to select molecules based on a range of properties, in a sequential or branched fashion. Filters may be based on a wide range of properties as described in the previous paragraph. As an example, a scenario is illustrated where the user is interested in finding all *P. falciparum* proteins matching the text term "synth*" where the effect of SNPs may be predicted on a 3D level. An initial query may be performed by selecting all proteins containing the annotation "synth*". The user is then presented with a graphical view of his query results, showing the number of initial results (119 in this case). An additional intersect filter may then be added to only show proteins where SNP information is available (68 genes). This may then be further filtered to only show proteins where predicted 3D-structures are also available (12 genes). The complete search strategy is visualized graphically as a pipeline (Figure 2), where the user interactively may alter points in the search strategy, create branches and set weighting for different aspects of the search. In a search strategy, unions and intersects will sum the weights, giving higher scores to items found in multiple searches. This interface is regarded as one of the most powerful, user-friendly and intuitive for all biological databases.

Users may create a personal account on the site, and search strategies as well as results may be saved in this way. In addition to the database searches, a series of tools are also available at PlasmoDB. These tools enable the user to perform BLAST searches against the malaria data, retrieve sequences by lists of gene IDs, access links to the PubMed and Entrez sites, access the malaria genome data in the GBrowse genome browser interface (Stein *et al.*, 2002), predict apicoplast-targeting signals, predict mitochondrial transit peptides and access the PlasmoCyc metabolic pathway annotations. Additionally, a web services WADL (Web Application Description Language) specification for searches against PlasmoDB is provided.

PlasmoDB is carefully curated, highly quality controlled and updated at a very regular frequency. Information about the available data is easily accessed from the data summary section on the front page of the resource. PlasmoDB would be the first resource to visit for a researcher embarking on a malaria drug discovery project, to obtain data about the availability of genes and proteins of interest, together with the relevant annotations and value-added information.

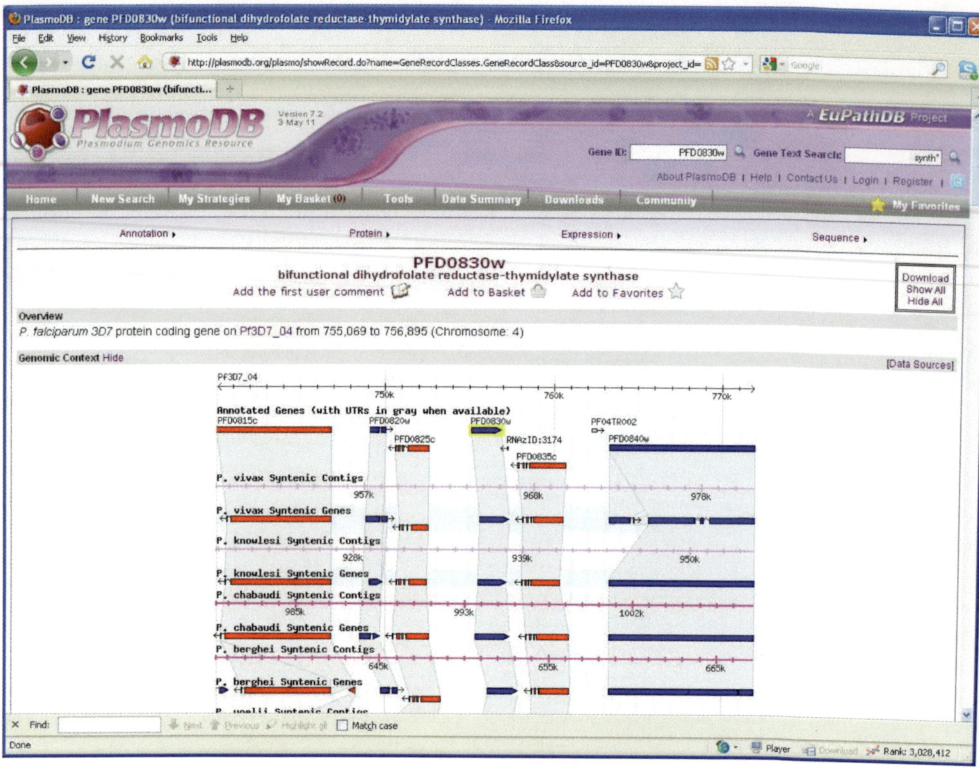

Fig. 1. The result view for the protein PFD0830w (bifunctional dihydrofolate reductase-thymidylate synthase from *P. falciparum*) in the PlasmoDB, showing the genomic context together with syntenic genes in other species. The rest of the detailed gene information mentioned in the text is not visible in this figure but continues lower down the browser screen.

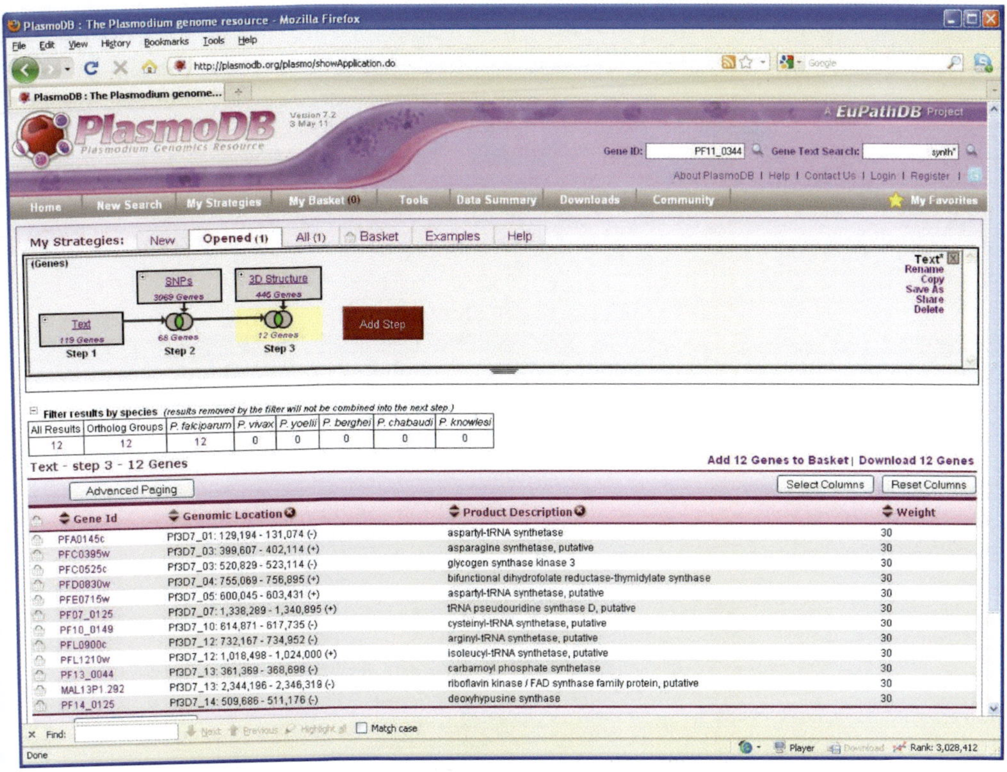

Fig. 2. The advanced result display interface of PlasmoDB, at the top graphically showing the data query pipeline with filtering steps performed using an initial text query followed by the availability of SNP information and 3D structural information. The resulting hits from the query are shown at the bottom. These steps may be edited again, or further branched and expanded.

3. Malaria metabolism databases

3.1 Malaria Parasite Metabolic Pathways (MPMP)

URL: http://sites.huji.ac.il/malaria

The Malaria Parasite Metabolic Pathways resource is maintained by Hagai Ginsburg, and is the most complete and up-to-date source of information for metabolic pathways in malaria (Ginsburg, 2009). Researchers may be interested in exploring information about the different enzymes in a pathway together with their characteristics, or alternatively in seeing the role that a specific enzyme plays in one or more pathways. MPMP has been constructed based on enzymes annotated in the parasite and on pathways known to occur in unicellular eukaryotes. While the pathways have been cross-checked against PlasmoDB, not all enzymes and reactions have been validated in malaria. The site also includes information related to cell-cell interactions, invasion of the erythrocyte and transport functions. The site provides information in a hierarchical fashion, starting with grouped pathways based on chemical component or biological process. This is followed by specific pathways or process, chemical structures and enzymes together with their genes. To browse the site, the user selects a primary category, such as carbohydrates. This is followed by the selection of a specific category. In this example, first carbohydrate metabolism and then specifically the glycolysis pathway was selected for visualization. A graphical overview of the glycolysis pathway is displayed. The overview shows the enzyme names, EC numbers, co-factors and metabolites of the pathway, as well as links to other metabolic pathways (Figure 3). The site may also be searched using enzyme names, EC numbers, other protein names or the names of metabolites.

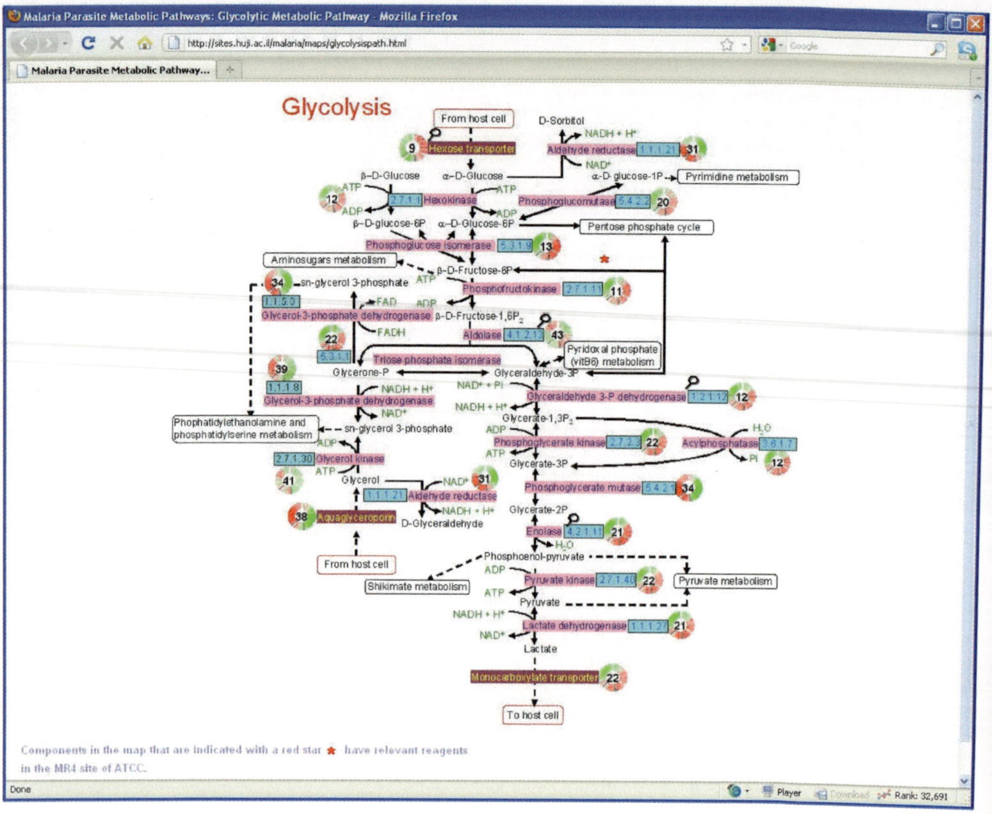

Fig. 3. The glycolysis pathway, as shown in Malaria Parasite Metabolic Pathways. The enzymes and well as chemical compounds and co-factors are visible. A small glyph showing stage-specific expression information is also shown where available.

From each enzyme, links are available to a set of other metabolic pathways databases including BRENDA (http://www.brenda.uni-koeln.de), ExPASy ENZYME (http://www.expasy.org/enzyme) and the IUBMB reaction schemes (http://www.chem.qmul.ac.uk/iubmb/enzyme/reaction). Links are also provided to PlasmoDB (http://plasmodb.org), and *P. falciparum* GeneDB (http://www.genedb.org). From metabolites, links are provided to KEGG (http://www.genome.jp/kegg) which provides chemical structures and formulas. The links provide access to a wealth of information including enzymatic activity, enzyme assays, kinetic parameters and inhibitors. Stage-dependent trancription of each enzyme is also shown as a pie-chart, based on the DeRisi/UCSF transcriptome database (http://malaria.ucsf.edu).

3.2 PlasmoCyc

URL: http://plasmocyc.stanford.edu

PlasmoCyc (Yeh *et al.*, 2004) forms part of the larger MetaCyc resource, where metabolic pathways for a range of organisms have been modeled. PlasmoCyc was initially constructed automatically using annotated EC terms as input to the PathoLogic tools (Caspi *et al.*, 2006). Additional enzymes and reactions were then manually added afterwards based on information obtained from literature. The pathways constructed in this fashion were then further expanded using data from the Malaria Parasite Metabolic Pathways resource. The PlasmoCyc site additionally hosts a set of potentially-interesting drug target proteins, together with motivations for their choice and literature references. PlasmoCyc may be accessed by searching for an enzyme name or EC number, using an ontology browser, or choosing from a list of pathways, proteins or compounds. Pathways may be viewed at different levels of detail. The initial view shows enzyme names, and the next level adds PlasmoDB IDs, EC numbers, compounds and co-factors. The subsequent level provides chemical structures of the compounds. In this example, the glycolysis pathway was selected for display (Figure 4). A useful functionality is the species comparison tool, where metabolic pathways may be compared between several different species to test for differences in the presence of pathway components and to identify unique enzymes for target selection.

3.3 Kyoto Encyclopedia of Genes and Genomes (KEGG)

URL: http://www.genome.jp/kegg

KEGG is a very comprehensive database on metabolism in many species, and includes malaria. KEGG includes information for pathways, diseases, drugs, orthology, genes, genomes, compounds and reactions (Kanehisa & Goto, 2000; Kanehisa *et al.*, 2010; Kanehisa *et al.*, 2006). KEGG contains pathway representations for *P. falciparum, P. vivax, P. yoelii, P. berghei, P. chabaudi* and *P. knowlesi*. KEGG may be accessed using various approaches. A common approach for browsing pathways is to select the KEGG pathway entry point, followed by a reference pathway of interest. Subsequently, an organism may be selected. Enzymes identified in the organism are then highlighted using color coding. In this example, the glycolysis pathway was selected for display (Figure 5). Selecting an enzyme on the pathway will provide a detailed page of information on the enzyme, including the sequence, known motifs and links to other databases such as SSDB, GenBank, PlasmoDB, GeneDB and UniProt. Selecting a compound will provide a detailed page including physical-chemical properties, the structure, reactions linked to the compound, pathways linked to the compound, enzymes linked to the compound and links to other databases such as CAS (http://www.cas.org), PubChem (http://pubchem.ncbi.nlm.nih.gov/), ChEBI (http://www.ebi.ac.uk/chebi/), KNApSAcK (http://kanaya.naist.jp/KNApSAcK/) and PDB (http://www.pdb.org).

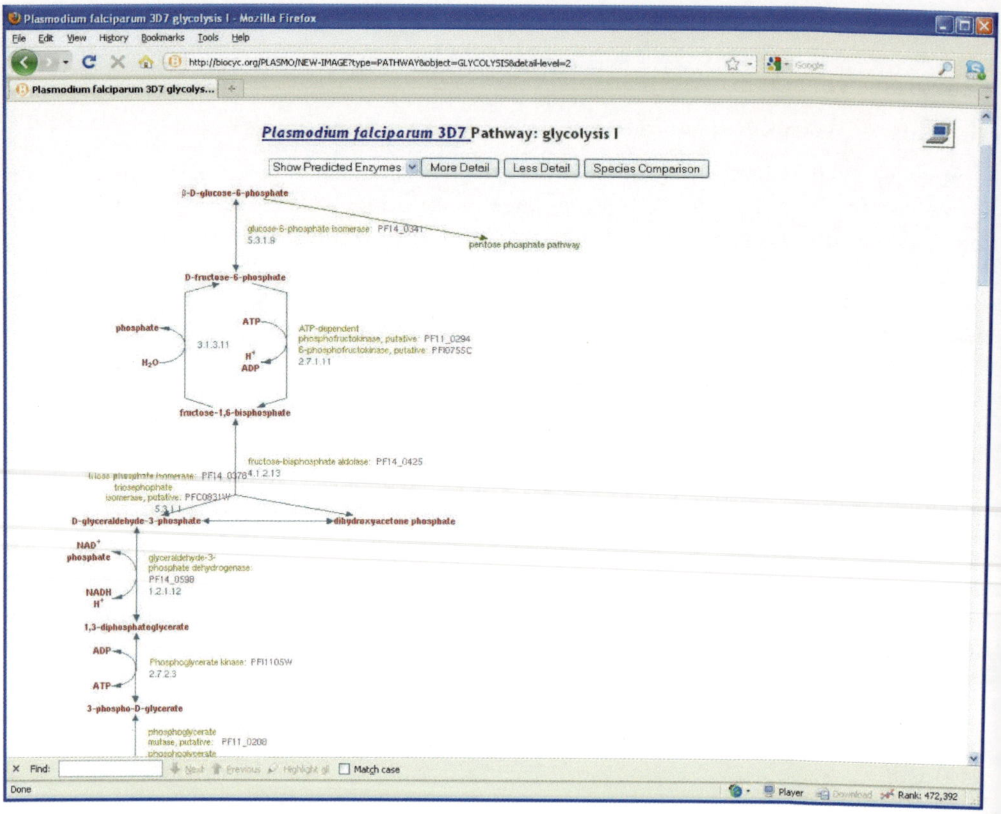

Fig. 4. The glycolysis pathway, as shown in PlasmoCyc. Enzymes, chemical compounds and co-factors are shown at this level. Multiple levels of detail may be selected for visualization.

Additionally, KEGG provides a series of analysis functionalities such as tools for mapping molecules to pathways and generating graphical representations, predicting metabolic pathways, annotation tools, sequence similarity searching and chemical similarity searching. A particularly useful feature is the ability to display gene expression data onto the KEGG pathways using the KEGG expression resource. A downloadable application is also provided for detailed analysis of gene expression data together with KEGG pathways and KEGG genomes. Many of the KEGG features may be accessed as a web service using the provided WSDL specifications. The KEGG pathways are also available for download in XML format.

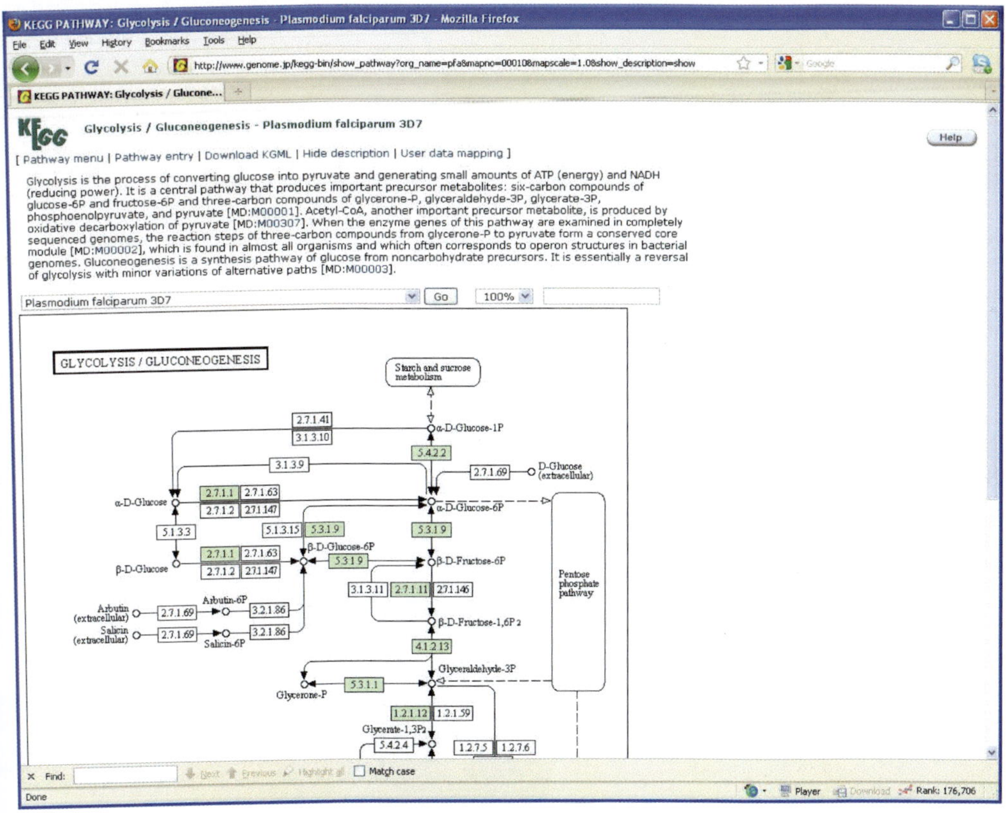

Fig. 5. The glycolysis pathway, as shown in KEGG. EC numbers and chemical compounds names are shown.

4. Protein-protein interaction databases

4.1 PlasmoMAP

URL: http://www.cbil.upenn.edu/plasmoMAP

PlasmoMAP is focussed at functional interactions between proteins in *P. falciparum* (Date & Stoeckert, 2006), with the goal of eventually illustrating a complete interactome. It is based on the reconstruction of functional genomics and computational data using a Bayesian framework. The interaction network covers around 68% of the parasite genome and infers information for nearly 2000 uncharacterized proteins. PlasmoMAP contains data for *P. falciparum* strains HB3, 3D7 and Dd2. The resource allows the user to access the data by either generating a complete protein-protein interaction dataset at a specified cut-off value, or by specifying a protein name for which to generate interaction partners. The PlasmoMAP network data is made available for download in LGL format, so that the networks may be viewed using the LGLView application. Additionally, the raw functional genomics data may be downloaded, as well as various subsets of the interaction data by confidence, by KEGG category, by GO category and by linkages detected in other apicomplexan organisms.

5. Gene expression databases

5.1 Malaria IDC strain comparison database

URL: http://malaria.ucsf.edu

The IDC site presents the data from the DeRisi lab studies on the transcriptome analysis of *P. falciparum* (Bozdech *et al.*, 2003; Llinás *et al.*, 2006). Queries may be executed using a variety of terms, including PlasmoDB ID, ORF description, oligonucleotide ID, automated prediction, automated description, GO annotation, GO number, common gene name, functional group, chromosome or by providing a list of ORFs or oligonucleotides. Strain, time, Fourier, amplitude and CGH constraints may be set for queries. In this example of viewing the expression of a specific gene, a query was performed for the PlasmoDB ID PFD0830w (bifunctional dihydrofolate reductase-thymidylate) and the expression data for the d33539_76 oligonucleotide was visualized for the 3D7 isolate (Fig 6). The chromosomal

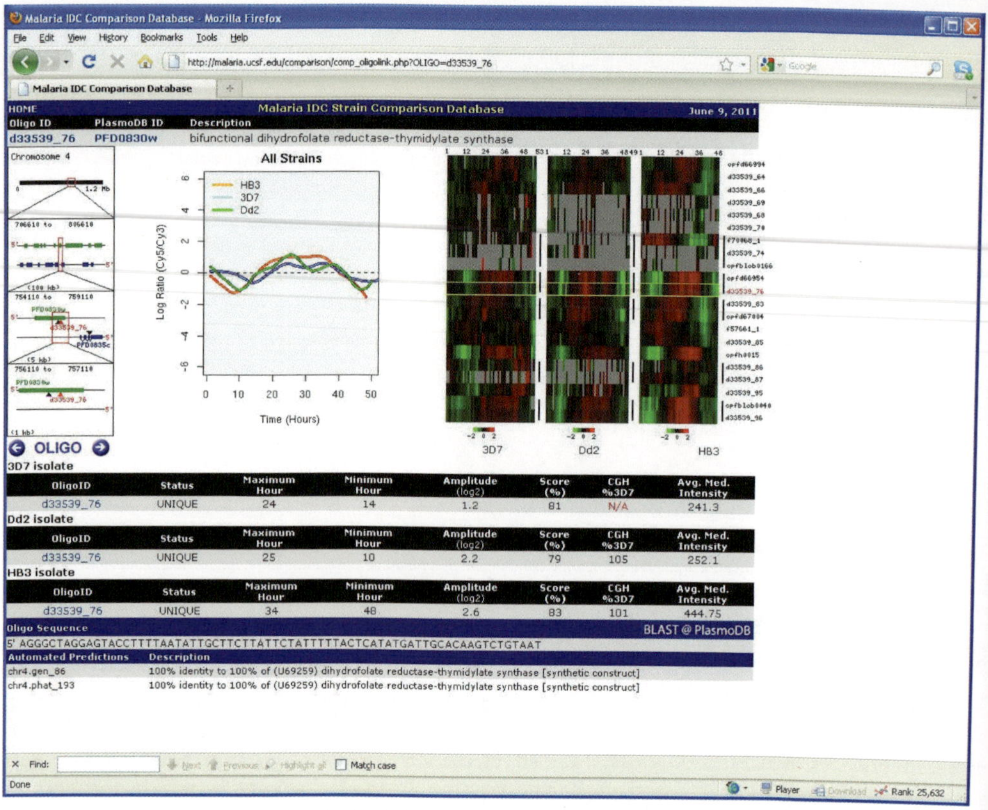

Fig. 6. The expression profile of PFD0830w (bifunctional dihydrofolate reductase-thymidylate synthase from *P. falciparum*) visualized in the Malaria IDC Strain Comparison Database as measured using the d33539_79 oligonucleotide probe. The chromosomal position is shown on the left. The expression of the gene over time is visible as a graph for the different parasite trains, and a heat map of expression measured by other probes are shown on the right. Detailed information is provided at the bottom.

location, log-ratio of expression over time and strain comparison heat map are shown together with a table providing more detailed time, median and scoring information. When a search is performed using specific constraints over the complete dataset, matching genes are shown in a tabular fashion, together with a miniaturized heatmap of the expression profile. The IDC data is also made available for download in normalized as well as non-normalized formats. Furthermore, the raw image files from the study may also be obtained.

6. Functional prediction databases

6.1 PlasmoDraft

URL: http://www.atgc-montpellier.fr/PlasmoDraft

The PlasmoDraft database predicts GO terms for genes from *P. falciparum*. It is based on a Guilt By Association (GBA) predictor named Gonna, measuring the profile of a gene's similarity using data from transcriptome, proteome and interactome studies to genes in the GeneDB database (Bréhélin *et al.*, 2008). The database may be viewed globally for each gene ontology category (Molecular Function, Biological Process and Cellular Component). The GO term is displayed, followed by its parameters for a series of parasite strains. These include prior probability (indicating term frequency), the best global degree of belief (GDB) and its confidence (TDR: True Discovery Rate). These are indicated using a color code varying from green to red (Figure 7). The database may also be searched using a gene, a GO term identifier or a keyword. This approach to functional prediction is complementary to the classical sequence based-approaches. Around 60% of genes lacking annotations are included, in addition to genes already annotated in GeneDB. Particularly useful is the ability to identify GO terms attached to a specific gene, and also genes attached to a specific GO term.

7. Protein structure databases

7.1 PDB

URL: http://www.pdb.org

Although not malaria-specific, the PDB database is the global repository for all protein structure information, derived primarily from X-ray crystallography and NMR studies (Bernstein *et al.*, 1977). At the time of writing, there were 59 structures from Plasmodia, of which some were duplicates of the same protein with different ligands or with single / multiple mutations. The PDB database may be searched using an extensive range of criteria, but the main approaches are using a text term search or performing a BLAST search using a protein sequence to find homologous proteins. The results view of a protein structure includes a preview of the protein structure, literature information, a molecular description, information about related PDB entries and information about associated ligands (Figure 8). The structure may be interactively viewed using JMol (http://www.jmol.org). The structural and sequence data may be downloaded in a range of formats for further investigation.

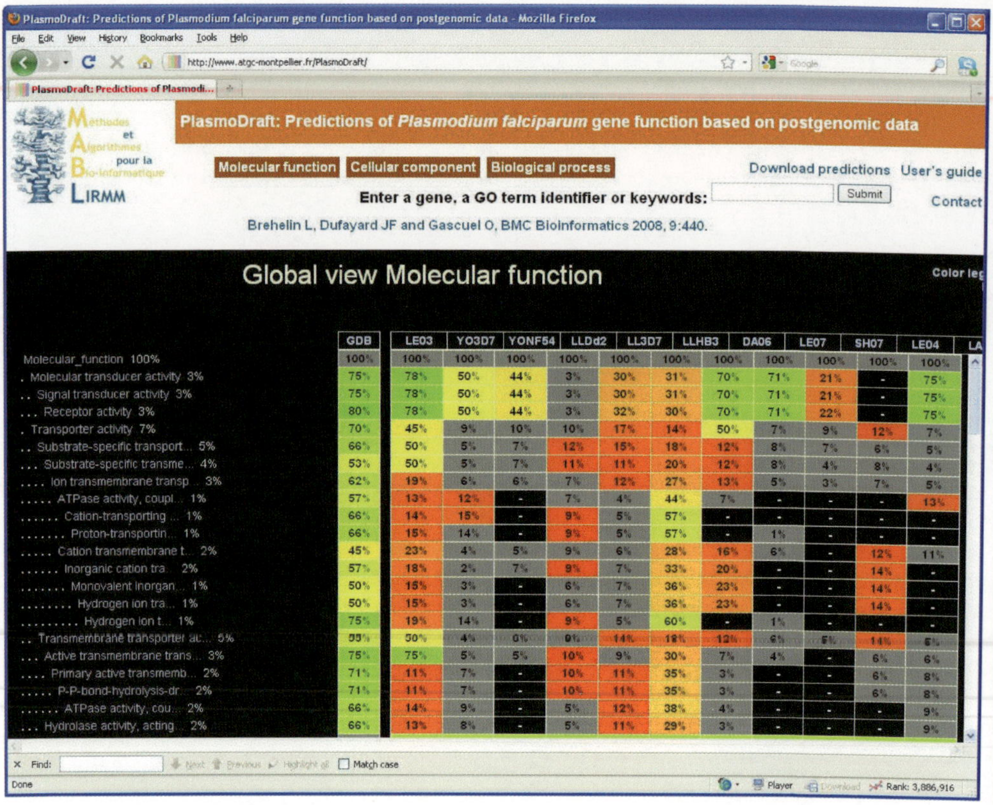

Fig. 7. A global view for a series of parasite strains based on the GO Molecular Function classification in PlasmoDraft. GO categories are listed on the left of the table, and the results are shown in columns for a series of different parasite strains.

7.2 TDI Kernel

URL: http://tropicaldisease.org/kernel

The TDI Kernel strongly supports the Open Source approach to drug discovery, and is aimed at the prediction of binding sites and ligand interactions through homology modeling approaches (Ortí *et al.*, 2009). Targets may be searched by organism, which includes *C. hominis*, *C. parvum*, *L. major*, *M. leprae*, *M. tuberculosis*, *P. falciparum*, *P. vivax*, *T. brucei*, *T. cruzi* and *T. gondii*. Further search criteria include keywords, UniProt IDs, DrugBank IDs, PDB Ligand ID and homology modeling parameters. At the time of writing, 28 templates had been analyzed for *P. falciparum*. The detailed view of a target shows the templates used for homology modeling, provides the generated models and shows the ligand predictions for the selected target (Figure 9). Each of these may be investigated further through links to PDB, MSD (http://www.ebi.ac.uk/msd) and DrugBank (Wishart *et al.*, 2008). For each prediction, the result may be expanded to further show a figure of the ligand bound in the active site, drug category information for the ligand, and current uses of the drug.

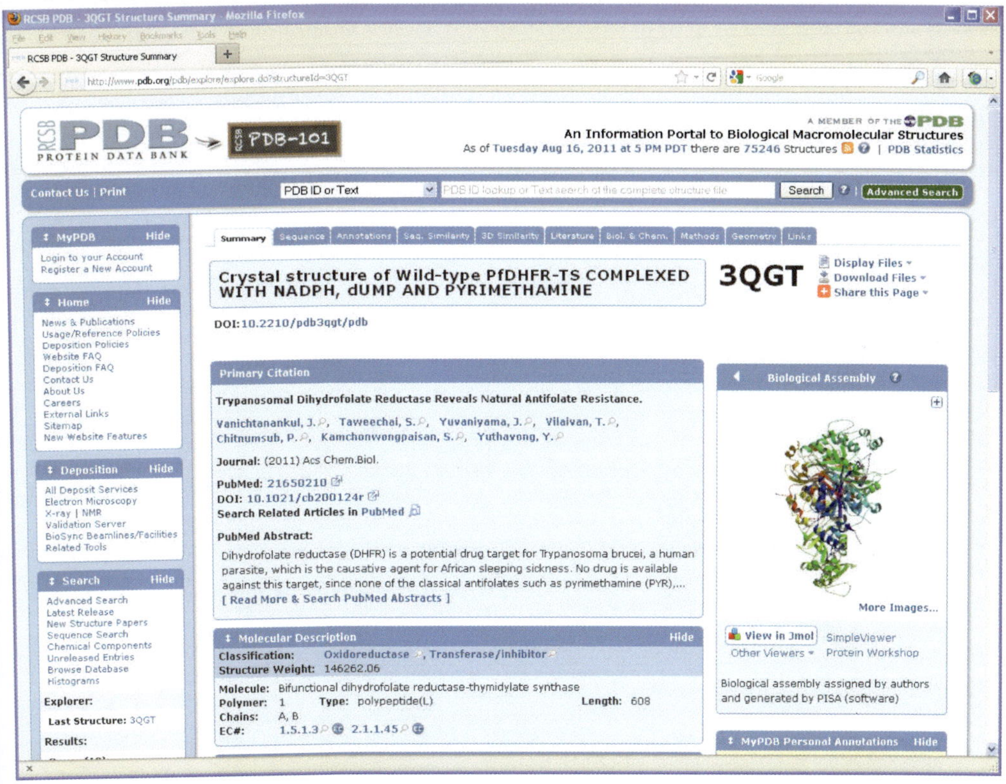

Fig. 8. The PDB results page for a structure of PFD0830w (bifunctional dihydrofolate reductase-thymidylate synthase from *P. falciparum*). A summary of the protein's information is shown in the centre, with a structural overview on the right.

7.3 ModBase

URL: http://modbase.compbio.ucsf.edu

ModBase is an extensive collection of homology models for a variety of species, including *P. falciparum* and *P. vivax* (Pieper *et al.*, 2009). The homology models have been constructed using ModPipe, a pipeline which uses mainly PSI-BLAST (Altschul *et al.*, 1997) and Modeler (Eswar *et al.*, 2006) for model building. At the time of writing, ModBase contained models for 2599 *P. falciparum* and 2359 *P. vivax* proteins. Searches may be performed using text terms or protein sequence, and results may be displayed as either a model overview, detail regarding the model or a sequence overview. The detailed view contains information about the model coverage of the protein sequence, model quality parameters, graphical representations of the protein structure and a wide range of external links to other relevant databases (Figure 10). Where available, SNP information and ligand binding sites may also be viewed.

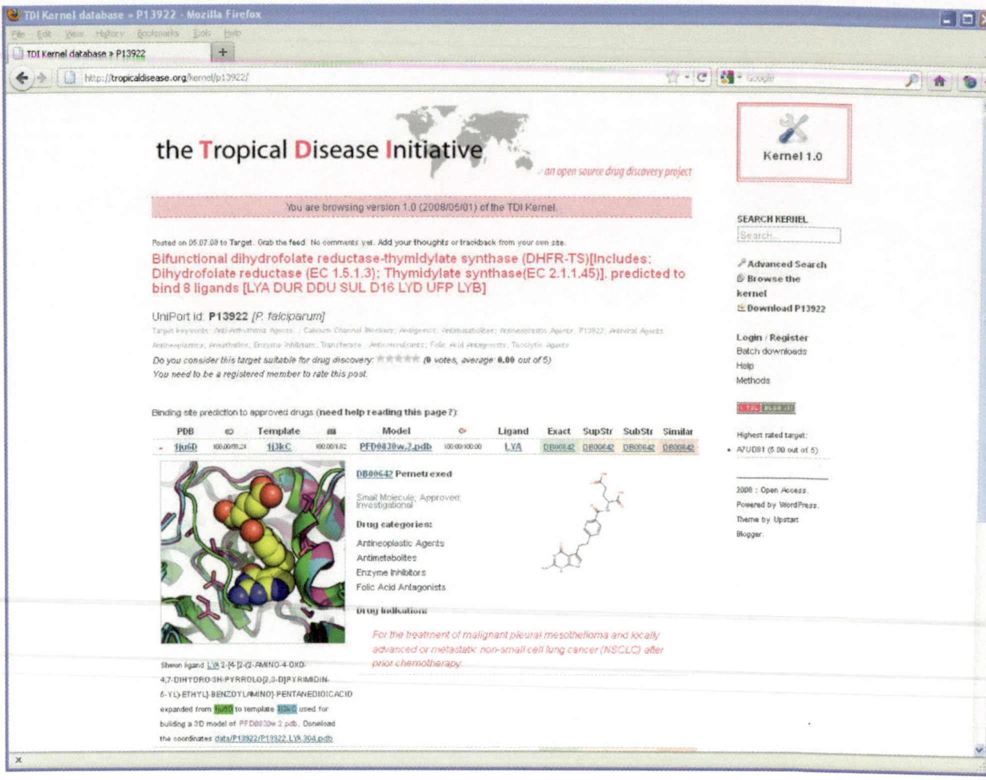

Fig. 9. The result view for PFD0830w (bifunctional dihydrofolate reductase-thymidylate synthase from *P. falciparum*) with LYA in the TDI Kernel resource. A structural view of the ligand in binding site is shown, as well as additional information about the protein and ligand.

8. Literature databases

8.1 The malaria literature database

URL: http://carrier.gnf.org/publications/Py

The Malaria Literature Database is compiled by the Genomics Institute of the Novartis Research Foundation. Whereas most literature searches focus only on abstracts, Google Scholar and Scirus is used to search in the body of Open Access papers for the presence of gene names. Gene name - publication pairs are then collected and indexed. Additionally, searches may be performed for genes, orthologs and published papers. Gene results are displayed with PlasmoDB links, and ortholog results are shown. Literature results are shown together with PubMed PMID links for easy access to the abstracts and papers. It is also possible to download all data in batch format.

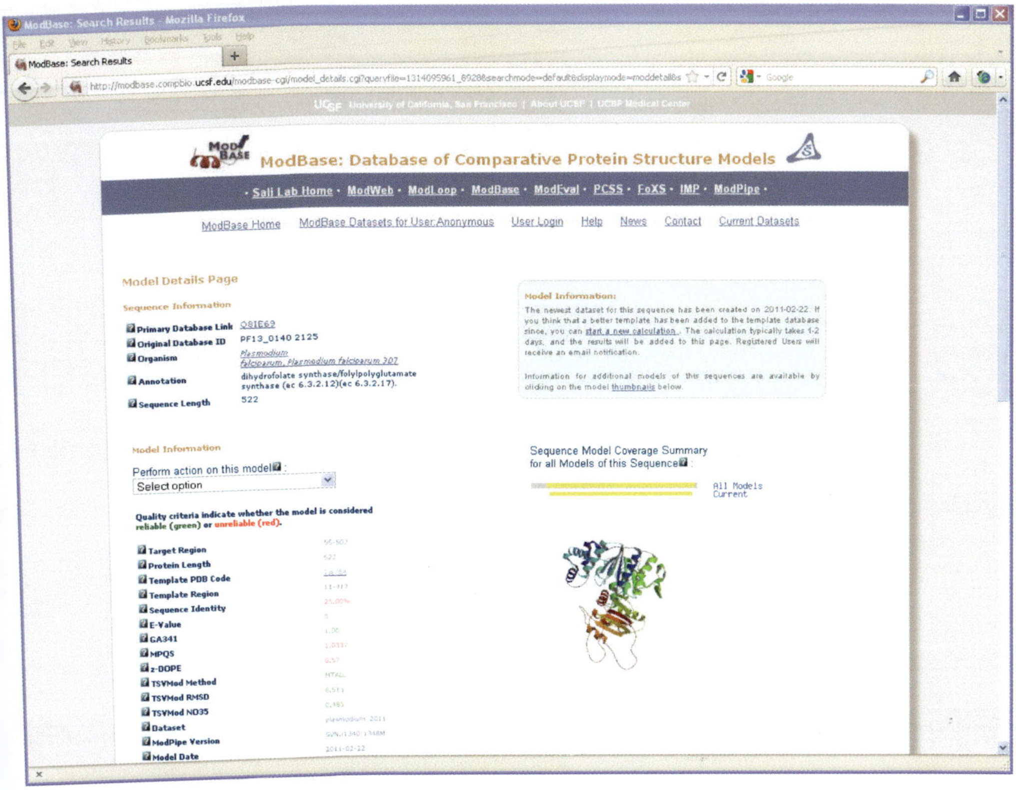

Fig. 10. A detailed view of a homology model of PFD0830w (bifunctional dihydrofolate reductase-thymidylate synthase from *P. falciparum*). Model parameters are shown on the left, with an alignment overview and graphical representation of the protein structure on the right.

9. Drug discovery databases

9.1 ChEMBL

The ChEMBL database is primarily a database of bioactive small molecules, and provides access to a wide range of targets and chemical compounds, including industry-generated datasets such as the GSK TCAMS malaria dataset and the Novartis-GNF malaria box set in the ChEMBL-NTD section (Overington, 2009). The targets section may be searched using either a keyword, protein sequence or a ChEMBL ID. The results for a specific target include bioactivity data, assay categories and parameters available for the target and a chemical classification of the related compounds by molecular weight, logP and PSA (Figure 11).

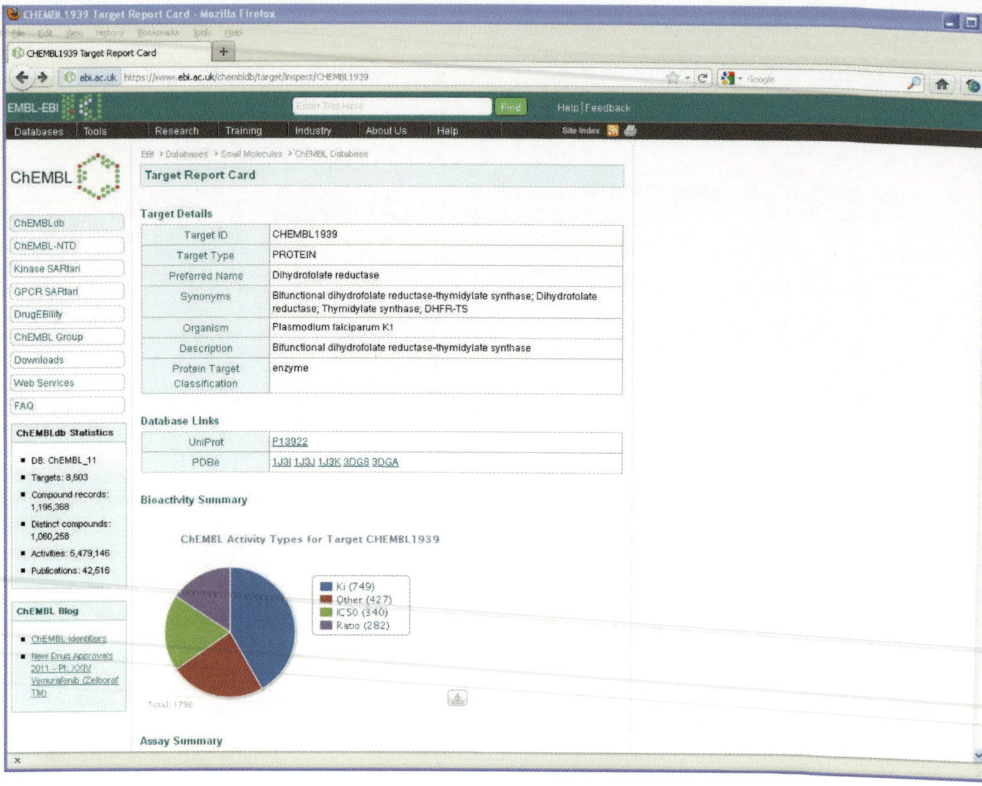

Fig. 11. The result view for PFD0830w (bifunctional dihydrofolate reductase-thymidylate synthase from *P. falciparum*) in ChEMBL. The protein's details are shown at the top, with database links followed by a graphical summary of available binding data at the bottom.

These are presented as a graphical summary view, where each section may be explored further. The next level of results is a table showing the compound structure, bioactivity, assay type, assay source, results and literature reference (Figure 12). Links between proteins and compounds are established through manual literature curation.

Chemicals may be searched using text-based queries or chemical structures. Results are returned in a tabular format with chemical structures and detailed chemical properties. When a compound is selected for further exploration, clinical trials relevant to the compound, bioactivity, assay and protein target information are also shown together with links to external databases. A search functionality for assays is also available. The ChEMBL database additionally contains specific resource areas for kinases (Kinase SARfari) and for G protein-coupled receptors (GPCR SARfari). It also contains the DrugEBIlity resource focussed on structure-based drugability.

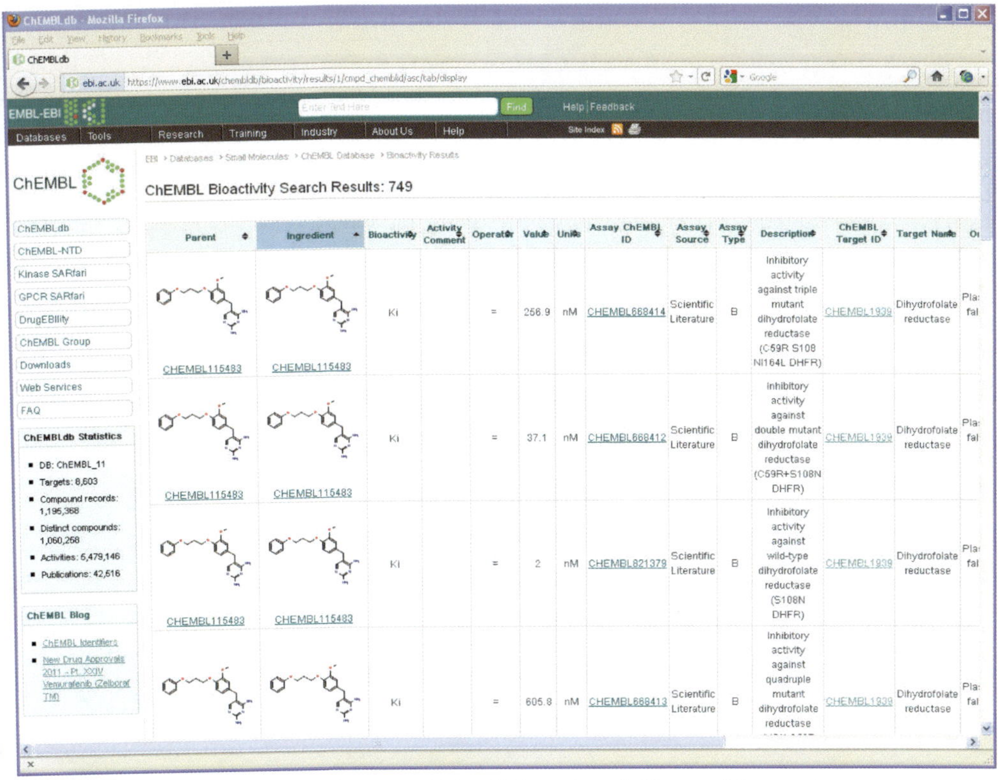

Fig. 12. A more detailed view for PFD0830w (bifunctional dihydrofolate reductase-thymidylate synthase from *P. falciparum*)-related compounds in ChEMBL. The chemical structures of the parent compound (if applicable) and the specific chemical ingredient are shown on the left, followed by columns containing detailed assay and target information.

9.2 TDR Targets

URL: http://tdrtargets.org

The TDR Targets database is a comprehensive integrated resource for the selection of drug targets and lead compounds in several different infectious diseases. It is the product of a collaboration of many research groups, and contains very extensive data for *P. falciparum* and *P. vivax*, but also for *T. gondii*, *M. tuberculosis*, *M. leprae*, *T. brucei*, *T. cruzi*, *L. major*, *B. malayi*, *S. mansoni* and *W. bancrofti* (Crowther *et al.*, 2010). It also contains chemical compounds. The TDR Targets database provides pre-compiled lists of targets, but also allows users to perform their own target selection based on a series of molecular properties. Gene information includes a series of fields such as gene ID, gene name, gene product name, exon count, length of gene, length of the protein, molecular weight of protein, isoelectric point of protein, hydrophobicity of proteins, number of transmembrane domains and presence of a signal peptide. Genes are additionally classified into enzymes, transporters and receptors. Functional annotation data includes InterPro domains (Hunter *et al.*, 2009), Pfam domains (Bateman *et al.*, 2004), GO data (Ashburner *et al.*, 2000) and EC numbers.

Structural data contains links to experimentally-derived 3D structures but also to homology models generated as part of the ModBase project. Expression data contains links to a series of microarray experiments. Antigenicity data was generated using the Kolaskar and Tongaonkar method (Kolaskar & Tongaonkar, 1990) as implemented in the EMBOSS antigenic module (Rice *et al.*, 2000). Phyletic distribution information was obtained from the OrthoMCL database (Li *et al.*, 2003). Essentiality data is based on gene knockout and knockdown studies in selected organisms. Drugability data is based on orthology to proteins in the Inpharmatica SAR database which is maintained by the ChEMBL group at the EBI. Drug-to-gene association data is mined from DrugBank and ChEMBL using orthology approaches. Assayability data is primarily obtained from the BRENDA database (Scheer *et al.*, 2011). Literature data originates from PubMed or from curators.

The chemical datasets in TDR Targets is a combination of small molecule data from a variety of sources. This includes properties such as names, synonyms, structure, InChi keys, molecular weight, LogP, hydrogen-bonding donors and acceptors, pharmacological activity and rating according to the Lipinski Rule-of-Five (Lipinski *et al.*, 2001). Bioactivity data is also available.

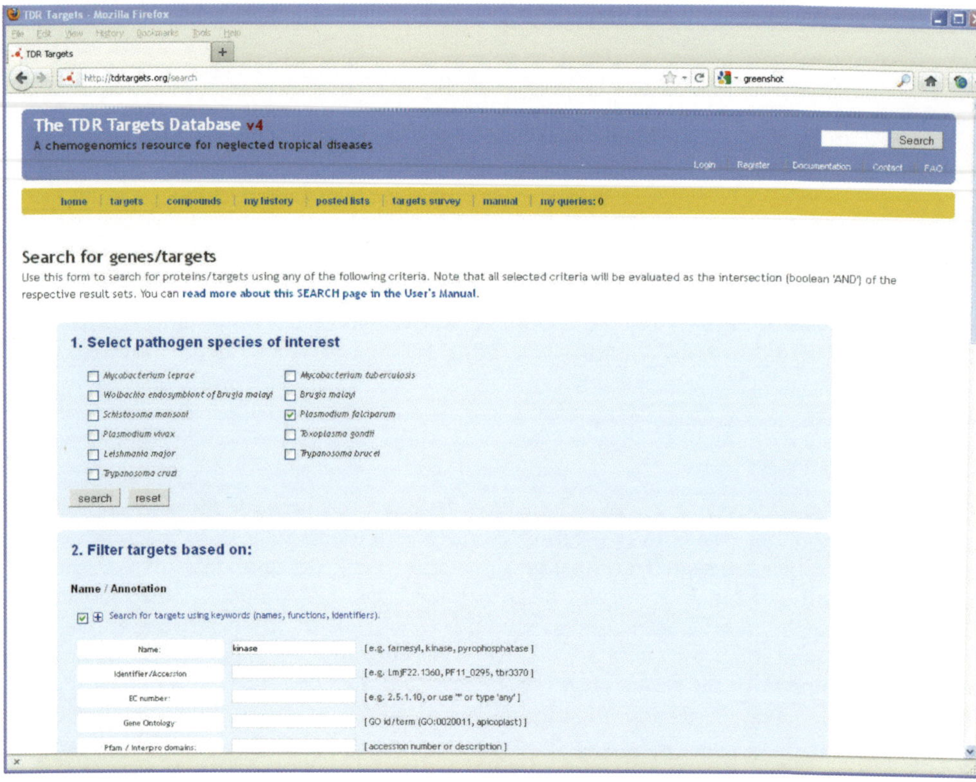

Fig. 13. The target search interface of the TDR Targets database. The different organisms available for searching are shown at the top, followed by possible search parameters at the bottom.

The target search functionality allows users to select proteins from the pathogen genome based on the very extensive criteria mentioned above, and queries may be saved for future reference. Searches are performed by first selecting the pathogen of interest, and this is followed by the addition of filtering criteria (Figure 13). Multiple queries may be executed, and subsquently cumulative search results may be generated by specifying unions, intersects or subtractions of the results. Weights and names may be associated with the different queries. When a target is explored, the view provides extensive information in all the categories listed above, sorted by category. Compound searches may be performed using text- or structure-based queries. Additionally, compound searches may be done based on chemical properties, activities and associated genes. A summary of resulting chemical structures is displayed together with basic properties, and a highly-detailed report for each compound may be obtained, including putative protein targets, activities and external resources for the compound (Figure 14). The TDR resource further provides a posted list feature for the sharing of data within the scientific community, as well as a targets survey page for gathering curated information from community experts.

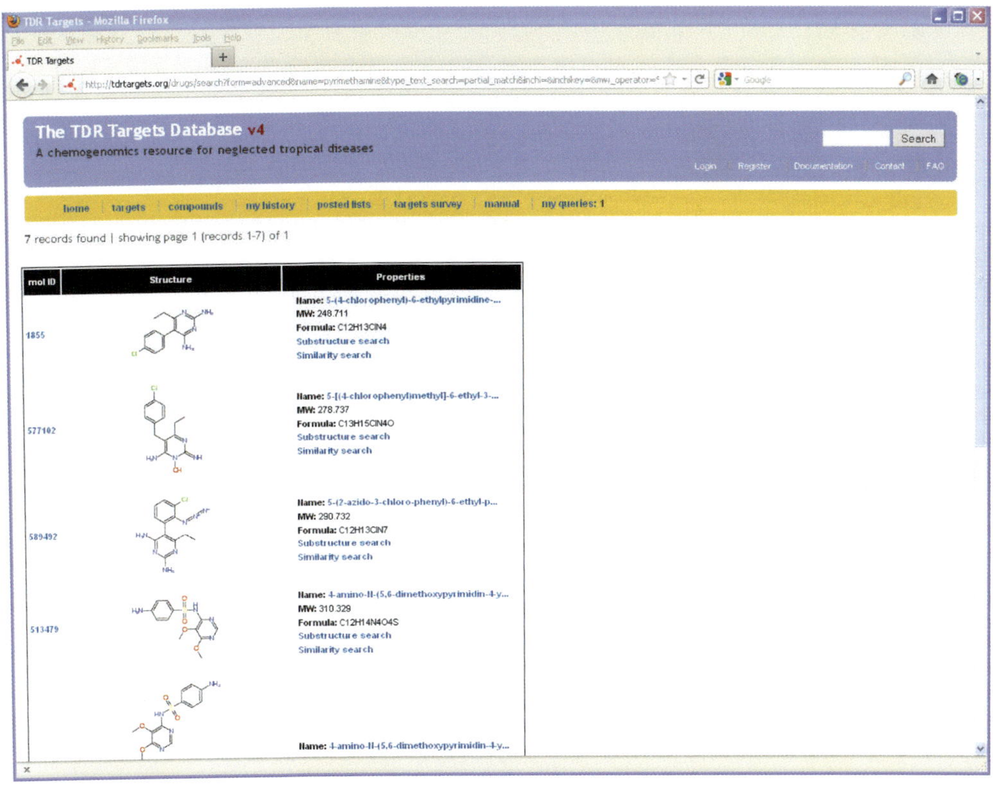

Fig. 14. The compound search results display of the TDR Targets database. Chemical identifiers and structures are shown on the left, with more detailed compound information on the right.

9.3 Discovery

URL: http://discovery.bi.up.ac.za

The Discovery resource is aimed at scientists who would like to explore primarily the *P. falciparum* genome for the selection of drug target proteins and lead compounds (Joubert *et al.*, 2009). Other parasite genomes included are *P. vivax*, *P. vivax*, *P. bergei*, *P. chabaudi* and *P. yoelii*. Also included for comparative purposes are the the human and mosquito genomes. The resource may be accessed by querying proteins or ligands. Proteins may be searched using simple keywords, combined terms or accession numbers. Protein data displayed includes orthology and sequence comparisons, ontology terms, functional annotations, metabolic pathways, structural information and possible ligand interactions based on orthology to sequences from DrugBank, PDB Ligand and KEGG. The new version of Discovery adds extensive data from ChEMBL, as well as literature mining and user annotation functionality (Figure 15).

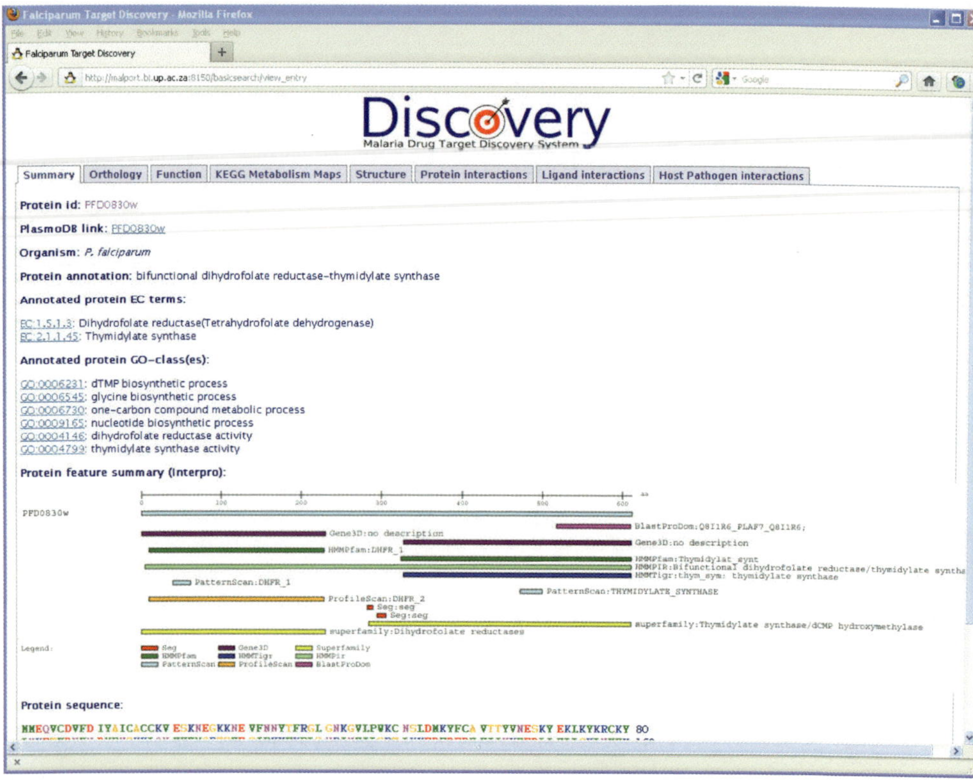

Fig. 15. The Discovery protein results view for PFD0830w (bifunctional dihydrofolate reductase-thymidylate synthase from *P. falciparum*). A summary of protein annotations is shown at the top, followed by a graphical representation of sequence motifs in the molecule. The other types of results that may be viewed can be seen as tabs at the top of the screen.

Chemical compounds may be searched using text terms or chemical structures, and searches are powered using the ChemAxon JChemBase software (http://www.chemaxon.com). Several different types of searches are available. Results are displayed in a tabular fashion, and compounds may be selected for further inspection. Additional detail is then provided, including the structure, ADMET properties and putative protein interactions (Figure 16).

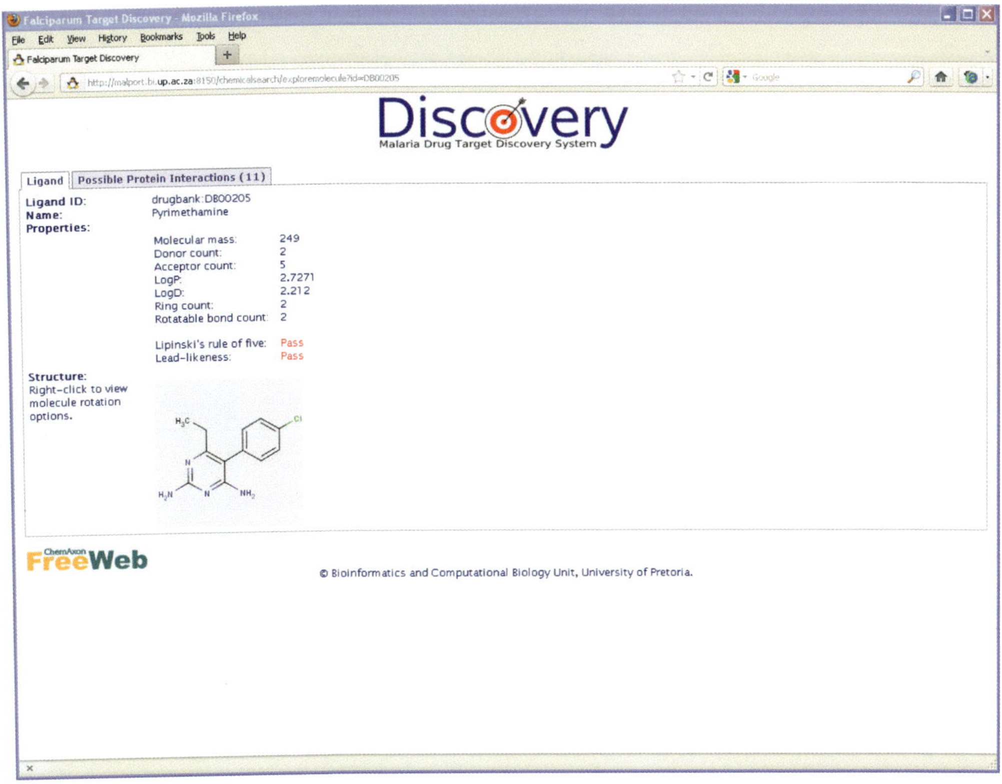

Fig. 16. The Discovery chemical results view for pyrimethamine. The chemical properties are shown at the top, followed by the structure of the compound at the bottom. The tab for viewing possible protein interactions is visible at the top of the page.

10. Conclusion

Researchers face many different challenges when embarking on the discovery of new drug targets. Here we provide an overview on valuable resources that will enable scientists to perform comprehensive searches and make numerous comparisons between targets prior to selection. In addition these tools can be used in the evaluation and data mining of existing targets, which can easily be overlooked using conventional methods and should therefore be used before committing expensive and time-consuming resources. Of primary concern is the properties that need to be taken into account when selecting putative drug proteins or lead compounds. The term "drugability" is widely used for describing the suitability of both proteins and compounds as targets and leads, but specific properties and parameters related to this can be difficult to formalize. Various examples of studies proposing drugability properties and possible scoring systems are available in the literature (Crowther *et al.*, 2010; Fauman *et al.*, 2011; Halgren, 2009; Hasan *et al.*, 2006; Nicola *et al.*, 2008; Schneider, 2004).

Whereas the resources discussed in the first part of the chapter mostly address resources with single specialized foci, the latter two resources have attempted to integrate the most relevant properties related to protein and compound suitability for drug design during the design of the search strategies. These resources make it possible for researchers to start out with a large number of proteins or compounds, and filter them sequentially based on a series of properties related to "drugability", therefore producing a smaller list of candidate molecules that may be explored further in greater detail using the more focussed sites, and through experimental approaches. These integrated resources make it possible for researchers to in effect start out with all proteins encoded by a genome or all compounds in a database, and rapidly decrease the potential candidate list to a manageable number using the rational application of filters to properties of their choice.

11. Glossary

A brief glossary of some terms that may not be familiar to all readers:

Bayesian:	A method employing Bayes' theorem on conditional probability
BLAST:	Basic Local Alignment Search Tool which is used for searching sequences vs. databases
EC number:	Enzyme Commission number defining the type of reaction catalyzed by an enzyme
Essentiality:	An indication of whether the organism can survive after an enzyme has been knocked out or inhibited
Homology model:	A model of a protein structure calculated by using the structure of another homologous protein as template
Lipinksi rule-of-five:	A rule of five parameters proposed by Lipinski and colleagues which is used predict the pharmacological or biological activity of a chemical compound
Ontology:	A biological ontology term or identifier forms part of the Gene Ontology (GO) Consortium classification which provides a vocabulary describing gene product characteristics
ORF:	An Open Reading Frame in a nucleic acid sequence which potentially encodes a peptide region
Orthologs:	Sequences which are related to a common evolutionary ancestor but have diverged due to speciation
Paralogs:	Sequences which are related to a common evolutionary ancestor but have diverged due to gene duplication
Proteome:	The complete set of proteins produced by an organism or tissue

12. References

Altschul, S. F.; Madden, T. L.; Schäffer, A. A.; Zhang, J.; Zhang, Z.; Miller, W., & Lipman, D. J. (1997). Gapped BLAST and PSI-BLAST: a new generation of protein database search programs. Nucleic Acids Res, Vol. 25(17), pp. 3389-3402.

Ashburner, M.; Ball, C. A.; Blake, J. A.; Botstein, D.; Butler, H.; Cherry, J. M.; Davis, A. P.; Dolinski, K.; Dwight, S. S.; Eppig, J. T.; Harris, M. A.; Hill, D. P.; Issel-Tarver, L.; Kasarskis, A.; Lewis, S.; Matese, J. C.; Richardson, J. E.; Ringwald, M.; Rubin, G. M., & Sherlock, G. (2000). Gene ontology: tool for the unification of biology. The Gene Ontology Consortium. Nat Genet, Vol. 25(1), pp. 25-29.

Aurrecoechea, C.; Brestelli, J.; Brunk, B. P.; Dommer, J.; Fischer, S.; Gajria, B.; Gao, X.; Gingle, A.; Grant, G.; Harb, O. S.; Heiges, M.; Innamorato, F.; Iodice, J.; Kissinger, J. C.; Kraemer, E.; Li, W.; Miller, J. A.; Nayak, V.; Pennington, C.; Pinney, D. F.; Roos, D. S.; Ross, C.; Stoeckert, C. J.; Treatman, C., & Wang, H. (2009). PlasmoDB: a functional genomic database for malaria parasites. Nucleic Acids Res, Vol. 37(Database issue), pp. D539-D543.

Aurrecoechea, C.; Brestelli, J.; Brunk, B. P.; Fischer, S.; Gajria, B.; Gao, X.; Gingle, A.; Grant, G.; Harb, O. S.; Heiges, M.; Innamorato, F.; Iodice, J.; Kissinger, J. C.; Kraemer, E. T.; Li, W.; Miller, J. A.; Nayak, V.; Pennington, C.; Pinney, D. F.; Roos, D. S.; Ross, C.; Srinivasamoorthy, G.; Stoeckert, C. J.; Thibodeau, R.; Treatman, C., & Wang, H. (2010). EuPathDB: a portal to eukaryotic pathogen databases. Nucleic Acids Res, Vol. 38(Database issue), pp. D415-D419.

Bateman, A.; Coin, L.; Durbin, R.; Finn, R. D.; Hollich, V.; Griffiths-Jones, S.; Khanna, A.; Marshall, M.; Moxon, S.; Sonnhammer, E. L. L.; Studholme, D. J.; Yeats, C., & Eddy, S. R. (2004). The Pfam protein families database. Nucleic Acids Res, Vol. 32(Database issue), pp. D138-D141.

Bernstein, F. C.; Koetzle, T. F.; Williams, G. J.; Meyer, E. F.; Brice, M. D.; Rodgers, J. R.; Kennard, O.; Shimanouchi, T., & Tasumi, M. (1977). The Protein Data Bank: a computer-based archival file for macromolecular structures. J Mol Biol, Vol. 112(3), pp. 535-542.

Bozdech, Z.; Llinás, M.; Pulliam, B. L.; Wong, E. D.; Zhu, J., & DeRisi, J. L. (2003). The transcriptome of the intraerythrocytic developmental cycle of *Plasmodium falciparum*. PLoS Biol, Vol. 1(1), pp. E5.

Bréhélin, L.; Dufayard, J.-F., & Gascuel, O. (2008). PlasmoDraft: a database of *Plasmodium falciparum* gene function predictions based on postgenomic data. BMC Bioinformatics, Vol. 9, pp. 440.

Caspi, R.; Foerster, H.; Fulcher, C. A.; Hopkinson, R.; Ingraham, J.; Kaipa, P.; Krummenacker, M.; Paley, S.; Pick, J.; Rhee, S. Y.; Tissier, C.; Zhang, P., & Karp, P. D. (2006). MetaCyc: a multiorganism database of metabolic pathways and enzymes. Nucleic Acids Res, Vol. 34(Database issue), pp. D511-D516.

Crowther, G. J.; Shanmugam, D.; Carmona, S. J.; Doyle, M. A.; Hertz-Fowler, C.; Berriman, M.; Nwaka, S.; Ralph, S. A.; Roos, D. S.; Voorhis, W. C. V., & Agüero, F. (2010). Identification of attractive drug targets in neglected-disease pathogens using an *in silico* approach. PLoS Negl Trop Dis, Vol. 4(8), pp. e804.

Date, S. V., & Stoeckert, C. J. (2006). Computational modeling of the *Plasmodium falciparum* interactome reveals protein function on a genome-wide scale. Genome Res, Vol. 16(4), pp. 542-549.

Eswar, N.; Webb, B.; Marti-Renom, M. A.; Madhusudhan, M. S.; Eramian, D.; Shen, M.-Y.; Pieper, U., & Sali, A. (2006). Comparative protein structure modeling using Modeller. Curr Protoc Bioinformatics, Vol. Chapter 5, pp. Unit 5.6.

Fauman, E. B.; Rai, B. K., & Huang, E. S. (2011). Structure-based druggability assessment-identifying suitable targets for small molecule therapeutics. Curr Opin Chem Biol, Vol. 15(4), pp. 463-468.

Gardner, M. J.; Hall, N.; Fung, E.; White, O.; Berriman, M.; Hyman, R. W.; Carlton, J. M.; Pain, A.; Nelson, K. E.; Bowman, S.; Paulsen, I. T.; James, K.; Eisen, J. A.; Rutherford, K.; Salzberg, S. L.; Craig, A.; Kyes, S.; Chan, M.-S.; Nene, V.; Shallom, S. J.; Suh, B.; Peterson, J.; Angiuoli, S.; Pertea, M.; Allen, J.; Selengut, J.; Haft, D.; Mather, M. W.; Vaidya, A. B.; Martin, D. M. A.; Fairlamb, A. H.; Fraunholz, M. J.; Roos, D. S.; Ralph, S. A.; McFadden, G. I.; Cummings, L. M.; Subramanian, G. M.; Mungall, C.; Venter, J. C.; Carucci, D. J.; Hoffman, S. L.; Newbold, C.; Davis, R. W.; Fraser, C. M., & Barrell, B. (2002). Genome sequence of the human malaria parasite *Plasmodium falciparum*. Nature, Vol. 419(6906), pp. 498-511.

Ginsburg, H. (2009). Caveat emptor: limitations of the automated reconstruction of metabolic pathways in Plasmodium. Trends Parasitol, Vol. 25(1), pp. 37-43.

Halgren, T. A. (2009). Identifying and characterizing binding sites and assessing druggability. J Chem Inf Model, Vol. 49(2), pp. 377-389.

Hasan, S.; Daugelat, S.; Rao, P. S. S., & Schreiber, M. (2006). Prioritizing genomic drug targets in pathogens: application to *Mycobacterium tuberculosis*. PLoS Comput Biol, Vol. 2(6), pp. e61.

Hunter, S.; Apweiler, R.; Attwood, T. K.; Bairoch, A.; Bateman, A.; Binns, D.; Bork, P.; Das, U.; Daugherty, L.; Duquenne, L.; Finn, R. D.; Gough, J.; Haft, D.; Hulo, N.; Kahn, D.; Kelly, E.; Laugraud, A. I.; Letunic, I.; Lonsdale, D.; Lopez, R.; Madera, M.; Maslen, J.; McAnulla, C.; McDowall, J.; Mistry, J.; Mitchell, A.; Mulder, N.; Natale, D.; Orengo, C.; Quinn, A. F.; Selengut, J. D.; Sigrist, C. J. A.; Thimma, M.; Thomas, P. D.; Valentin, F.; Wilson, D.; Wu, C. H., & Yeats, C. (2009). InterPro: the integrative protein signature database. Nucleic Acids Res, Vol. 37(Database issue), pp. D211-D215.

Joubert, F.; Harrison, C. M.; Koegelenberg, R. J.; Odendaal, C. J., & de Beer, T. A. P. (2009). Discovery: an interactive resource for the rational selection and comparison of putative drug target proteins in malaria. Malar J, Vol. 8, pp. 178.

Kanehisa, M., & Goto, S. (2000). KEGG: kyoto encyclopedia of genes and genomes. Nucleic Acids Res, Vol. 28(1), pp. 27-30.

Kanehisa, M.; Goto, S.; Furumichi, M.; Tanabe, M., & Hirakawa, M. (2010). KEGG for representation and analysis of molecular networks involving diseases and drugs. Nucleic Acids Res, Vol. 38(Database issue), pp. D355-D360.

Kanehisa, M.; Goto, S.; Hattori, M.; Aoki-Kinoshita, K. F.; Itoh, M.; Kawashima, S.; Katayama, T.; Araki, M., & Hirakawa, M. (2006). From genomics to chemical genomics: new developments in KEGG. Nucleic Acids Res, Vol. 34(Database issue), pp. D354-D357.

Kolaskar, A. S., & Tongaonkar, P. C. (1990). A semi-empirical method for prediction of antigenic determinants on protein antigens. FEBS Lett, Vol. 276(1-2), pp. 172-174.

Li, L.; Stoeckert, C. J., & Roos, D. S. (2003). OrthoMCL: identification of ortholog groups for eukaryotic genomes. Genome Res, Vol. 13(9), pp. 2178-2189.

Lipinski, C. A.; Lombardo, F.; Dominy, B. W., & Feeney, P. J. (2001). Experimental and computational approaches to estimate solubility and permeability in drug discovery and development settings. [Review]. Adv Drug Deliv Rev, Vol. 46(1-3), pp. 3-26.

Llinás, M.; Bozdech, Z.; Wong, E. D.; Adai, A. T., & DeRisi, J. L. (2006). Comparative whole genome transcriptome analysis of three *Plasmodium falciparum* strains. Nucleic Acids Res, Vol. 34(4), pp. 1166-1173.

Nicola, G.; Smith, C. A., & Abagyan, R. (2008). New method for the assessment of all drug-like pockets across a structural genome. J Comput Biol, Vol. 15(3), pp. 231-240.

Ortí, L.; Carbajo, R. J.; Pieper, U.; Eswar, N.; Maurer, S. M.; Rai, A. K.; Taylor, G.; Todd, M. H.; Pineda-Lucena, A.; Sali, A., & Marti-Renom, M. A. (2009). A kernel for the Tropical Disease Initiative. Nat Biotechnol, Vol. 27(4), pp. 320-321.

Overington, J. (2009). ChEMBL. An interview with John Overington, team leader, chemogenomics at the European Bioinformatics Institute Outstation of the European Molecular Biology Laboratory (EMBL-EBI). Interview by Wendy A. Warr. J Comput Aided Mol Des, Vol. 23(4), pp. 195-198.

Pieper, U.; Eswar, N.; Webb, B. M.; Eramian, D.; Kelly, L.; Barkan, D. T.; Carter, H.; Mankoo, P.; Karchin, R.; Marti-Renom, M. A.; Davis, F. P., & Sali, A. (2009). MODBASE, a database of annotated comparative protein structure models and associated resources. Nucleic Acids Res, Vol. 37(Database issue), pp. D347-D354.

Rice, P.; Longden, I., & Bleasby, A. (2000). EMBOSS: the European Molecular Biology Open Software Suite. Trends Genet, Vol. 16(6), pp. 276-277.

Scheer, M.; Grote, A.; Chang, A.; Schomburg, I.; Munaretto, C.; Rother, M.; Söhngen, C.; Stelzer, M.; Thiele, J., & Schomburg, D. (2011). BRENDA, the enzyme information system in 2011. Nucleic Acids Res, Vol. 39(Database issue), pp. D670-D676.

Schneider, M. (2004). A rational approach to maximize success rate in target discovery. Arch Pharm (Weinheim), Vol. 337(12), pp. 625-633.

Stein, L. D.; Mungall, C.; Shu, S.; Caudy, M.; Mangone, M.; Day, A.; Nickerson, E.; Stajich, J. E.; Harris, T. W.; Arva, A., & Lewis, S. (2002). The generic genome browser: a building block for a model organism system database. Genome Res, Vol. 12(10), pp. 1599-1610.

Wishart, D. S.; Knox, C.; Guo, A. C.; Cheng, D.; Shrivastava, S.; Tzur, D.; Gautam, B., & Hassanali, M. (2008). DrugBank: a knowledgebase for drugs, drug actions and drug targets. Nucleic Acids ResPDBLIgand, Vol. 36(Database issue), pp. D901-D906.

Yeh, I.; Hanekamp, T.; Tsoka, S.; Karp, P. D., & Altman, R. B. (2004). Computational analysis of *Plasmodium falciparum* metabolism: organizing genomic information to facilitate drug discovery. Genome Res, Vol. 14(5), pp. 917-924.

14

Human Genetic Contribution to the Outcome of Infection with Malaria Parasites

Alison Machado, Cheikh Loucoubar, Laura Grange,
Jean-François Bureau, Anavaj Sakuntabhai and Richard Paul
Unité de Génétique Fonctionnelle des Maladies Infectieuses,
Institut Pasteur
France

1. Introduction

The study of the contribution of human genetics to the risk of severe malaria has a long history, with Haldane in the 1950s reporting a major role of the sickle cell mutation (HbS), in the protection against severe disease (Haldane, 1949). Since then, genetic variants of β-globin (HbE: Hutagalung et al., 1999; HbC: Agarwal et al., 2000; HbS: Aidoo et al., 2002), α-globin (Mockenhaupt et al., 2004), Band 3 protein (Foo et al., 1992), HLA (Hill et al., 1991) and several cytokine loci (Tumor Necrosis Factor-alpha: Knight et al., 1999; Interleukin-12: Morahan et al., 2002a; Interferon-alpha receptor-1: Aucan et al., 2003; Interleukin-4: Gyan et al., 2004) have been demonstrated to confer protection to severe malaria. To date, the majority of studies have been case/control association studies, comparing severe malaria to uncomplicated cases. Due to the fact that *Plasmodium falciparum* is the etiological agent of severe malaria, all studies have consequently focussed on this parasite. The other congeneric species and notably *Plasmodium vivax*, can, however, cause severe disease, albeit at a much lower incidence, and warrant an increased research effort (Price et al., 2007).

Here we argue that for infectious diseases in general and for malaria parasites in particular, more attention should be paid to the "biological" course and outcome of infection in addition to severe disease. This is for several reasons: (i) the majority of infections in endemic settings do not cause severe disease. Indeed, severe disease is a collective term that englobes multiple pathologies (including cerebral malaria, severe malaria anaemia, metabolic acidosis, multiple organ failure) that likely involve very different biological pathways and thus should not be analysed as a single phenotype; (ii) the progression from clinical malaria to asymptomatic infection defines the acquisition of clinical immunity and identifying the mechanisms underlying this tipping point is central to the development of disease control methods; (iii) *P. falciparum* is remarkable in that sterilising anti-parasite immunity is never achieved. Although the parasite has a variety of mechanisms enabling this, the human also plays a part. Identifying pathways that "enable" the parasite to persist without elimination will provide insight into this apparent immune defence dysfunction; (iv) the biology of the parasite within the host will be informative as to how the parasite optimises its exploitation of and subsequent transmission from the human host. The parasite must persist and transmit to mosquitoes in the face of very differing immune environments. The differential impact of human genetics according to the clinical outcome of infection will throw light on how the parasite manages its strategy for survival and reproduction (transmission).

Focussing on infection enables implementation of a family-based study design that controls for population sub-structure and admixture. Such an approach would be impractical for the study of severe disease because of its relative infrequency. Longitudinal family-based studies enable a more detailed real-time analysis of the human response to infection. Thus, as well as controlling for population sub-structure, they can (i) reveal how the same individual responds at different times in his life and thus generate insight into the acquisition of clinical and anti-parasite immunity; (ii) enable incorporation of parasite genetics both with respect to the long-term co-evolutionary trajectory of the host-parasite duo and the short-term impact of intervention (Loucoubar et al., 2011a).

Evidence for a contribution of host genetic factors to mild clinical malaria and biological phenotypes, such as number of clinical episodes, parasite density, immune responses to *P. falciparum* antigens has progressed with the development of increasingly sophisticated techniques. Population level differences in susceptibility to malaria have been observed between sympatric ethnic groups (Modiano et al., 1996) and, at a finer scale, differential phenotypic expression was observed in monozygotic and dizygotic twins; there was greater phenotypic similarity in monozygotic twins, strongly suggesting genetic control as such twins are genetically more similar than dizygotic twins (Jepson et al., 1995). Segregation studies that assess the extent of phenotypic similarity in families demonstrated co-segregation of parasite density and of prevalence of mild malaria in families (Rihet et al., 1998a). Microsatellite typing of family-based cohorts enabled this segregation to be narrowed down to chromosomal regions (Flori et al., 2003; Garcia et al., 1998; Rihet et al., 1998b; Sakuntabhai et al., 2008; Timmann et al., 2007). Candidate gene approaches have also shown association of specific genetic polymorphisms with mild clinical malaria (Kun et al., 2001; Walley et al., 2004; Williams et al., 1996). Emphasis has understandably been placed on clinical malaria and very few studies have considered asymptomatic malaria and only to a limited extent (Flori et al., 2003; Garcia et al., 1998; Mombo et al., 2003; Rihet et al., 1998a, 1998b; Timmann et al., 2007).

This chapter presents a summary of the achievements in the field of genetic analysis to date, the benefits of examining biological parasite phenotypes and the practical aspects of sampling and analysis. Firstly, we discuss in some detail issues concerning phenotype choice, the pros and cons of case/control vs. family based methods, the importance of context-dependency and of taking into account covariates. We then expand upon the utility of heritability analyses and describe the novel methods that should be a requisite for performing a genetic analysis of quantitative malaria parasite phenotypes. We then discuss our own findings using heritability and genome wide analyses that have led us to propose a novel hypothesis concerning the role of allergy in malaria. Finally we outline the future direction that genetic studies should take, most notably concerning the need to develop tools to examine gene-gene and gene-environment interactions.

2. Malaria parasite course and outcome of infection

2.1 Quantitative malaria-related phenotypes

The malaria parasite spp. lifecycles will undoubtedly be known to readers or covered in associated chapters. Here, we place the life-cycle within a perspective useful for human genetic studies. Although differing in the details, different *Plasmodium* spp. broadly share three distinct life cycle parts within the human host: invasion and asexual proliferation within the liver, invasion and asexual proliferation within red blood cells and the production of sexual stages, gametocytes, from a proportion of these asexually proliferating haploid parasites within the red blood cells. These gametocytes are essential for successful transmission to mosquitoes and subsequent infection of new human hosts. The parasite, as with any other sexually reproducing eukaryote, will, to the best of its capacity, have evolved to optimally exploit its host and maximise its reproductive rate through infection of new hosts. In turn, the human is expected to have evolved to minimise the damage caused by the parasite. The course of infection and the outcome of the human-parasite interaction are thus quantifiable by measurement of the density of asexual and sexual circulating parasites and the frequency of clinical episodes.

Placing the in-host biology of the parasite within the context of the clinical outcome of the infection is central to unravelling how human genetics impacts upon the pathophysiology of malaria. The clinical outcome of infection ranges from severe through mild disease to asymptomatic infection. Less well documented is the progression of clinical expression during the course of a single infection. Early treatment, thanks to considerable public health efforts, has now reduced the burden of disease and in study cohorts we do not know whether an individual with mild malaria would have progressed to severe disease if left untreated and/or eventually control but not eliminate the infection, leading to a chronic long-term asymptomatic infection. Thus, our focus is on parasite biological phenotypes in the context of symptomatic or asymptomatic infection outcomes, with no division into mild *vs.* severe disease. Thus, we ask why is there variation in the density of asexual parasite stages that individuals can withstand before becoming symptomatic and once symptomatic, why do only some infections attain very high densities. Transmission is a crucial part of the lifecycle for the parasite and there is good evidence that the parasite has evolved to optimise its transmission to mosquitoes with respect to the host response to infection (Paul et al., 2003). We thus examine the human factors that influence gametocyte production and whether they differ in symptomatic and asymptomatic infections. Some biological phenotypes, most notably those pertaining to the exo-erythrocytic stages, are beyond our current ability to measure in sufficient detail but do warrant increased research effort. Preventing liver stage infection and eliminating latent hypnozoites in relapsing species are clear targets for reducing the prevalence of infection.

Major differences in certain life-cycle aspects do exist amongst the *Plasmodium* spp. infecting man and surprisingly little is known about the biology or the acquired immune response to species other than *P. falciparum*. The major apparent differences include the capacity to form relapsing latent hypnozoite stages that reside in the liver (*P. vivax* and *Plasmodium ovale*), the rate of development of the asexually replicating erythrocytic stages (48hours for *P. falciparum*, *P. vivax* and *P. ovale vs.* 72 hours for *P. malariae*), the capacity for asexual stage parasites to cytoadhere (*P. falciparum*) and the predilection for invading red blood cells of differing ages (broadly *P. vivax* and *P. ovale* preferentially invade reticulocytes, *P. malariae* mature red blood cells and *P. falciparum* has a more catholic taste). The duration of a single infection varies significantly: *P. malariae* seemingly lasts up to 30 years despite no evidence of the existence of exo-erythrocytic latent stages, *P. vivax* and most probably *P. ovale* have latent hypnozoite stages and thus although a single blood stage infection may be short-lived (less than a year), relapse extends the duration of a single infection; *P. falciparum* infections can last up to 2 years. Thus, whilst the current emphasis on *P. falciparum* has led to the identification of genetic factors controlling certain clinical and biological phenotypes, their relevance to other species may not be certain and there is much to be done with respect to the three non-falciparum species infecting man (Louicharoen et al., 2009). *Plasmodium knowlesi*, although shown to infect man, has yet to be sufficiently studied to be amenable for human genetic study.

2.2 The phenotype problem

Just as the grouped nature of severe disease yields a poorly resolved phenotype, precise definition of mild clinical malaria and biological phenotypes is equally important and yet arguably more difficult. Defining what is a clinical episode in an endemic setting where malaria co-exists with sundry other infectious diseases is, for the most part, rather *ad hoc.* There are various statistical methods that attempt to define the proportion of fevers attributable to malaria (Smith et al., 1994), but at an individual level body temperature, symptoms associated with malaria and the presence of parasites define a clinical episode. In more studied populations a threshold of parasite density is used in an attempt to account for the high prevalence of asymptomatic infections and the similarity of malaria symptoms with those of other diseases. In practice, local clinicians tend to know when a clinical presentation is a clinical malaria episode but attempts to quantify this and determine quantifiable measurable criteria lead to highly variable definitions. Indeed, within site variation in symptoms and threshold densities will exist not only according to age, but also as a result of human genetics. Biological phenotypes are as complex to define. Although we can measure, for example, asexual and sexual stage parasite densities, the extent to which such data represent any meaningful measure of the host-parasite interaction needs to be considered. Asexual parasite density can alter rapidly and this is especially the case for *P. falciparum,* which has the capacity to sequester. Sexual stage parasite density will to some extent depend on the asexual parasite density, but the added significance of variation in gametocyte density rather than simply gametocyte positivity for transmission to mosquitoes is debatable (Paul et al., 2007). Moreover, at each step (exo-erythrocytic, asexual erythrocytic and sexual erythrocytic), there will likely be variation among parasite clones in the timing and extent of progression through the life-cycle. Specifically, the pre-patent and the asexual growth periods prior to the production of sexual stages will vary among clones. If timing varies so will the densities of parasite stages. On top of this parasite-specific variation, there will be variation resulting from the host-parasite interaction. This will reflect the extent of parasite-specific immunity developed by the host, the general "condition" of the host and "fixed" host genetic factors. Implicit within such host influence is the notion that the phenotypic expression of human genetic variation impacting upon the parasite will vary for an individual depending on that individual's age and history. Independently of any exposure to the specific parasite species in question, an individual's immune response matures over time and can be shaped by exposure (or lack thereof) to non-infectious agents.

Allergy is the paradigm of such immune system maturation. The maturation of the immune system, both innate and acquired, will in turn impact upon the influence of genetic factors that potentially confer protection to malaria parasites. In short, we advocate taking repeated measures from the same individual, as a single snap-shot will not only miss any variability due to the parasite, but also provide no context within which to characterise the individual, beyond obvious factors such as age and gender.

Despite all this noise and natural variation, however, the genetic signal is seemingly strong enough to be detected for many of malaria-related phenotypes. Fine-tuning of the phenotypes may generate more power in more detailed genetic analyses, and one of the simplest methods to assess the strength of the fine-tuning is to perform heritability analyses (see section 4).

2.3 Environmental influence and context-dependency

Acquired immunity is a major factor determining the outcome of an infection. The epidemiology of *P. falciparum* is characterised by premunition and the slow development of acquired immunity. In areas of very intense transmission, there is a relatively rapid development of premunition, whereby the individual can tolerate the presence of the parasite without expressing symptoms. Such clinical immunity thus generates a sub-population who are infected but asymptomatic. As the intensity of transmission decreases, the degree of exposure and age at which premunition develops is progressively later until in areas with low transmission intensity every infection leads to symptoms. The acquisition of immunity that clears the parasite is rarely achieved and only in regions of very intense transmission in old age groups. Acquired clinical and anti-parasite immunity is short-lived and leave of absence of an individual from an endemic area will decrease what little immunity had developed. Thus, human mobility at an individual level is an important confounding factor. In addition, in many areas malaria transmission is seasonal. This seasonal absence/reduction of infectious bites is akin to a period of absence from exposure and can alter the state of the individual and how they respond to an infection in the transmission and "non"-transmission seasons. The epidemiology of *P. falciparum* malaria varies according to the number of infectious bites an individual receives per unit time; importantly, although obvious, the same number of infectious bites spread over two months *vs.* over a year will not yield the same epidemiological profile. The temporal heterogeneity in exposure is a key confounding factor for phenotypic analysis. This will of course be the case for the other species to some extent, but the long duration of *P. malariae* infection and the capacity to relapse for *P. vivax*/*P. ovale* will uncouple the tight link between infectious mosquito bites and the prevalence of infection observed for *P. falciparum*.

A second highly important and often neglected context-dependency is the impact of other co-circulating infectious pathogens. It is widely recognised that multiple co-infecting *Plasmodium* spp. affect each other (Bruce et al., 2000) and the debate over the importance of helminth infections for malaria remains unresolved (Nacher et al., 2000; Spiegel et al., 2003). Whilst concomitant infections can be accounted for, the long term impact of *Plasmodium* spp. on each other is an entirely different problem. There is increasing evidence that there is cross-immunity among *Plasmodium* spp. and accounting for this requires longitudinal sampling. Whilst birth cohorts would be optimal, the investment is considerable. As a proxy, the development of serological methods that could stratify populations according to level of exposure to all co-circulating would provide a useful tool to examine the long term effects of infection by the community of pathogens on the pathogen of interest.

3. Study populations – Who and how many

A major requisite in any epidemiological study design is defining the sample size that can give the power to detect the effect of interest. For genetic studies, the response traditionally given is "as many as possible" and generally Genome Wide Association studies (GWAS) aim for sample sizes in the thousands. Sample size requirements impose a huge burden and constraint on research and for genetic studies, it is customary that the identified candidate genes are confirmed in a replicate study. The cost of such an endeavour is prohibitive and available to very few laboratories world-wide. Moreover, such large numbers will necessarily include populations from different environments and thus be immediately confounded. For complex diseases, such as malaria, single large effect genes are few and far between. Detecting small effect genes will require a large sample size, but reducing the stringency of the acceptance threshold for candidate gene nomination should be considered. This is especially true if the emphasis shifts from finding the gene, as in monogenic diseases, to identifying important biological pathways. There are multiple solutions to increasing resistance to parasites and repetitive identification of genes involved in specific biological pathways offers convergence towards understanding what governs the outcome of infection.

3.1 Replication

Genetic studies require that candidate genes are confirmed in separate populations. Replication is, however, frequently difficult and causal polymorphisms often have a low effect, increasing, for example, the risk of developing the disease by less than 5-10% (Wu et al., 2010). Moreover, whilst the assumption that there are a few key genes resulting in pathology for non-infectious diseases may be justifiable, this may not be the case for infectious diseases. Malaria is a good example where selective pressure on different populations has occurred relatively recently and thus different ethnicities have evolved different protective mechanisms. Replicating single genetic candidate polymorphisms may not therefore be an entirely appropriate approach and when performed should consider the ethnicities of the study populations. The focus should therefore be placed on the functional consequences of a mutation during an infection and this with reference to the biology of the pathogen and the normal host response. Malaria, on the face of it, is a prime example of this. Sickle cell trait confers protection and yet there are numerous other haemoglobin mutations selected in different ethnicities that potentially offer the same protective solution but via different mechanisms. Whilst some mutations may well exert their protective effect through the same mechanism (e.g. HbC), others may not. The co-occurrence of multiple putatively protective mutations introduces considerable analytical complexity that demands more rigorous consideration than has hitherto been enacted. Furthermore, the emphasis is necessarily shifting away from a pure candidate gene approach to one that considers all the single nucleotide polymorphisms (SNPs) at a locus of interest and focuses on the biological consequences of the mutation.

3.2 Family-based versus case control

Association studies allow identification of genes and their allelic variants involved in susceptibility to disease. They are indispensable for identifying susceptibility genes after candidate chromosomal regions have been revealed by genetic linkage study. The basic method of study compares the allele frequency of a genetic marker from affected (i.e. expressing phenotype) individuals and unaffected control individuals (case-control studies), chosen randomly from a population. The marker used may be a polymorphism without causal relationship to the phenotype or a mutation in a gene candidate. A positive result suggests that the marker studied is involved either directly or by virtue of being linked to the causal gene (i.e. the marker is in linkage disequilibrium with the causal gene whereby marker and causal alleles co-occur more frequently than they would by chance). The major problem with case-control studies is the possibility of false positive results due to differences in environmental factors that influence the development or the evolution of the phenotype being studied. The choice of the control population is one of the most important problems of case-control study: if the control group are not from the same population as the affected individuals, uncontrolled environmental factors or population stratification might induce false positive association. Family-based studies not only account for population stratification, but also increase environmental homogeneity. Classically the major advantage of case-control studies over family-based designs has concerned power. All individuals in case/control studies are unrelated and are thus independent data points, whereas families include individuals who are related and not independent. The non-independent nature of phenotypic data from related individuals can, in fact, be accounted for, as will be discussed in the next section. Moreover, not only is this received wisdom of contrasting power not likely to be as general as believed (Knight & Camp, 2011), but also improved sequencing technology will likely increase the power of family-based designs (Ott et al., 2011). The major limitation of family-based designs remains the identification of sufficient numbers of affected individuals *per se*. Although this may be a problem for extreme phenotypes (e.g. cerebral malaria), it is not for mild malaria and biological phenotypes. Finally, family-based designs offer the possibility of repeated measures, thereby providing a more detailed and complete picture of how an individual responds to an infection. The downside of such longitudinal studies, other than the cost, is the impact that increased access to treatment will have and the potential bias of studying a well-treated population.

4. Preliminary genetic analyses – Heritability

4.1 Application to natural populations

Heritability is an important parameter that indicates the genetic contribution underlying an observed phenotype and provides an indication of the power to detect the effect of individual genes when performing GWAS. A large heritability implies a strong correlation between phenotype and genotype, so that loci with an effect on the phenotype can be more easily detected (Visscher et al., 2008). Estimation of heritability in its broad sense in natural populations is not possible and hence narrow sense heritability, which estimates the additive genetic contribution, is calculated. Actual values of heritability are specific for a study population at a particular time and thus not strictly comparable among studies, although broad trends can be inferred.

Heritability analyses have until recently remained the quantitative tool of animal and plant breeders. They have been relatively ignored by human geneticists and the study of natural populations for several reasons. Firstly, to generate sufficient data, well-conducted longitudinal family-based epidemiological studies that take into account confounding environment factors are required (Ntoumi et al., 2007). This requires a considerable investment. Secondly, because the genetic component is not measured directly but is inferred from the resemblance between relatives and because relatives often live in the same house, differentiating genetic from the shared environment is problematical. Inadvertent exclusion of a key environmental factor would erroneously lead to substantial over-estimates of heritability. Thirdly, the statistical methods that can manage repeated measures inherent in longitudinal surveys for robust heritability analyses have only recently been developed. Finally, given the relative inaccuracy of heritability estimates and the increasing ease with which genome wide analyses can be performed, the added value of calculating heritability has been considered questionable.

This view of the utility of heritability analyses has been largely colored by its extensive historical use in breeding programs where projections of selection experiments are invaluable. For the study of complex infectious diseases, the value of heritability lies elsewhere and goes beyond the simple question of evaluating the potential genetic contribution to a phenotype. This "novel" value of heritability is well exemplified by the recent observation that there is considerable missing heritability in GWAS of more complex diseases (Manolio et al., 2009); only a fraction of estimated heritability can be accounted for by the genes identified in GWAS. Without initial estimation of heritability, this anomaly would not have been identified. The potential causes for this, include potentially important roles of epistasis, gene-environmental interaction and the confounding effect of population specific genetic architecture (Eichler et al., 2010). In addition to genetic explanations, one potential source contributing to the missing heritability concerns the phenotype; poorly resolved phenotypes lower the power to detect genetic variants (van der Sluis et al., 2010). One important point often misunderstood is that the absence of heritability of a phenotype implies no genetic contribution – this is not true. Narrow sense heritability measures the proportion of the variance in the phenotype explained only by additive genetics and there can be non-additive genetic effects. Furthermore, a causal variant that has an effect on a phenotype, but which is present at 100% allelic frequency will have zero heritability. Conversely, a large heritability does not imply that only a few genes are involved.

4.2 Repeated measures, complex pedigrees and statistical analyses

Historically, heritability analyses have used single measures of the phenotype or a summary variable when repeated measures were performed. Such summary measures tend to lead to over-inflated estimates of heritability and in the advent of available statistical methods, should be avoided. Likewise, heritability analyses used to analyse the residual of the phenotype after having taken into account other covariates. Such an approach assumes that there is no interaction between the genetic factors and these other covariates, an assumption that is likely to be invalid. Statistical methods now exist whereby simultaneous analysis of the genetic and environmental contribution to a phenotype is possible.

Heritability analyses of phenotypes gathered through repeated measurements of individuals from a community with a complex pedigree structure must take into account the bias introduced by multiple measures from the same individual and the fact that individuals are related. The individual observations are not independent. Although taking a single measure for an individual can overcome the first issue, multiple measures from the same individual are informative as they provide a notion of the repeatability of the phenotype and enables calculation of the intra-individual or permanent environment effect. This intra-individual variation contains features that are particular to each individual. This will include house effects, maternal effects, individual behaviour and non-additive genetic effects. The house and maternal effect can be taken into account by using appropriate matrices; each pair of individuals either do (1) or do not (0) share the same house or mother.

Creating a genetic relatedness matrix of the study population is not only central for heritability calculations, but extremely useful to take into account the non-independence of individuals when performing classical regression analyses. The genetic covariance (the familial relationship) among all pairs of individuals in the study cohort can be simply calculated using the pedigree information as follows:

For A and B, a given pair in a pedigree, the genetic covariance is computed as r(A,B) = 2x coancestry(A,B) where the coancestry between A and B is calculated using the method presented in Falconer and Mackay (1996): $coancestry(A,B) = \Sigma_p(1/2)^{n(p)} \times (1 + I_{Common\ Ancestor})$ where p is the number of paths in the pedigree linking A and B, n(p) the number of individuals (including A and B) for each path p and IX is the inbreeding coefficient of an individual X, which is equal to the coancestry between the two parents of X. IX is set to 0 if X is a founder. The consequent Pedigree-based genetic relatedness matrix has dimensions KxK, where K is the total number of individuals in the pedigree including those with missing phenotypes. This matrix can be built using INBREED procedure of SAS. A house matrix can also be constructed whereby a value of 1 is ascribed if the relative pair shares the same house or 0 otherwise. Likewise, to examine the extent that there are maternal effects that are passed onto offspring, a maternal matrix can be established.

Repeated measures analyses are best handled using Generalized Linear Mixed Models (GLMM). Mixed models enable fitting of random effects. Random effects are assumed to be normally distributed, and conditional on these random effects, data can have any distribution in the exponential family (e.g. Gaussian, Binomial, or Poisson). For repeated measures of unrelated individuals the random variable would simply be the individual identity. For related individuals, the genetic relatedness matrix will take into account the individual repeated measures plus the bias introduced by the non-independence of observations from related individuals.

Heritability analyses seek to decompose the total variance of the phenotype in question into components explained by additive genetic, intra-individual, house effects. Heritability is the proportion of the phenotypic variance that is due to additive genetics. Other covariates, such as age, gender etc, can also be taken into account. Although there are several programs able to perform such analyses, we have found that SAS offers a complete and yet flexible library of procedures (version 9.1.3, SAS Institute Inc., Cary, NC, USA), notably GLIMMIX, MIXED and INBREED. For count outcome variables (e.g. parasite density, number of clinical episodes per unit time), a Poisson regression model is fitted, which explicitly takes into account the non-negative integer-valued aspect of the dependent count variable. Therefore a GLMM with a Poisson distribution can be fitted using GLIMMIX and *log* as the link function between E(*variable* | *covariates*). For binary outcome variables (e.g. presence or absence of gametocytes), GLMM are fitted with a Binomial distribution with a *logit* link function. A maximal model with all covariates is fitted and a minimal adequate model including only significant covariates obtained. The effect of each covariate on the outcome variable is estimated taking into account inbreeding, via the genetic relatedness matrix integrated in GLIMMIX using the LDATA option, repeated measures and house effects.

5. Heritability analyses of malaria phenotypes in longitudinal family-based cohorts

5.1 Study sites and populations

Our study sites include three family-based cohorts that have been followed for over ten years. Two of the cohorts occur in Senegal but differ by an order of magnitude in transmission intensity; in addition to *P. falciparum*, both *P. malariae* and *P. ovale* co-circulate. The third cohort is a large Karen community in Thailand with low transmission intensity but equal incidence of *P. vivax* and *P. falciparum*.

The Dielmo and Ndiop longitudinal surveys in Senegal have been described in detail elsewhere (Rogier et al., 1999; Sakuntabhai et al., 2008; Trape et al., 1994). Briefly, a longitudinal cohort study of malaria has been carried out since 1990 in Dielmo and 1993 in Ndiop. In Dielmo there are 594 individuals forming 190 nuclear families and in Ndiop 653 in 208 nuclear families. In each cohort, the majority of individuals form one large complex family: 453 individuals in Dielmo and 503 in Ndiop. Overall there are 10 completely independent families in Dielmo and 21 in Ndiop. The ethnic composition differs between the two cohorts. In Dielmo, the ethnic groups consisted of 79% Serere, 11% Mandinka and 10% miscellaneous, whereas in Ndiop, there were 76% Wolof, 19% Fulani and 5% miscellaneous. Family structures were constructed by using a questionnaire, interviewing each individual or key representatives of the household to obtain both demographic information such as birth date, age, sex and genetic relationships between children, their parents, and sometimes their grandparents or non-relatives in the same household, and other households. Previous typing with microsatellites enabled the construction of a pedigree based on Identity-by-Descent (IBD) using MERLIN (Abecasis et al., 2001; Sakuntabhai et al., 2008), thereby enabling constitution of the genetic relatedness matrix.

Malaria transmission is perennial in Dielmo, where a river maintains larval breeding sites for the mosquitoes even in the dry season. The number of infective bites per person per year (Entomological Inoculation Rate, EIR) is of the order of 200. By contrast, malaria transmission is strictly seasonal in Ndiop and dependent upon the rainy season that occurs from July-September and the EIR is approximately 20. Such differing transmission has marked consequences on the epidemiology of malaria in the villages. This is most evident in the higher *P. falciparum* prevalence rates of infection in Dielmo (80%) compared to the seasonal rates in Ndiop that change from 20% in the dry season to 70% in the rainy season (Sakuntabhai et al., 2008). Peak incidence of clinical *P. falciparum* infections occurs in the 1-4 year old age group in Dielmo and in the 8-12 year old age group in Ndiop.

In Thailand, a community-based cohort study has been on-going since 1998 (Phimpraphi et al., 2008a), situated in a mountainous area of Ratchaburi province, Thailand near the Thai-Myanmar border. Suan Phung has a total population of 5,368 living in 7 hamlets. The ethnic composition of this community is majoritarily Karen (85%), with Thai (14%) and the rest are Mon and Burmese (1%). The total pedigrees are comprised of 2,427 individuals, including absent or deceased relatives. There are 238 independent families containing 603 nuclear families; the majority are 2 generation-families with family size range from 3 to 958. The epidemiology of malaria has been described elsewhere (Phimpraphi et al., 2008a). Briefly, the incidence of malaria is highly seasonal with annual peaks in May-June. Incidence was low, peaking at 141 episodes of *P. falciparum* per 1000 person-years and 70 for *P. vivax* over the 6-year intense study period. In this site, virtually all infections lead to febrile episodes and thus there is no information on asymptomatic infections. Peak incidence occurs in an earlier age group (5-9 years old) for *P. vivax* than for *P. falciparum* (10-15 years old). Parasite densities of either species peak in the <10 years old age group. Microsatellite genotyping again enabled the construction of a pedigree based on IBD (Phimpraphi et al., 2008b).

5.2 Heritability of malaria-related phenotypes with differing transmission intensity

Heritability analyses were conducted on several clinical and biological malaria-related phenotypes. The major non-genetic factors included age and variables concerned with differential extent of exposure on both a temporal (season, year) and spatial scale (hamlet, house). Figure 1 summarises the differential impact of the non-genetic and genetic factors on the number of clinical episodes (*P. falciparum* and *P. vivax*), the asexual parasite density

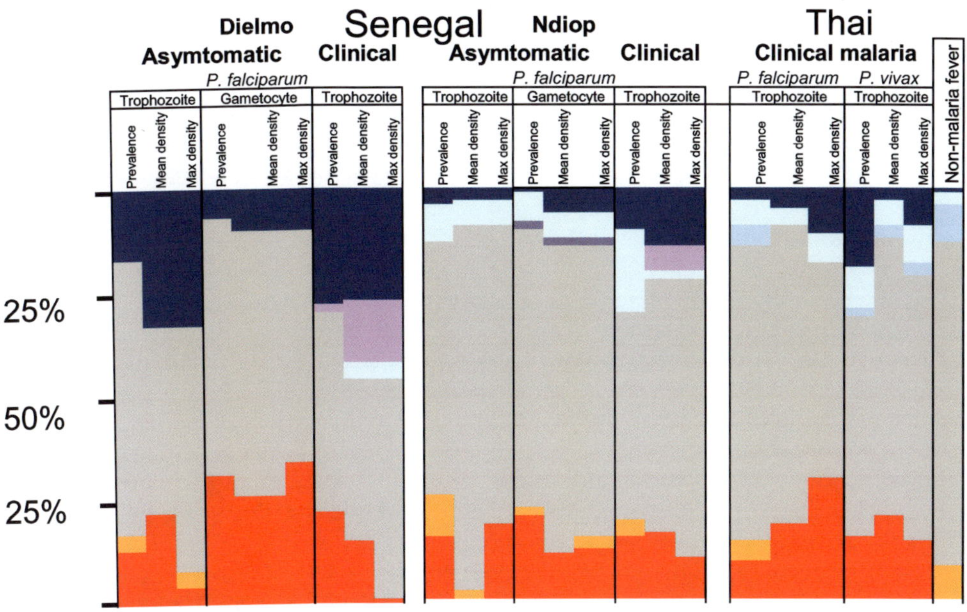

Fig. 1. Percentage of variance in malaria-related phenotypes explained by additive genetics (red), house (orange), hamlet (light blue), age (dark blue), date (turquoise), days in village (mauve), asexual parasite density (dark grey) and unknown (light grey). Malaria-related phenotypes include the prevalence of asymptomatic and clinical episodes and the mean and maximum asexual parasite density (trophozoite) during asymptomatic and clinical episodes.

during both clinical and asymptomatic infections and gametocyte prevalence and density, but only during asymptomatic infections; there was no significant heritability for gametocyte phenotypes during symptomatic infections. Non-malaria fever is included in the Thai study despite an absence of any genetic contribution, because of its significant correlation with malaria phenotypes.

5.2.1 Impact of non-genetic factors

Overall, it can be seen that age is more important in the highest transmission cohort (Dielmo) and decreases in importance as transmission intensity drops. This reflects the acquisition of clinical and anti-parasite immunity with exposure. A finer measure of exposure is given by the number of days present in the cohort, which has a significant impact on the number of clinical episodes. This effect not only reflects the probability of being infected, but also the well-recognised short-lived nature of clinical immunity: despite a history of exposure, absence from a malaria endemic setting can reduce the extent of clinical immunity developed. Temporal variation in the number of clinical episodes and in parasite density during both clinical and asymptomatic parasite density is notable for the Senegal cohort of highly seasonal transmission (Ndiop). Whilst seasonal variation in clinical episodes is expected, a seasonal effect on parasite density is less easily explained, especially for asymptomatic infections. This same effect is present for the production of gametocytes and we have recently shown that variation in mosquito biting rate has an impact on both asexual parasite density and gametocyte production (unpubl. data). This effect is seemingly linked to immune status of the individual, notably the levels of IgE.

Spatial variation is evident among the seven hamlets in the Thai site, but has little impact at the finer scale of house. In zones of high transmission intensity, where there is effectively saturating transmission and thus homogeneous exposure, fine scale spatial differences may not exist. The relatively small effect of house, even at lower transmission intensities, may be the result of the biting behaviour of the mosquitoes. In the Thai study site, the two mosquito vector species are *Anopheles minimus* and *Anopheles maculatus*, which are predominantly exophilic, thereby explaining the lack of a house level effect (Somboon et al., 1994). In Ndiop, Senegal, the major vector is *Anopheles arabiensis*, which will bite both indoors and outdoors and will also bite cattle. This non-specialist host choice may result in a biting distribution that is less house-oriented, being also affected by the distribution of animal enclosures. Although the occurrence of a small house effect in all three sites for several phenotypes, including parasite density, might reflect very local scale variability in biting rate, the confounded relationship of genetic relatedness and house may not be sufficiently resolved. Analysis of the heritability in the Thai study site with and without taking into account house led to estimates of the genetic contribution of 12% (with house) *vs.* 20% (without house) for the number of clinical episodes. The absence of any house effect for clinical *P. vivax* cases but the presence of such an effect for *P. falciparum* in the Thai site is likely because of relapse rather than differential biting habits of different mosquito vectors, although there may be differential transmission of the two species by different mosquito spp. (Somboon et al., 1994). There is no analytical approach to enable complete differentiation of the genetic and share house effects, especially in the case where there are no relatives in the cohort living in different houses. In our case, the cohorts all contain relatives living in different houses and non-relatives sharing households and thus the genetic relatedness and house matrices will enable both effects to be estimated, even though they are clearly confounded. Parasite density phenotypes during clinical episodes were not influenced by house in any site, consistent with the hypothesis that although house can contribute to the tendency to become infected, it does not impact upon the parasite once the infection has started.

5.2.2 Impact of genetic factors

Examination of the genetic contribution among the study sites reveals evidence for a strong genetic contribution to the number of *P. falciparum* clinical attacks: 12%, 16% and 22% with increasing transmission intensity. Interestingly, excluding household effects, results in contributions of approximately 20% in all 3 sites. The similarity of these values is remarkable given the very differing transmission intensities observed and the differing ethnicities. The marginal decrease in heritability with the decrease in transmission intensity likely reflects the increased heterogeneity in exposure at lower transmission intensities. The difference in the contribution of genetics is, however, small given the very large difference in transmission intensity. Moreover, the heritability of the number of clinical episodes is quite conserved irrespective of the phenotypic definitions used, the geographical region and even the *Plasmodium* species implicated. Similar values were observed in a study in Kenya (20%; Mackinnon et al., 2005) and a study in Sri Lanka (15%; Mackinnon et al., 2000) and for *P. vivax* (19% in Thailand (Phimpraphi et al., 2008b) and 15% in Sri Lanka).

A striking feature is the extensive differences in the impact of genetics on the mean *vs.* maximum parasite density. Parasite density has been recognised for a long time to be under human genetic control (Garcia et al., 1998; Rihet et al., 1998a), but the biological meaning of measures of parasite density requires contextual interpretation. The maximum parasite densities in both clinical and asymptomatic infections clearly indicate the extent to which the parasite can be controlled during and prior to the onset of a clinical episode. However, whilst the latter intuitively pinpoints the density at which an individual will clinically express the infection, a run-away symptomatic infection may attain exaggerated densities that are poorly informative of the biological pathways involved. The mean parasite density provides at least some replicated measure of how the individual controls a single infection, being less reliant on the extreme values. Although inherited blood disorders might result in generally lower parasite densities, the major pathways influencing parasite density will certainly be those of the immune system. Age has often been used as a proxy for the acquisition of immunity and accounting for age should reduce the contribution of that arm of the immune system to the genetic effect. It should be noted, however, that there may be a genetic contribution to acquired immunity (Stirnadel et al., 1999) and there is now some evidence that the inherited blood disorders operate interactively with the acquired immune response (Amaratunga et al., 2011). Nevertheless, our analyses would suggest that there is a contribution to the genetic effect from the innate arm of the immune system.

Gametocyte carriage has been associated with a worsening blood environment for the parasite (e.g. fever responses, anaemia) (Nacher et al., 2002; Price et al., 1999). However, such cues are only associated with symptomatic episodes of malaria and it is now well established that asymptomatic infections can also generate gametocytes and infect mosquitoes (Bousema & Drakeley, 2011). Differences in the tendency of sympatric ethnic groups to carry gametocytes have been noted for a long time (Perry 1914; Paganotti et al.

2006). We found a significant human genetic contribution associated with gametocyte prevalence in asymptomatic *P. falciparum* infections. By contrast, there was no heritability associated with the production of gametocytes for *P. falciparum* or *P. vivax* symptomatic infections. Increased gametocyte carriage has been observed in individuals with HbC (Gouagna et al., 2010) and HbS, although its contribution was small (Lawaly et al., 2010). Clearly there are other genes implicated in eliciting gametocyte production by the parasite. Thus, a proportion of the population is susceptible to carry gametocytes and be super-spreaders. Targeting such individuals with specific intervention methods is an intriguing option.

5.3 Correlation among phenotypes

Examining the correlations among phenotypes can be extremely informative in characterising the outcome of infection. The number of clinical episodes and maximum parasite density were positively associated with each other in the Senegalese cohorts (Dielmo r=0.54; Ndiop r=0.34) but not in Thailand. The correlation was strongest in the cohort of highest transmission intensity (Dielmo). In Thailand, there was comparatively little variation in the number of clinical episodes experienced by any individual (1-13). The positive correlation between these two phenotypes is consistent with the interpretation that individuals experiencing many *P. falciparum* clinical attacks have a poor capacity to control parasite density, which thus frequently reaches the high threshold density necessary to elicit a clinical attack (Rogier et al., 1996). As immunity develops, the human will be increasingly capable of controlling the proliferation of the parasite and keep the densities at sub-clinical levels. However, there was a negative correlation between the ability to harbour high parasite loads without symptoms and the number of clinical malaria attacks. Our results point to a genetic influence on the control of parasite density governing the occurrence of clinical attacks. In other words, higher asymptomatic parasite loads seemingly protect against occurrence of clinical episodes. One possible mechanism is through maintenance of an efficient concomitant clinical immunity reducing the risk of developing clinical malaria despite the presence of a relatively elevated parasite load. This is the first indication for a genetic basis to premunition acquired by individuals living in endemic areas (Sergent & Parrot, 1935). The immunological basis of such premunition remains elusive. Interestingly, high parasite specific IgE levels in asymptomatic infected individuals have been shown to be reduce the odds of a clinical episode (Bereczky et al., 2004), thus suggesting the Th1/Th2 balance and hence the relative cytophilic IgG1/3 and IgE titres produced in response to parasite density determine the progression to clinical disease.

The Thai analyses demonstrated a strong negative correlation between the number of non-malaria fevers and *P. falciparum* cases, suggesting that illness due to non-malaria pathogens may protect from *P. falciparum* infection or disease and vice versa. That there was no genetic contribution to non-malarial fever would suggest that there is no genetic trade-off generating susceptibility to *P. falciparum* with protection from non-malaria fever. However, the non-malaria fever phenotype is very imprecise and thus absence of a genetic effect may be a phenotype problem. Nevertheless, the negative correlation underlines the importance of considering malaria infections in context of other circulating pathogens. In contrast, there was evidence of between *Plasmodium* spp. interactions. There was a positive correlation between the number of *P. vivax* episodes and maximum *P. falciparum* parasite density, suggesting that common mechanisms are involved in determining these phenotypes. Individuals previously infected with *P. vivax* during the early years of study (1998-2000) had higher maximum *P. falciparum* parasite densities in 2001-2004. They also had a greater number of *P. vivax* episodes, but did not have significantly different maximum *P. vivax* parasite densities from those not previously infected with *P. vivax*. This suggests that common mechanisms do govern susceptibility to infection by *P. vivax* and control of *P. falciparum* density but not control of *P. vivax* density. Given the differences in red blood cell tropism, although blood disorders may be implicated, the involvement of shared immunological mechanisms is likely, supporting the hypothesis that there is significant cross-species protective immunity (Loucoubar et al., 2011b).

6. Linkage analyses of malaria phenotypes identifies regions associated with atopy

Linkage analyses are the classical statistical genetic analyses testing for co-segregation between a chromosomal region and a phenotype of interest. Prior to the high density genotyping now available for genome wide association, linkage analysis was the preferred method for gene discovery, enabling chromosomal regions of interest to be identified with relatively low genotyping coverage.

6.1 Genome wide linkage analysis of *P. falciparum* in Senegal

Our genome wide linkage analysis in the two Senegalese cohorts identified three novel regions of linkage in addition to the 5q31 region that has been previously reported to be linked to asymptomatic parasite density (Flori et al., 2003; Garcia et al., 1998; Rihet et al., 1998b). All of the regions have been previously found to be linked to asthma/atopic disease or related phenotypes, such as IgE titres (Iyengar et al., 2001; Jang et al., 2005; Kurz et al., 2006; Xu et al., 2001; Zhang et al., 2003). The novel regions of linkage were chromosome 5p15-p13 and 13q13-q22 linked with the number of *P. falciparum* clinical malaria attacks in Dielmo, and chromosome 12q21-q23 with the maximum parasite density during asymptomatic carriage in Ndiop. The linkage results differ for the two cohorts, likely reflecting the important differences both in the ethnic backgrounds and in the prevailing transmission conditions. Interestingly, the 5q31 locus has been linked to several immune related disorders, including asthma/atopy (Meyers et al., 1994), inflammatory bowel disease (Lee et al., 2002), Crohn disease (Peltekova et al., 2004), Celiac disease (Latiano et al., 2007) and psoriasis (Friberg et al., 2006). Moreover, genes within the 5q31 locus have been suggested to regulate delayed-type hypersensitivity responses associated with Leishmania chagasi infection (Jeronimo et al., 2007). This region contains a cluster of cytokines, among which IL12B may play a critical role since it has been associated with some immune-related diseases. An insertion/deletion polymorphism in the promoter region of IL12B has been reported to be associated with psoriasis (Cargill et al., 2007) and cerebral malaria (Morahan et al., 2002a) while two intronic SNPs were associated with asthma (Morahan et al., 2002b; Randolph et al., 2004).

With the exception of the β-globin locus, there was no overlap of the regions of linkage that we detected and the location of the genes that have been previously reported to be associated with severe/cerebral malaria. This apparent discordance between genes responsible for severe malaria and those controlling the response to *Plasmodium* infection in our study may also indicate that the mechanisms (and genes) involved in the protection against severe malaria are largely independent of those involved in the response to mild clinical malaria and/or the control of blood parasitemia.

6.2 Role of allergy in malaria

The acquisition of immunity to the human lethal malaria parasite *P. falciparum* develops very slowly and is not sterilising. Even in zones where the transmission intensity is high, the development of immunity only results in a premunition leading to a reduction in the number of clinical episodes and the progressive control of parasite density. Cytophilic immunoglobulins (IgG1 & IgG3), which are capable of eliminating the parasites by opsonisation, play an important role in this premunition (Wilson & McGregor, 1973). An important role of the Th1/Th2 balance in the development of clinical malaria has been suggested by numerous studies (e.g. Elghazali et al., 1997). Orientation of the immune response towards a Th1 versus a Th2 profile, will respectively promote IgG *vs.* IgE proliferation. The role of IgE in clinical and severe malaria is still poorly documented and results are controversial. *P. falciparum*-specific IgE is elevated in malaria patients and has been proposed to play a pathogenic role in severe malaria (Elghazali et al., 1997; Perlmann et al., 1997), although high levels in individuals with asymptomatic infections were associated with protection (Bereczky et al., 2004). The induction of a Th2 biased immune response by *P. falciparum* may generate a tendency to develop a Th2 type immune response to other antigens. Dendritic cells that are oriented to a Th2 phenotype by an antigen are more susceptible to orient the immune response towards a Th2 profile when confronted by a second antigen (de Jong et al., 2002). It has been suggested that the Th2 bias induced by *P. falciparum* may exacerbate allergy and explain the higher than normal frequency of several cancers in malaria endemic populations (Taylor-Robinson, 1998).

Direct evidence has been found for a pathogenic role of histamine (a major effector molecule in allergy response) in mouse malaria models using both genetic and pharmacological approaches; histamine binding to Histamine receptor-1 (H1R) and receptor-2 (H2R) increases the susceptibility of mice to infection with *Plasmodium* and histidine decarboxylase–deficient mice, which are free of histamine were highly resistant to severe malaria (Beghdadi et al., 2008). H1R mediates most of the proinflammatory effects of histamine (Bryce et al., 2006). The anti-inflammatory and immunosuppressive effects of histamine are largely dependent on stimulation of H2R. In addition, there is suggestion that histamine might influence the polarization of T-helper cell development through inhibitory effects on dendritic cells (Idzko et al., 2002). Reports indicate that specific components of the innate immune system, including eosinophils (Kurtzhals et al., 1998), basophils (Nyakeriga et al., 2003), and Mast cells (MCs) (Furuta et al., 2006), could play important roles in the pathogenesis of malaria. Increased levels of histamine in plasma and tissue, derived from basophils and MCs, notably following stimulation by IgE through the high affinity receptor FcεR1, are associated with the severity of disease in humans infected with *P. falciparum* and in animal malaria models (Bhattacharya et al., 1988; Srichaikul et al., 1976). Chlorpheniramine, a histamine receptor-1 agonist reversed resistance to chloroquine and amodiquine both in vivo and in vitro (Sowunmi et al., 2007). Moreover, astemizole, another HR1 agonist, was identified as an antimalarial agent in a clinical drug library screen (Chong et al., 2000). Finally, *P. falciparum* produces translationally controlled tumor protein, which is a homolog of the mammalian histamine-releasing factor that causes histamine release from human basophils (MacDonald et al., 2001). How this could benefit the parasite is not known, but the vasodilatory effects of histamine might permit the parasites to circulate more readily and histamine might increase endothelial cell-surface expression of thrombomodulin, which is both a tissue anticoagulant and a receptor for parasitized erythrocyte sequestration.

Our heritability, correlation and genome wide linkage study results are consistent with there being a relationship between malaria and allergy and raise the hypothesis that the development of clinical malaria may be due to an allergic reaction to malaria parasites or by-products of parasite infection, or that allergy/atopy and the response to malaria infection may share common mechanisms. Thus, clinical immunity to malaria may indeed be immunotolerance and absence of allergic-type responses rather than the presence of neutralising antibodies to malaria "toxins" as previously suggested (Jakobsen et al., 1995). Several lines of additional evidence support the concept that susceptibility to malaria and atopy may be related to the same immunological defect. In Ethiopia, atopic children had a higher prevalence of malaria attacks (Haileamlak et al., 2005), while in Tanzania maternal malaria had a protective effect on wheezing in children age of four (Sunyer et al., 2001). Finally, a mouse model for human atopic disease (NC/Jic) was found to be susceptible to murine malaria (Ohno et al., 2001) and a major quantitative trait locus (derm1) for atopic disease mapped close to the region controlling parasitemia (Kohara et al., 2001).

7. Genetic association studies and the post-genomic era

Most of the protective variants are thought to have emerged in populations living in regions endemic for malaria as a result of the high selective pressure due to the parasite (Kwiatkowski, 2005). The past decade has seen growing evidence of ethnic differences in susceptibility to malaria and of the diverse genetic adaptations to malaria that have arisen in different populations. The fact that different malaria-resistance alleles have arisen in different places suggests that a great deal of selection by malaria has happened relatively recently in human history and certainly since human migration out of Africa (Eid et al., 2010). Such population differences in susceptibility to malaria are becoming more amenable to study since the development of high through-put genetic technology, thereby allowing us to genetically dissect the outcome of infection.

7.1 Candidate and genome wide association studies

Association studies are used for identifying genes and their common allelic variants involved in predisposition to a disease. Such studies are performed after localization of susceptible loci by linkage analysis. This method compares the allele frequency of a genetic marker of affected and non-affected individuals, chosen at random in a population (case-control study). The marker might be the causal polymorphism or any polymorphism in linkage disequilibrium (LD) with the causal one. A positive association with one marker suggests that this marker is in LD with the causal polymorphism. The LD between two markers is defined by the existence of a combination of alleles of these markers more often than expected by chance. The choice of the control population is one of the most important problems of case-control studies: if the control group is not from the same population as the affected individuals, uncontrolled environmental factors or population stratification might induce false positive association. Association studies are the most widely used contemporary approach to relate genetic variation to phenotypic diversity. This is due to their higher power and lower cost to detect a susceptibility locus than linkage analysis.

The genome era has heralded unparalleled possibilities to identify genetic variants that underpin disease (http://www.genome.gov/gwastudies). The majority of these initial studies have concerned non-infectious diseases and, for the most part, examined dichotomous disease phenotypes, nominally affected and unaffected. Application to infectious diseases has only been relatively recent (Thye et al., 2010; Zhang et al., 2009) and for malaria has focussed on severe disease (Jallow et al., 2009). Genome wide association studies of clinical malaria and biological phenotypes are currently underway in our laboratory and whilst certain to reveal many novel candidate genes of importance, we know this is not enough. It is widely recognized that common multifactorial diseases are caused by multiple genetic and environmental factors and interactions among all these factors.

7.2 Multiple loci and gene x environment interactions

Following the success of identifying genes underlying diseases resulting from single locus mutations and inherited in a Mendelian fashion, it has become clear that there are many complex diseases that are inherited in a non-Mendelian fashion. That there are many loci affecting a trait is no surprise, but the simultaneous analysis of many loci is problematic for several reasons, especially when searching for novel genes as in the case of GWAS. The first is the curse of dimensionality - there are more candidate loci than there are observations. The second is the extent to which genes exert their effects independently, or whether there exist interactions among genes with respect to the phenotype. Thirdly, there is the question of whether there exists gene x environment interactions.

With the development of genotyping technologies, GWAS have become the method of choice to identify complex disease associated genes using SNPs as biomarkers (Hardy & Singleton, 2009). In the past three years, about 400 GWAS have successfully identified more than 531 genetic variants associated with various traits or diseases (Manolio et al., 2009). Standard analytical approaches in GWAS have proceeded by individually testing each SNP of the hundreds of thousands of genotyped SNPs. Thus, only SNPs that have a relatively strong marginal effect have been detected, explaining only a small part of the heritability. Hence, other SNPs that have weaker association with disease and/or act primarily through a complex mechanism involving interactions with other genetic variants and environmental factors have yet to be discovered. There is an increasing number of statistical methods and software that are being proposed to allow analysing multiple genetic markers and their interactions simultaneously (Cordell, 2009), but the identification of these interactions remain very challenging. Powerful methods for conducting genome-wide interactions studies are therefore needed. One of the interesting features of GWAS is that the same loci were found associated with several diseases (e.g. cancers, cardio-vascular diseases, auto-immune diseases), suggesting that genes with a pleiotropic effect may be more frequent than anticipated and may play a key role in basic physiopathological mechanisms underlying a number of diseases. The identification of pleiotropic genes which are likely to influence master regulators of biological processes is therefore of major importance. Studying together diseases that are supposed to share common genetic determinants can facilitate the characterization of such genes.

8. Conclusion

The ultimate goal of studying the human genetics underlying infectious disease is to identify key biological pathways that determine the outcome of infection. Human genetics studies of malaria have, to date, almost exclusively focussed on severe disease caused by *P. falciparum* and yet this is a relatively rare event that regroups many pathologies. The majority of infections cause mild clinical symptoms or are asymptomatic. Asymptomatic infections are evidence for the development of clinical immunity (premunition), acquired at a rate proportional to exposure. Quantifying the frequency of a symptomatic *vs.* an asymptomatic outcome of infection and the parasite densities during such outcomes provides a measure of the host-parasite interaction. More detailed parasite phenotypes, such as those looking at particular parasite stages, provide additional insight into how the human response to infection determines the phenotype. Longitudinal family-based cohort studies offer the opportunity to generate non-severe malaria-related phenotypes for individuals over time, allowing the progression towards premunition to be examined. Family-based studies offer the possibility of assessing the robustness of phenotypes through simple heritability analysis. Fine-tuning phenotypes as such will save time and money during the human genotyping stage and subsequent analysis. Our cohort studies revealed surprisingly similar human genetic contributions to the clinical outcome of infection despite very large differences in transmission intensity. Identifying and accounting for confounding factors and covariates is essential and the similarity of the heritability values is reassuring for the robustness of the phenotype and implicitly suggest that covariates have been correctly accounted for. However, the potential that such covariates interact with human genes of interest should not be forgotten and future focus on gene-environment interactions is paramount. In addition, we identified for the first time a human genetic contribution to the transmission of the parasite. This opens up exciting possibilities for targeting transmission as well as disease. From our subsequent linkage studies, we found evidence that similar biological pathways govern the clinical outcome of a *P. falciparum* infection and allergy. In addition to the potential therapeutic possibilities, that common biological pathways govern multiple diseases offers the huge potential for combining efforts across multiple domains.

9. Acknowledgements

We are grateful to the villagers of Dielmo, Ndiop and Suan Phung for their participation and continued collaboration in this project. We thank the administrative authority of Institut Pasteur of Dakar, Senegal and Mahidol University, Thailand for their continuous support. Funding by provided by Institut Pasteur and the Ecole des Hautes Etudes en Santé Publique.

10. References

Abecasis, G.R., Cherny, S.S., Cookson, W.O., & Cardon, L.R. (2001) Merlin-- rapid analysis of dense genetic maps using sparse gene flow trees. *Nat Genet*, 30, 97-101.

Agarwal, A., Guindo, A., Cissoko, Y., Taylor, J.G., Coulibaly, D., et al. (2000) Hemoglobin C associated with protection from severe malaria in the Dogon of Mali, a West African population with a low prevalence of hemoglobin S. *Blood*, 96, 2358-2363.

Aidoo, M., Terlouw, D.J., Kolczak, M.S., McElroy, P.D., ter Kuile, F.O., et al. (2002) Protective effects of the sickle cell gene against malaria morbidity and mortality. *Lancet*, 359, 1311-1312.

Amaratunga, C., Lopera-Mesa, T.M., Brittain, N.J., Cholera, R., Arie, T., et al. (2011) A role for fetal hemoglobin and maternal immune IgG in infant resistance to *Plasmodium falciparum* malaria. *PLoS ONE*, 6, e14798.

Aucan, C., Walley, A.J., Hennig, B.J., Fitness, J., Frodsham, A., et al. (2003) Interferon-alpha receptor-1 (IFNAR1) variants are associated with protection against cerebral malaria in the Gambia. *Genes Immun*, 4, 275-282.

Beghdadi, W., Porcherie, A., Schneider, B.S., Dubayle, D., Peronet, R., et al. (2008) Inhibition of histamine-mediated signaling confers significant protection against severe malaria in mouse models of disease. *J Exp Med*, 205, 395-408.

Bereczky, S., Montgomery, S.M., Troye-Blomberg, M., Rooth, I., Shaw, M.A., et al. (2004) Elevated antimalarial IgE in asymptomatic individuals is associated with reduced risk for subsequent clinical malaria. *Int J Parasitol*, 34, 935-942.

Bhattacharya, U., Roy, S., Kar, P.K., Sarangi, B., & Lahiri, S.C. (1988) Histamine & kinin system in experimental malaria. *Indian J Med Res*, 88, 558–563.

Bousema, T., & Drakeley, C. (2011) Epidemiology and infectivity of *Plasmodium falciparum* and *Plasmodium vivax* gametocytes in relation to malaria control and elimination. *Clin Microbiol Rev*, 24, 377-410.

Bruce, M.C., Donnelly, C.A., Alpers, M.P., Galinski, M.R., Barnwell, J.W., et al. (2000) Cross-species interactions between malaria parasites in humans. *Science*, 287, 845-848.

Bryce, P.J., Mathias, C.B., Harrison, K.L., Watanabe, T., Geha, R.S., et al. (2006) The H1 histamine receptor regulates allergic lung responses. *J Clin Invest*, 116, 1624 - 1632.

Cargill, M., Schrodi, S.J., Chang, M., Garcia, V.E., Brandon, R., et al. (2007) A large-scale genetic association study confirms IL12B and leads to the identification of IL23R as psoriasis-risk genes. *Am J Hum Genet*, 80, 273-290.

Chong, C.R., Chen, X., Shi, L., Liu, J.O., & Sullivan, D.J. (2006) A clinical drug library screen identifies astemizole as an antimalarial agent. *Nat Chem Biol*, 2, 415-416.

Cordell, H.J. (2009) Detecting gene-gene interactions that underlie human diseases. *Nat Rev Genet*, 10, 392-404.

de Jong, E.C., Vieira, P.L., Kalinski, P., Schuitemaker, J.H., Tanaka, Y., et al. (2002) Microbial compounds selectively induce Th1 cell-promoting or Th2 cell-promoting dendritic cells *in vitro* with diverse Th cell-polarizing signals. *J Immunol*, 168, 1704–1709.

Eichler, E.E., Flint, J., Gibson, G., Kong, A., Leal, S.M., et al. (2010) Missing heritability and strategies for finding the underlying causes of complex disease. *Nat Rev Genet*, 11, 446-450.

Eid, N.A., Hussein, A.A., Elzein, A.M., Mohamed, H.S., Rockett, K.A., et al. (2010) Candidate malaria susceptibility/protective SNPs in hospital and population-based studies: the effect of sub-structuring. *Malaria Journal*, 9, 119-129.

Elghazali, G., Perlmann, H., Rutta, A.S., Perlmann, P., & Troye-Blomberg, M. (1997) Elevated plasma levels of IgE in *Plasmodium falciparum*-primed individuals reflect an increased ratio of IL-4 to interferon gamma (IFN-gamma)-producing cells. *Clin Exp Immunol*, 109, 84-89.

Falconer, D.S., & Mackay, T.F.C. (1996) *Introduction to Quantitative Genetics* (4th Edn.) Longman, London.

Friberg, C., Bjorck, K., Nilsson, S., Inerot, A., Wahlstrom, J., et al. (2006) Analysis of chromosome 5q31-32 and psoriasis: confirmation of a susceptibility locus but no association with SNPs within SLC22A4 and SLC22A5. *J Invest Dermatol*, 126, 998-1002.

Flori, L., Kumulungui, B., Aucan, C., Esnault, C., Traore, A.S., et al. (2003) Linkage and association between *Plasmodium falciparum* blood infection levels and chromosome 5q31-q33. *Genes Immun*, 4, 265-268.

Foo, L.C., Rekhraj, V., Chiang, G.L., & Mak, J.W. (1992) Ovalocytosis protects against severe malaria parasitemia in the Malayan aborigines. *Am J Trop Med Hyg*, 47, 271-275.

Furuta, T., Kikuchi, T., Iwakura, Y., & Watanabe, N. (2006) Protective roles of mast cells and mast cell-derived TNF in murine malaria. *J Immunol*, 177, 3294–3302.

Garcia, A., Marquet, S., Bucheton, B., Hillaire, D., Cot, M., et al. (1998) Linkage analysis of blood *Plasmodium falciparum* levels: interest of the 5q31-q33 chromosome region. *Am J Trop Med Hyg*, 58, 705-709.

Gouagna, L.C., Bancone, G., Yao, F., Yameogo, B., Dabiré, K.R., et al. (2010) Genetic variation in human HBB is associated with *Plasmodium falciparum* transmission. *Nat Genet*, 42, 328-331.

Gyan, B.A., Goka, B., Cvetkovic, J.T., Kurtzhals, J.L., Adabayeri, V., et al. (2004) Allelic polymorphisms in the repeat and promoter regions of the interleukin-4 gene and malaria severity in Ghanaian children. *Clin Exp Immunol*, 138, 145-150.

Haileamlak, A., Dagoye, D., Williams, H., Venn, A.J., Hubbard, R., et al. (2005) Early life risk factors for atopic dermatitis in Ethiopian children. *J Allergy Clin Immunol*, 115, 370-376.

Haldane, J.B. (1949) The association of characters as a result of inbreeding and linkage. *Ann Eugen*, 15, 15-23.

Hardy, J., & Singleton, A. (2009) Genomewide association studies and human disease. *N Engl J Med*, 360, 1759–1768.

Hill, A.V., Allsopp, C.E., Kwiatkowski, D., Anstey, N.M., Twumasi, P., et al. (1991) Common west African HLA antigens are associated with protection from severe malaria. *Nature*, 352, 595-600.

Hutagalung, R., Wilairatana, P., Looareesuwan, S., Brittenham, G.M., Aikawa, M., et al. (1999) Influence of hemoglobin E trait on the severity of Falciparum malaria. *J Infect Dis*, 179, 283-286.

Idzko, M., la Sala, A., Ferrari, D., Panther, E., Herouy, Y., et al. (2002) Expression and function of histamine receptors in human monocyte derived dendritic cells. *J Allergy Clin Immunol*, 109, 839–846.

Iyengar, S.K., Jacobs, K.B., & Palmer, L.J. (2001) Improved evidence for linkage on 6p and 5p with retrospective pooling of data from three asthma genome screens. *Genet Epidemiol*, 21 Suppl 1, S130-135.

Jakobsen, P.H., Bate, C.A., Taverne, J., & Playfair, J.H. (1995) Malaria: toxins, cytokines and disease. *Parasite Immunol*, 17, 223-231.

Jallow, M., Teo, Y.Y., Small, K.S., Rockett, K.A., Deloukas, P., et al. (2009) Wellcome Trust Case Control Consortium; Malaria Genomic Epidemiology Network. Genome-wide and fine-resolution association analysis of malaria in West Africa. *Nat Genet*, 41, 657-665.

Jang, N., Stewart, G., & Jones, G. (2005) Polymorphisms within the PHF11 gene at chromosome 13q14 are associated with childhood atopic dermatitis. *Genes Immun*, 6, 262-264.

Jepson, A.P., Banya, W.A., Sisay-Joof, F., Hassan-King, M., Bennett, S., et al. (1995) Genetic regulation of fever in *Plasmodium falciparum* malaria in Gambian twin children. *J Infect Dis*, 172, 316-319.

Jeronimo, S.M., Holst, A.K., Jamieson, S.E., Francis, R., Martins, D.R., et al. (2007) Genes at human chromosome 5q31.1 regulate delayed-type hypersensitivity responses associated with *Leishmania chagasi* infection. *Genes Immun*, 8, 539-551.

Knight, J.C., Udalova, I., Hill, A.V., Greenwood, B.M., Peshu, N., et al. (1999) A polymorphism that affects OCT-1 binding to the TNF promoter region is associated with severe malaria. *Nat Genet*, 22, 145-150.

Knight, S., & Camp, N.J. (2011) Validity and power of association testing in family-based sampling designs: evidence for and against the common wisdom. *Genet Epidemiol*, 35, 174-181.

Kohara, Y., Tanabe, K., Matsuoka, K., Kanda, N., Matsuda, H., et al. (2001) A major determinant quantitative-trait locus responsible for atopic dermatitis-like skin lesions in NC/Nga mice is located on Chromosome 9. *Immunogenetics*, 53, 15-21.

Kun, J.F., Mordmuller, B., Perkins, D.J., May, J., Mercereau-Puijalon, O., et al. (2001) Nitric oxide synthase 2 (Lambarene) (G-954C), increased nitric oxide production, and protection against malaria. *J Infect Dis*, 184, 330-336.

Kurtzhals, J.A., Reimert, C.M., Tette, E., Dunyo, S.K., Koram, K.A., et al. (1998) Increased eosinophil activity in acute *Plasmodium falciparum* infection – association with cerebral malaria. *Clin Exp Immunol*, 112, 303–307.

Kurz, T., Hoffjan, S., Hayes, M.G., Schneider, D., Nicolae, R., et al. (2006) Fine mapping and positional candidate studies on chromosome 5p13 identify multiple asthma susceptibility loci. *J Allergy Clin Immunol*, 118, 396-402.

Kwiatkowski, D.P. (2005) How malaria has affected the human genome and what human genetics can teach us about malaria. *Am J Hum Genet*, 77, 171-192.

Latiano, A., Mora, B., Bonamico, M., Megiorni, F., Mazzilli, M.C., et al. (2007) Analysis of candidate genes on chromosomes 5q and 19p in celiac disease. *J Pediatr Gastroenterol Nutr*, 45, 180-186.

Lawaly, Y.R, Sakuntabhai, A., Marrama, L. Konaté, L., Phimpraphi, W., et al. (2010) Heritability of the human infectious reservoir of malaria parasites. *PLoS ONE*, 5, e11358.

Lee, J.K., Park, C., Kimm, K., & Rutherford, M.S. (2002) Genome-wide multilocus analysis for immune mediated complex diseases. *Biochem Biophys Res Commun*, 295, 771-773.

Loucoubar, C., Goncalves, B., Tall, A., Sokhna, C., Trape, J.F., et al., (2011a) Impact of changing drug treatment and malaria endemicity on the heritability of malaria phenotypes in a longitudinal family-based cohort study. *PLoS ONE*, 6, e26364.

Loucoubar, C., Paul, R., Bar-Hen, A., Huret, A., Tall, A., et al. (2011b) An Exhaustive, Non-Euclidean, Non-Parametric Data Mining Tool for Unraveling the Complexity of Biological Systems – Novel Insights into Malaria. *PLoS ONE*, 6, e24085.

Louicharoen, C., Patin, E., Paul, R., Nuchprayoon, I., Witoonpanich, B., et al. (2009) Positively selected G6PD-Mahidol mutation reduces *Plasmodium vivax* density in South-East Asians. *Science*, 326, 1546-1549.

MacDonald, S.M., Bhisutthibhan, J., Shapiro, T.A., Rogerson, S.J., Taylor, T.E., et al. (2001) Immune mimicry in malaria: *Plasmodium falciparum* secretes a functional histamine-releasing factor homolog in vitro and in vivo. *Proc Natl Acad Sci USA*, 98, 10829-10832.

Mackinnon, M.J., Gunawardena, D.M., Rajakaruna, J., Weerasingha, S., Mendis, K.N., et al. (2000) Quantifying genetic and nongenetic contributions to malarial infection in a Sri Lankan population. *Proc Natl Acad Sci U S A*, 97, 12661–12666.

Mackinnon, M.J., Mwangi, T.W., Snow, R.W., Marsh, K., & Williams, T.N. (2005) Heritability of malaria in Africa. *PLoS Med*, 2, e340.

Manolio, T.A., Collins, F.S., Cox, N.J., Goldstein, D.B., Hindorff, L.A., et al. (2009) Finding the missing heritability of complex diseases. *Nature*, 461, 747-753

Meyers, D.A., Postma, D.S., Panhuysen, C.I., Xu, J., Amelung, P.J., et al. (1994) Evidence for a locus regulating total serum IgE levels mapping to chromosome 5. *Genomics*, 23, 464-470.

Mockenhaupt, F.P., Ehrhardt, S., Gellert, S., Otchwemah, R.N., Dietz, E., et al. (2004) Alpha(+)-thalassemia protects African children from severe malaria. *Blood*, 104, 2003-2006.

Modiano, D., Petrarca, V., Sirima, B.S., Nebie, I., Diallo, D., et al. (1996) Different response to *Plasmodium falciparum* malaria in west African sympatric ethnic groups. *Proc Natl Acad Sci U S A*, 93, 13206-13211.

Mombo, L.E., Ntoumi, F., Bisseye, C., Ossari, S., Lu, C.Y., et al. (2003) Human genetic polymorphisms and asymptomatic *Plasmodium falciparum* malaria in Gabonese schoolchildren. *Am J Trop Med Hyg*, 68, 186-190.

Morahan, G., Boutlis, C.S., Huang, D., Pain, A., Saunders, J.R., et al. (2002a) A promoter polymorphism in the gene encoding interleukin-12 p40 (IL12B) is associated with mortality from cerebral malaria and with reduced nitric oxide production. *Genes Immun*, 3, 414-418.

Morahan, G., Huang, D., Wu, M., Holt, B.J., White, G.P., et al. (2002b) Association of IL12B promoter polymorphism with severity of atopic and non-atopic asthma in children. *Lancet*, 360, 455-459.

Nacher, M., Gay, F., Singhasivanon, P., Krudsood, S., Treeprasertsuk, S., et al. (2000) *Ascaris lumbricoides* infection is associated with protection from cerebral malaria. *Parasite Immunol*, 22, 107-113.

Nacher, M., Singhasivanon, P., Silachamroon, U., Treeprasertsuk, S., Tosukhowong, T., et al. (2002) Decreased hemoglobin concentrations, hyperparasitemia, and severe malaria are associated with increased *Plasmodium falciparum* gametocyte carriage. *J Parasitol*, 88, 97–101.

Ntoumi, F., Kwiatkowski, D.P., Diakité, M., Mutabingwa, T.K., & Duffy, P.E. (2007) New interventions for malaria: mining the human and parasite genomes. *Am J Trop Med Hyg*, 77, 270-275.

Nyakeriga, M.A., Troye-Blomberg, M., Bereczky, S., Perlmann, H., Perlmann, P., et al. (2003) Immunoglobulin E (IgE) containing complexes induce IL-4 production in human basophils: effect on Th1-Th2 balance in malaria. *Acta Trop*, 86, 55–62.

Ohno, T., Ishih, A., Kohara, Y., Yonekawa, H., Terada, M., et al. (2001) Chromosomal mapping of the host resistance locus to rodent malaria (*Plasmodium yoelii*) infection in mice. *Immunogenetics*, 53, 736-740.

Ott, J., Kamatani, Y., & Lathrop, M. (2011) Family-based designs for genome-wide association studies. *Nat Rev Genet*, 12, 465-474.

Paganotti, G.M., Palladino, C., Modiano, D., Sirima, B.S., Raberg, L., et al. (2006) Genetic complexity and gametocyte production of *Plasmodium falciparum* in Fulani and Mossi communities in Burkina Faso. *Parasitology*, 132, 607-614.

Paul, R.E.L., Ariey, F., & Robert, V. (2003) The evolutionary ecology of *Plasmodium*. *Ecol Letters*, 6, 866-880.

Paul, R.E.L., Bonnet, S., Boudin, C., Tchuinkam, T., & Robert, V. (2007) Upper and lower limits of gametocyte allocation in *Plasmodium falciparum*. *Inf Genet Evol*, 7, 577–586.

Peltekova, V.D., Wintle, R.F., Rubin, L.A., Amos, C.I., Huang, Q., et al. (2004) Functional variants of OCTN cation transporter genes are associated with Crohn disease. *Nat Genet*, 36, 471-475.

Perlmann, P., Perlmann, H., Flyg, B.W., Hagstedt, M., Elghazali, G., et al. (1997) Immunoglobulin E, a pathogenic factor in *Plasmodium falciparum* malaria. *Infect Immun*, 65, 116-121.

Perry, E.L. (1914) Endemic malaria of the Jeypore hill tracts of the Madras Presidency. *Indian J Med Res*, 2, 456-491.

Phimpraphi, W., Paul, R.E.L., Yimsamran, S., Puangsa-art, S., Thanyavanich, N., et al. (2008) Longitudinal study of *Plasmodium falciparum* and *Plasmodium vivax* in a Karen population in Thailand. *Malaria J*, 7, 99.

Phimpraphi, W., Paul, R.E.L., Witoonpanich, B., Turbpaiboon, C., Peerapittayamongkol, C., et al. (2008) Heritability of *P. falciparum* and *P. vivax* malaria in a Karen population in Thailand. *PLoS ONE*, 3, e3887.

Price, R., Nosten, F., Simpson, J.A., Luxemburger, C., Phaipun, L., et al. (1999) Risk factors for gametocyte carriage in uncomplicated falciparum malaria. *Am J Trop Med Hyg*, 60, 1019–1023.

Price, R.N., Tjitra, E., Guerra, C.A., Yeung, S., White, N.J., et al. (2007) Vivax malaria: neglected and not benign. *Am J Trop Med Hyg*, 77, 79-87.

Randolph, A.G., Lange, C., Silverman, E.K., Lazarus, R., Silverman, E.S., et al. (2004) The IL12B gene is associated with asthma. *Am J Hum Genet*, 75, 709-715.

Rihet, P., Abel, L., Traore, Y., Traore-Leroux, T., Aucan, C., et al. (1998a) Human malaria: segregation analysis of blood infection levels in a suburban area and a rural area in Burkina Faso. *Genet Epidemiol*, 15, 435-450.

Rihet, P., Traore, Y., Abel, L., Aucan, C., Traore-Leroux, T., et al. (1998b) Malaria in humans: *Plasmodium falciparum* blood infection levels are linked to chromosome 5q31-q33. *Am J Hum Genet*, 63, 498-505.

Rogier, C., Commenges, D., & Trape, J.F. (1996) Evidence for an age-dependent pyrogenic threshold of *Plasmodium falciparum* parasitemia in highly endemic populations. *Am J Trop Med Hyg*, 54, 613-619.

Rogier, C., Tall, A., Diagne, N., Fontenille, D., Spiegel, A., et al. (1999) *Plasmodium falciparum* clinical malaria: lessons from longitudinal studies in Senegal. *Parassitologia*, 41, 255-259.

Sakuntabhai, A., Ndiaye, R., Casademont, I., Peerapittayamongkol, C., Rogier, C., et al. (2008) Genetic determination and linkage mapping of *Plasmodium falciparum* malaria related traits in Senegal. *PLoS ONE*, 3, e2000.

Sergent, E., & Parrot, L. (1935) L'immunité, la prémunition et la résistance innée. *Arch Inst Pasteur Algérie*, XIII, 279.

Smith, T., Schellenberg, J.A., & Hayes, R. (1994) Attributable fraction estimates and case definitions for malaria in endemic areas. *Statistics in Medicine*, 13, 2345–2358.

Somboon, P., Suwonkerd, W., & Lines, J.D. (1994) Susceptibility of Thai zoophilic Anophelines and suspected malaria vectors to local strains of human malaria parasites. *Southeast Asian J Trop Med Public Health*, 25, 766-770.

Sowunmi, A., Gbotosho, G.O., Happi, C.T., Adedeji, A.A., Bolaji, O.M., et al. (2007) Enhancement of the antimalarial efficacy of amodiaquine by chlorpheniramine in vivo. *Mem Inst Oswaldo Cruz*, 102, 417-419.

Spiegel, A., Tall, A., Raphenon, G., Trape, J.F., & Druilhe, P. (2003) Increased frequency of malaria attacks in subjects co-infected by intestinal worms and *Plasmodium falciparum* malaria. *Trans R Soc Trop Med Hyg*, 97, 198-199.

Srichaikul, T., Archararit, N., Siriasawakul, T., & Viriyapanich, T. (1976) Histamine changes in *Plasmodium falciparum* malaria. *Trans R Soc Trop Med Hyg*, 70, 36–38.

Stirnadel, H.A., Beck, H.P., Alpers, M.P., & Smith, T.A. (1999) Heritability and segregation analysis of immune responses to specific malaria antigens in Papua New Guinea. *Genet Epidemiol*, 17, 16-34.

Sunyer, J., Mendendez, C., Ventura, P.J., Aponte, J.J., Schellenberg, D., et al. (2001) Prenatal risk factors of wheezing at the age of four years in Tanzania. *Thorax*, 56, 290-295.

Taylor-Robinson, A.W. (1998) Malaria-specific IgE as a risk factor for cancer and atopy. *Am J Trop Med Hyg*, 59, 181.

Thye, T., Vannberg, F.O., Wong, S.H., Owusu-Dabo, E., Osei, I., et al. (2010) Genome-wide association analyses identifies a susceptibility locus for tuberculosis on chromosome 18q11.2. *Nat Genet*, 42, 739-41.

Timmann, C., Evans, J.A., Konig, I.R., Kleensang, A., Ruschendorf, F., et al. (2007) Genome-wide linkage analysis of malaria infection intensity and mild disease. *PLoS Genet*, 3, e48.

Trape, J.F., Rogier, C., Konate, L., Diagne, N., Bouganali, H., et al. (1994) The Dielmo project: a longitudinal study of natural malaria infection and the mechanisms of protective immunity in a community living in a holoendemic area of Senegal. *Am J Trop Med Hyg*, 51, 123-137.

van der Sluis, S., Verhage, M., Posthuma, D., & Dolan, C.V. (2010) Phenotypic complexity, measurement bias, and poor phenotypic resolution contribute to the missing heritability problem in genetic association studies. *PLoS ONE*, 5, e13929.

Visscher, P.M., Hill, W.G., Wray, N.R. (2008) Heritability in the genomics era--concepts and misconceptions. *Nat Rev Genet*, 9, 255-266.

Walley, A.J., Aucan, C., Kwiatkowski, D., & Hill, A.V. (2004) Interleukin-1 gene cluster polymorphisms and susceptibility to clinical malaria in a Gambian case-control study. *Eur J Hum Genet*, 12, 132-138.

Williams, T.N., Maitland, K., Bennett, S., Ganczakowski, M., Peto, T.E., et al. (1996) High incidence of malaria in alpha-thalassaemic children. *Nature*, 383, 522-525.

Wilson, R.J., & McGregor, I.A. (1973) Immunoglobulin characteristics of antibodies to malarial S-antigens in man. *Immunology* 25, 385-398.

Wu, M. C., Kraft, P., Epstein, M. P., Taylor, D. M., Chanock, S. J., et al. (2010) Powerful SNP-Set Analysis for Case-Control Genome-wide Association Studies. *Am J Hum Genet*, 86, 929-942.

Xu, J., Meyers, D.A., Ober, C., Blumenthal, M.N., Mellen, B., et al. (2001) Genome wide screen and identification of gene-gene interactions for asthma-susceptibility loci in three U.S. populations: collaborative study on the genetics of asthma. *Am J Hum Genet*, 68, 1437-1446.

Zhang, F.R., Huang, W., Chen, S.M., Sun, L.D., Liu, H., et al. (2009) Genome wide association study of leprosy. *N Engl J Med*, 361, 2609-2618.

Zhang, Y., Leaves, N.I., Anderson, G.G., Ponting, C.P., Broxholme, J., et al. (2003) Positional cloning of a quantitative trait locus on chromosome 13q14 that influences immunoglobulin E levels and asthma. *Nat Genet*, 34, 181-186.

Part 7

Malaria Drug Evaluation

15

Advances in Antimalarial Drug Evaluation and New Targets for Antimalarials

Grellier Philippe, Deregnaucourt Christiane and Florent Isabelle
National Museum of Natural History, UMR 7245 CNRS, Team APE, Paris, France

1. Introduction

Parasitic infections due to the protozoa *Plasmodium* are responsible for malaria, a severe disease that still caused about 225 million cases and 781,000 human deaths in 2009, despite the efforts developed during the last decade to fight this disease (Alonso et al., 2011). The international funding allocated to antimalarial strategies has increased regularly since 2003 from about 0.3 billions to 1.7 billion dollars in 2009 (Collier, 2009), allowing many countries to undertake or strengthen effective fights against the parasite, the disease and the vectors. Nonetheless, more than half of the world population still lives in area where there is a risk of malaria transmission. The difficulty in fighting malaria is that five species of *Plasmodium,* namely *P. ovale, P. malariae, P. vivax, P. falciparum* and *P. knowlesi* (until recently considered as a nonhuman primate parasite) transmitted by over 30 species of *Anopheles* female mosquitoes are known to cause human malaria. The most virulent, *P. falciparum,* is responsible for severe clinical malaria and death. Furthermore, an increasing prevalence of resistance of vectors to insecticides, and of parasites to the standard antimalarial drugs has been observed for decades.

Today, the chemotherapeutic arsenal for malaria treatment is limited to three main families of compounds: quinolines, antifolates and artemisinin derivatives. Recommended chemotherapy is based on combinations of existing drugs with artemisinin derivatives (artemisinin combination therapies or ACT), the only antimalarial drug having no clear resistance recorded but for which alarming reports of tolerance in the field indicate it could be just a question of time (Noedl et al., 2008). From 2000 to 2008, the use of ACT combined with vector control allowed to reduce considerably the number of cases of malaria in a dozen African countries, so that nowadays, about 50 % of the total cases of malaria in Africa are found in mainly five countries (Enserink, 2010). However, no new class of antimalarials has been introduced into clinical practice since 1996 due to the intrinsic difficulties in discovering and developing new antimicrobials. A recent review of the global antimalarial drug development (Figure 1), including drugs at various clinical stage development and those expected to enter in phase I studies, showed that the pipeline is rather strong but novelty in terms of drug targets that is required to circumvent resistance is relatively low (Olliaro & Wells, 2009). This situation and the complexity in developing efficient vaccines require an urgent need for new drugs with original mechanisms of actions.

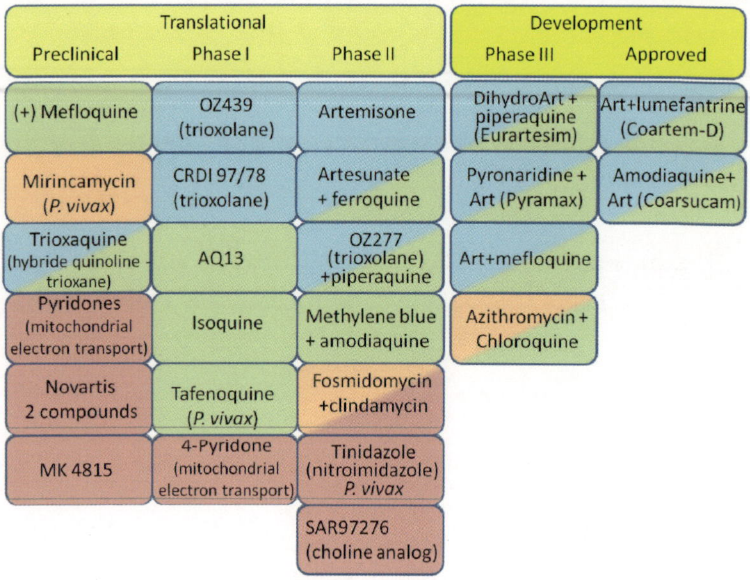

Fig. 1. Global antimalarial drug development pipeline (February 2009), after (Olliaro & Wells, 2009). Artemisinin (Art) derivatives or drugs containing the trioxane ring of artemisinin are illustrated in blue; aminoquinolines and structurally related compounds as well as aryl alcohols are in green; antibiotics are in orange; others drugs having different targets or mechanisms of action are in brown-red.

2. Development of bioassays for antimalarial activity

2.1 Malaria parasite life cycle

P. falciparum has a complex life cycle involving the *Anopheles* vector, where the sexual phase occurs, and humans where the parasite undergoes two phases of extensive asexual proliferation. After the bite by an infected *Anopheles*, the parasites at the sporozoite stage enter the blood and are carried to the liver where they traverse and invade hepatocytes initiating what is called the hepatic or exoerythrocytic phase. During this asymptomatic period, that lasts 5-7 days for *P. falciparum*, the sporozoites develop within the hepatocytes and, after several rounds of mitosis, produce several thousands of new infective forms called the merozoites that are released into the bloodstream and invade the red blood cells. During this intraerythrocytic cycle, which lasts 48 h for *P. falciparum* and causes the malaria disease, the parasite undergoes a successive development into the ring stage (0-20 h) and the trophozoite stage (20-36 h), which then undergoes several mitoses (schizont stage, 36-48 h) that lead to the differentiation of 16-24 infective merozoites. Erythrocyte lysis releases the merozoites into the bloodstream and a new intraerythrocytic cycle can be initiated. For some still not well understood reasons, some merozoites differentiate into male and female gametocytes that are taken up by the *Anopheles* during the blood meal. Gametogenesis resumes in the digestive tract of the mosquito and sexual reproduction occurs forming a zygote that produces, after a meiosis and several mitosis, thousands of haploid sporozoites under the basal lamina, which then migrate to the salivary glands and can be transmitted to humans during a bite. Different antimalarial bioassays have been developed based on the *in vitro* inhibition of parasite growth or, more recently, on the inhibition of potential parasite targets, allowing the screening of chemical compounds.

2.2 Bioassays against the erythrocytic stage

The intraerythrocytic cycle, being responsible for the symptoms of the disease, is still the main parasite stage against which drugs are tested. Initially, drug screenings were limited to the use of animal malaria models (rodent, chicken or monkey). The development of the continuous culture of *P. falciparum* on human erythrocytes (Trager & Jensen, 1976) was a critical advance, allowing drug evaluation on well established laboratory strains and on fresh isolates from patients. Typically, parasites are maintained on leucocyte-free erythrocytes at 2-5% haematocrit, in 4-(2-hydroxyethyl)-1-piperazineethanesulfonic acid (HEPES)-buffered Roswell Park Memorial Institute (RPMI) medium and supplemented with 5-10% human serum, at 37 °C, under a reduced percentage of oxygen. Hypoxanthine can be added to the culture medium to stimulate parasite growth and to sustain high parasitemia, and it is recommended for the culture of fresh isolates. Standardized protocols have been proposed e.g. (in *Methods in Malaria Research*, http://www.mr4.org/Publications/tabid/326/Default.aspx).

Plasmodium vivax is the most widespread species and, except in equatorial Africa, is responsible for the most prevalent malaria infection of humans, causing 70 to 80 million clinical cases per year. Although *P. vivax* infections are rarely fatal, they remain an important cause of morbidity, particularly in Asia Pacific region. Compared to *P. falciparum*, *P. vivax* can be considered as a neglected disease. Resistance of *P. vivax* to the antimalarial drug chloroquine, the reference drug for treating *P. vivax* infection, has been reported since the 90's. It is therefore of importance to develop tools for monitoring drug resistance and developing new drugs. In contrast to *P. falciparum*, establishment of continuous cultured lines of *P. vivax* has not yet been achieved limiting drug evaluation, particularly high throughput screening. *P. vivax* does not easily grow in culture, requiring removal of leucocytes and enrichment of the growth media. Parasite growth can only be performed for short periods, but maintaining cultures up to 4 weeks can be obtained by supplying reticulocytes from normal blood (Udomsangpetch et al., 2008). Drug assays developed for *P. falciparum* are transposable to fresh and cryopreserved *P. vivax* isolates (Kosaisavee et al., 2006). It is generally assumed that drugs active against *P. falciparum* blood stages will be also active against *P. vivax* blood stages; this has been shown in clinical studies for dihydroartemisinin–piperaquine and for artesunate–pyronaridine (Olliaro & Wells, 2009). Such assumption and the technical constraints to study *P. vivax* explain the limited interest for this species. For the other human malaria parasites, *P. knowlesi* has been adapted to long-term culture on monkey erythrocytes (Kocken et al., 2002) but no continuous cultivation of *P. ovale* and *P. malariae* has been set up.

Standard protocols of drug and resistance evaluation on *P. falciparum* are recommended by the World Health Organisation to facilitate comparison of data. They generally involve evaluation by using Giemsa-stained smears and counting parasitemia or parasite stage distribution in treated and non-treated cultures. These assays require minimal equipment and can be easily applied in the field. However they are time-consuming thereby preventing rapid, large-scale screening of molecules. Several methods have been developed for screening large numbers of compounds in 96-well plates, or even in 384-well plates.

2.2.1 Incorporation of radiolabelled precursors

These assays are based on the incorporation of metabolic precursors by the parasite that reflects its growth. They take advantage of the fact that the red blood cell possesses a reduced basic metabolism. Uptake of [^{3}H]-hypoxanthine, a precursor for nucleic acids, was the first described (Desjardins et al., 1979) and is still the most widely used but other precursors, such as [^{3}H]-amino acids or [^{3}H]-ethanolamine have also been described. Users must keep in mind that addition of hypoxanthine to the medium to sustain parasite development will interfere with the sensitivity of the isotopic assay using [^{3}H]-hypoxanthine, considered as the gold standard antimalarial drug assay. Although very sensitive and reproducible, applicable for high-throughput screening, these assays have several disadvantages. They are costly, involve radioactivity with the constraints associated to the manipulation of radioactive compounds and the treatment of radioactive wastes, and require special equipment (cell harvester, liquid-scintillation counter). They can thus be problematic to set up in locations with poor resources.

2.2.2 Colorimetric assays

Non-radioactive and low-cost alternative assays have been developed but are usually less standardized and often less sensitive than the [^{3}H]-hypoxanthine uptake method. Colorimetric assays include the detection of *Plasmodium* lactate dehydrogenase (pLDH) activity (Makler et al., 1993), by its preferential metabolism of the substrate 3-acetylpyridine adenine dinucleotide which is weakly metabolized by the human LDH, or by the tetrazolium assay (Delhaes et al., 1999). The assays require accessible equipments (spectrophotometers) and good correlations were observed with the radioactive assays. Sensitive immunocapture assays based on monoclonal antibodies directed against pLDH were developed for drug screening (Druilhe et al., 2001, Makler et al., 1998) and were miniaturized for assays in 384-well plates (Bergmann-Leitner et al., 2008). pLDH detection was also the basis of rapid immunoassays for malaria diagnostic from whole blood using strips (OptiMal®) (Palmer et al., 1998). ELISA based on the quantification of the *Plasmodium* histidine-rich protein II (HRP2) was also developed and commercialized (Noedl et al., 2002). Currently, both assays are as sensitive as the isotopic assay. However, reagents are not widely available and their stability in field conditions may be questioned; also the genetic variations encountered within these parasite proteins may lead to a decrease of the assay sensitivity.

2.2.3 Fluorometric and flow cytometry-based assays

Taking advantage that erythrocytes have no or only remnant DNA/RNA, fluorescence-based assays were developed for high-throughput drug assays using DNA-binding fluorophores. Fluorescence correlates parasitemia. The currently used fluorophores are Hoechst, DAPI, SYBRGreen I, PICO green and YOYO, the two former being less used because they exhibit excitation and emission properties not appropriate for current fluorescence plate readers and consumables, which is not the case for the latter. Protocols have been optimized and they propose one-step assays applicable to high-throughput screening and as sensitive as the isotopic and the immunocapture assays on laboratory strains or clinical isolates (Bacon et al., 2007, Baniecki et al., 2007, Bennett et al., 2004). The assays are cost-effective, requiring only a spectrofluorometer, and dyes are readily available worldwide. These fluorometric assays seem sufficiently sensitive to identify complex chemical mixtures with antiplasmodial activity such as plant extracts (Abiodun et al., 2010). Although several works observed similar results between the isotopic and fluorometric assays, users must have in mind that fluorescence intensity is highly dependent on its physico-chemical environment and that false positive responses due to fluorescence quenching by a chemical compound of the tested sample are not occasional.

Flow cytometry is currently used to study the biology of malaria parasites, but is still little used to evaluate parasite drug susceptibility, certainly because of the high cost of cytometers and a capacity restricted to moderate throughput assays (Grimberg, 2011). However, owing to the large range of fluorescent probes available having different biological or biochemical affinities that can be simultaneously analysed, flow cytometry allows the access to many more information than just parasite proliferation (DNA content). It opens a new way to analyse drug susceptibility by integrating the DNA content and a deeper investigation of biological and biochemical effects of the drug on the parasite. Quantum dot (QD) is a CdSe/ZnS semiconductor crystal widely used for bioimaging applications and diagnostics because of its high photostability, large stokes shift and narrow emission spectra. In a recent work, authors searched for QD chemicals that could label *P. falciparum*-infected erythrocytes and found a polyethylenglycolated cationic QD (PCQD) that specifically label erythrocytes infected by the late stage parasites and not the uninfected erythrocytes and the erythrocytes infected by the early stage parasites (Ku et al., 2011). They used PCQD to quantify the antimalarial effect of chloroquine in 96-well plates by flow cytometry and found the assays as sensitive as the pLDH assay with a comparable cost and its performance enabled high-throughput assays. Innovative advances were also recorded for the development of assays using flow cytometry for evaluating drugs active on the gametocyte stage (see section 2.3).

2.2.4 Interlaboratory variations

Discrepancies in the activity of a same compound are often observed between laboratories. They can be due to the type of antimalarial assay used or to the *P. falciparum* strains used as well as their drug resistance status. However, data may also be influenced by laboratory-specific modifications of screening conditions. One can report:

- The use of asynchronized or synchronized cultures. *P. falciparum* has an asynchronous intraerythrocytic development *in vitro*. The synchronous development that is observed *in vivo* in humans can be restored by specific treatments taking into account the biological properties of the erythrocytes infected by the different parasite stages: e.g. 5% sorbitol treatment or gelatine floatation to specifically lyse or concentrate, respectively, the erythrocytes infected by the trophozoite and schizont stages. Assays on synchronized cultures of early stage parasites aim to be generalized because they reflect the parasite synchronisation observed in humans. Synchronous cultures allow further studies of the drug effects on specific stages of the parasite development.
- The duration of the drug incubation. This can vary from the classical 48 h assays that are widely used, to assays of 24 h or 72 h or of a longer period, especially for evaluating fast or slow-acting drugs. That is particularly illustrated by drugs having a delayed-death effect such as the antibiotics tetracyclines and clindamycin. In the presence of clinically relevant concentrations of these antibiotics, parasites grow normally, divide and invade new erythrocytes. Inhibitory effects are only observed when parasites

develop during the second erythrocytic cycle. This delayed-death effect has been attributed to inhibition of mitochondrion or apicoplast targets (Dahl & Rosenthal, 2008). Activity of such molecules would be underestimated using synchronized cultures and assays of less than 48 h.

- The use of human serum or serum substitutes. Variability of quality of human serum batches as well as the difficulty to have access to non-immune human sera in endemic malaria countries can be serious problems for data reproducibility and has led to the evaluation of numerous serum substitutes or sera of other species to support *P. falciparum* growth in culture (Basco, 2003). Albumax® was proposed as a substitute for human serum and is now used routinely by many laboratories. Two types exist, Albumax® I and II, both are used, depending upon the authors, generally at a concentration of 5 g/l. Their composition is not well characterized, as well as the biochemical differences between both types. They are mainly composed of chromatographically purified fatty acid-rich bovine serum albumin and have a low IgG content. In addition to their high cost, batch-to-batch variability were observed in the past and *Plasmodium* strains must be adapted to culture with Albumax® (Grellier P., personal communication). This latter point can be problematic for evaluating drug resistance of fresh isolates, which have been reported to grow poorly in the presence of Albumax® (Basco, 2004). Furthermore, contrasted results were reported when comparing antimalarial drug efficacy in assays containing Albumax® or human serum. Some authors observed differences in the IC_{50} of antimalarials (Ringwald et al., 1999), others observed no difference (Singh et al., 2007). In our hands and in our search of natural products with antimalarial activity, differences of IC_{50} may be important between both conditions for some chemicals. This can be due in part to the differences in lipid and protein content of the two culture media and to the binding properties of the antimalarial that may influence the pharmacodynamic profile of the drug, as observed for halofantrine, a highly lipophilic drug which significantly associates to triglyceride rich plasma lipoproteins (Humberstone et al., 1998).
- The culture conditions. Initial parasitemia, haematocrit, as well as atmosphere under which cultures are maintained (e.g., a 5% CO_2 atmosphere versus a well-defined atmosphere such as 6% O_2, 3% CO_2, 91% N_2) are all factors that may be the cause of discrepancies. For example, it has been documented that IC_{50} values for chloroquine depend highly on the oxygen pressure during the assay. A *P. falciparum* strain may display chloroquine-resistance (IC_{50} >100nM) at 10% O_2 and behave as a sensitive strain at 21% O_2 (Briolant et al., 2007).

2.3 Bioassays against the gametocyte stages

The emergence of resistance has highlighted the importance to develop drugs against parasite transmission (from human to *Anopheles* and from *Anopheles* to human) that has been recognized to be a priority in the efforts to eradicate malaria. Sexual stages (gametocytes) are being investigated as targets for vaccines but few drugs have been developed against these transmission stages. The only available compounds known to efficiently eliminate gametocytes are 8-aminoquinolines (primaquine and tafenoquine), but their use is restricted due to serious haematological toxicity. They cause haemolysis in patients with G6PD deficiency and, in cases of severe forms of G6PD deficiency, the risks of primaquine treatment might exceed the benefits (Beutler & Duparc, 2007). Difficulties to culture and to obtain large amounts of gametocytes have limited research in this area. Gametocytes have a quite long maturation period *in vitro* (more than 10 days), gametocytogenesis is stimulated by stress conditions and sexual subpopulation represents a small percentage of infected red blood cells. Furthermore, *Plasmodium* strains have a tendency to lose their capacity to produce gametocytes over time in culture and gametocyte-infected erythrocytes are difficult to separate from erythrocytes infected by asexual stages. Until recently, there had been few significant advances in techniques for producing gametocytes for drug screening. These techniques were difficult to set up and required costly equipments. New protocols have now improved our capability to produce gametocytes *in vitro* in a reproducible way, and to enrich gametocytes with a high degree of purity using MACS® magnetic affinity columns (Baker, 2007). Those improvements associated to the ability to genetically manipulate parasites have allowed the recent setting-up of protocols for evaluating drug effects on sexual conversion and gametocyte maturation with high-throughput capacities. They are based on : 1) the discrimination by flow cytometry of asexual and sexual forms using hydroethine that is taken up by the parasite and metabolized into ethidium, a nucleic acid-binding fluorochrome (Chevalley et al., 2010); 2) the use of transgenic *P. falciparum* parasites expressing a green fluorescent protein chimera of the early sexual blood stage (protein Pfs16) as a marker for commitment to gametocytogenesis; this marker associated to hydroethine allows also to measure the direct activity of drugs against the late-stages gametocytes (Peatey et al., 2009). In a same way, the stage II or later stage marker (PF10_0164) fused to the green fluorescent protein was used associated with the nuclear dye Hoescht 33342 to quantify the drug effects on the asexual stages and on the sexual conversion and the gametocyte maturation in a same assay (Buchholz et al., 2011). In a general way, the application of transfection technology to malaria parasites paves the way to a new generation of assays targeting specific pathways or parasite stages.

2.4 Bioassays for the hepatic stage of *Plasmodium*

Drug development against the liver stage has two main advantages: 1) Such drugs could be used as prophylactic agents by preventing the access of the parasite to the blood and, in consequence, the development of the disease; 2) *P. vivax* and *P. ovale*, unlike *P. falciparum*, have latent forms (hypnozoites) in the liver responsible for relapsing infections, sometimes years after the primary infection. Hypnozoites are unaffected by the drugs acting on the erythrocytic stage. Thus, anti-hypnozoite drugs could be used as anti-relapse agents, limiting then recrudescences.

The number of available drugs that act against the hepatic phase is limited. The 8-aminoquinolines (primaquine and tafenoquine) are the main and the most efficient ones, but have serious haematological toxicity as already mentioned. Evaluation of drugs against the hepatic stage has been mainly performed using *in vivo* models of rodent parasites e.g., *P. berghei* and *P. yoelii*. However, such drug screening is time consuming and costly due to the need to reproduce the complete life-cycle of the parasite to obtain viable sporozoites. Difficulties increase greatly if screening is performed using monkey models for human malaria parasites. The ability to culture *Plasmodium* in hepatocytes has opened new perspectives in the research of drugs active against the hepatic stage (Mazier et al., 1985, Mazier et al., 2004). *In vitro* screenings are usually performed using sporozoites of rodent *Plasmodium* infecting primary rodent hepatocytes or hepatoma cell lines but assays based on primary culture of human hepatocytes infected with *P. falciparum* sporozoites were also reported. Recently, assay on liver stage of *P. vivax* was established using purified and cryopreserved sporozoites opening new perspectives for development of anti-relapse drugs (Chattopadhyay et al., 2010). The sporozoite development within the hepatocyte into a schizont stage is followed either by Giemsa staining or immunofluorescence assay using specific antibodies or a genetically-manipulated fluorescent parasite. Potential antimalarial drugs acting on the hepatic stage have emerged (Carraz et al., 2006, Mahmoudi et al., 2003, Mahmoudi et al., 2008, Parvanova et al., 2009, Singh et al., 2010, Tasdemir et al., 2010, Yu et al., 2008). A high-throughput *in vitro* screening of drug activity on *Plasmodium* liver stages was developed based on a sophisticated infrared fluorescence scanning system, which allows rapid, automatic counting of infected hepatocytes (Gego et al., 2006). The recent development of bioluminescent parasites allows now a non-invasive real time monitoring and quantitative analysis of liver stage development *in vitro* and *in vivo* in rodents that offers new tools for drug evaluation (Mwakingwe et al., 2009, Ploemen et al., 2009) (see section 4.3.2). Automated visual assay was also set up to follow the extracellular cell death of sporozoites (Hegge et al., 2010). Although promising, such assays are however greatly dependent upon the production of a large number of sporozoites in insects, a limiting step for high-throughput screening.

2.5 Bioassays for parasite targets

Our understanding of malaria parasite biochemistry has considerably increased over the past two decades and has allowed the identification of many potential targets for new drugs, even if half of the *P. falciparum* genes are still in search of a biological function (Florent et al., 2010). Progresses have been made possible thanks to the decrypted genomes of several *Plasmodium* species and other Apicomplexans (see www.eupathdb.org), that have enabled the rapid identification of putative targets that are homologous to validated targets in other organisms. Usually, target validation in *Plasmodium* requires demonstrating that a specific inhibitor, designed or identified as being active against this particular target, indeed shows antimalarial activity *in vitro* and/or *in vivo*. However, such an approach called "chemical-validation" has limits since it is often difficult to demonstrate that the inhibitor kills the parasite by indeed acting specifically on this target and not by inhibiting unrelated biochemical mechanisms. Thus, nowadays, "genetic-validation" of the selected target must also be achieved in parallel i.e., the deletion of the corresponding gene must seriously impair the parasite's growth or ideally prevent its survival.

Recent advances in genetic understanding of *Plasmodium* have greatly increased the ability to genetically validate potential drug targets (Limenitakis & Soldati-Favre, 2011). Methodologies able to transfect rodent *Plasmodium* and *P. falciparum* so as to modify or knock out genes that code for potential target proteins have been available for over a decade. They have been progressively improved and refined to now permit conditional knock out of the gene at a chosen parasite stage that may be different from the transfected stage (Lacroix et al., 2011), conditional elimination of the gene product by fusing a degradation domain and Shield ligand (Dvorin et al., 2010) or compensation of a lethal phenotype resulting from knock out of an essential gene by expression in trans of a wild-type version of this gene (Slavic et al., 2010). Phenotypic analysis of the resultant mutant parasites then allows to study the importance of a particular target in the different phases of development of the life-cycle of *Plasmodium*. Many putative targets, initially suspected to be essential to a given parasite stage turned out finally dispensable to this stage but essential to others (see few examples such as FabI or falcipain-1 below). Furthermore, access to transcriptomic and proteomic technologies offers new opportunities to study the impact of a drug treatment on the entire parasite metabolism either at the RNA or protein levels. This leads to a better understanding of the mechanism(s) of action of drugs and the biochemical pathways involved in killing the parasites (Sims & Hyde, 2006). Recently, the achievement of random mutagenesis of *P. berghei* and *P. falciparum* genome by PiggyBac transposable element opened the route towards systematic plasmodial gene invalidation, that will obviously speed up the genetic validation process of putative targets (Crabb et al., 2011).

These recent advances have allowed development of bioassays based upon validated targets for drug screening, or targets still in the process of validation (for review see (Grellier et al., 2008, Prabhu & Patravale, 2011, Sahu et al., 2008)) : haem polymerization (O'Neill et al., 2006), pyrimidine, purine, folate (Hyde, 2007), lipid (Wengelnik et al., 2002), shikimate (McRobert et al., 2005), non-mevalonate (Wiesner & Jomaa, 2007) and other apicoplast metabolisms (Sato & Wilson, 2005), mitochondrial electron transport (Mather et al., 2007), redox homeostasis (Bauer et al., 2006), protein prenylation (Van Voorhis et al., 2007), proteases (Wegscheid-Gerlach et al., 2010), kinases (Doerig & Meijer, 2007)... Some of them are detailed below.

Databases such as TDR targets (http://tdrtargets.org) gather information on putative targets for several pathogens including *Plasmodium*, providing tools for their prioritization in whole genomes depending on user queries (Aguero et al., 2008). The Protein Data Bank (www.pdb.org) is also a useful resource, providing data on proteins whose 3D-structures have been solved experimentally by using either X-Rays or NMR. As of September 2011, more than 300 entries correspond to plasmodial proteins, knowing that several structures involving different ligands may have been solved for a same protein.

2.5.1 Inhibition of haeme polymerization

Haeme polymerization (Figure 2) is a natural process that occurs in the acidic food vacuole of the parasite where haemoglobin, a major source of amino acids for the parasite, is degraded by specific proteases. Haeme, which is toxic for the parasite, is detoxified by polymerization into a pigment, the haemozoin. Inhibition of haemozoin formation is considered as an attractive target for antimalarial drugs and high-throughput assays are available (Biagini et al., 2003, Deharo et al., 2002, Huy et al., 2007, Ncokazi & Egan, 2005, Rush et al., 2009, Weissbuch & Leiserowitz, 2008). The 4-aminoquinolines such as chloroquine and amodiaquine act by interfering with this polymerization process. Cysteine and aspartic parasite proteases (falcipains and plasmepsins, respectively) involved in the degradation of haemoglobin are also potential targets (Wegscheid-Gerlach et al., 2010) (see section 2.5.2).

2.5.2 Proteases

Although none of the currently marketed antimalarials is targeting plasmodial proteases, this class of enzymes, which is involved in a wide diversity of biological pathways during the parasite life cycle, has been the subject of intense investigations for the last decades

(Wegscheid-Gerlach et al., 2010). The cystein and aspartyl endoproteases involved in the essential pathway of haemoglobin degradation now known as falcipain-2, 2′ and -3 and plasmepsin-I, -II, -III (or HAP, for histo-aspartyl protease) and –IV have first emerged as promising protease targets. Intensive research focused on these enzymes during the last decades has yielded inhibitors active down to the nM levels on the native or recombinant enzymes, inhibiting parasite growth in culture from the nM to μM levels and capable to cure *Plasmodium*-infected mice (McKerrow et al., 2008, Rosenthal, 2010). Gene disruption studies however clearly indicated that all of these enzymes besides falcipain-3 are highly redundant. In fact, falcipain-3 is the only for which gene disruption did not yield viable blood-stage parasites (Liu et al., 2006, Sijwali et al., 2006). The development of inhibitors targeting these enzymes but displaying improved properties in term of activity, selectivity, safety to the host nonetheless pertains, facilitated by their availability under recombinant active form, allowing both high-throughput screenings and experimental determination of their 3D-structures, including for the most recently described plasmepsin I (Bhaumik et al., 2011). A strong argument for maintaining such a development against these haemoglobinases is linked to the proposal to use combined protease inhibitor therapy based on the observation that cystein and aspartyl inhibitors demonstrated synergistic antimalarial effects (Semenov et al., 1998).

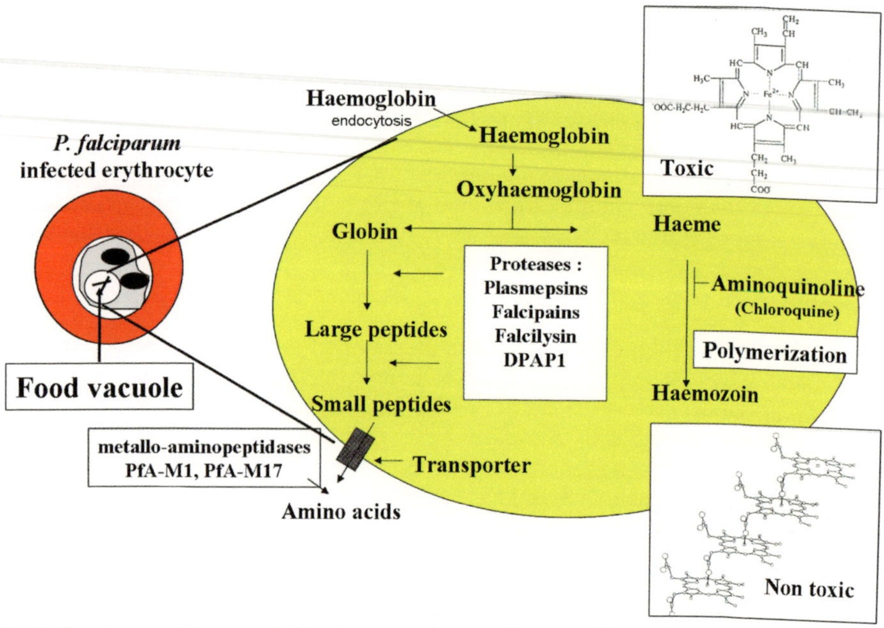

Fig. 2. Mechanisms of haemoglobin degradation and haeme detoxification in *Plasmodium falciparum*-infected red blood cell, after (Mambu & Grellier, 2008)

In parallel, the last decade has seen the emergence as promising targets of several new parasite proteases, among the ~100 that are encoded in the *P. falciparum* genome (Wu et al., 2003). Some are also involved in haemoglobin breakdown such as the cystein protease DPAP1 (Klemba et al., 2004), the metallo-endopeptidase falcilysin displaying however a dual activity, both able to process peptides in the food vacuole and to mature proteins imported to the apicoplast (Eggleson et al., 1999, Ponpuak et al., 2007), and the metallo-aminopeptidases PfA-M1 and PfA-M17 (McGowan et al., 2009, Skinner-Adams et al., 2009, Trenholme et al., 2010). Some have emerged from studies focusing on other key biological events such as erythrocyte egress/invasion and merozoite surface antigen maturation such as the subtilisin-like proteases -1 and -2 and the cystein proteases DPAP3, SERA-5 and SERA-6 (Blackman, 2008). Other proteases for which essential roles during the parasite asexual development have been demonstrated include Plasmepsin V, involved in maturation of proteins exported to the infected-red blood cell (Boddey et al., 2010, Russo et al., 2010). During these investigations, some proteases were found dispensable for the parasite asexual development in erythrocyte but important in other stages such as gametogenesis or the development of insect stages (Sologub et al., 2011). This is the case for the cystein proteases falcipain-1 and SERA-8. Gene deletion assays were determinant to indicate that falcipain-1, initially believed to be involved in haemoglobin breakdown then in red blood cell invasion, was in fact dispensable for the parasite blood-stage development but important for oocyst production (Eksi et al., 2004). Also, the *P. berghei* ortholog of SERA-8 appears involved in sporozoite egress from oocysts (Aly & Matuschewski, 2005).

2.5.3 Apicoplast-based targets

The apicoplast is a vestigial, non-phostosynthetic, plastid-like organelle inherited from the prokaryotic world by secondary endosymbiosis and found in most apicomplexan parasites including *Plasmodium* that is essential to their biology. In *P. falciparum*, it maintains a 35-kb circular genome and several particular biochemical pathways that are present in bacteria and plants but are absent in humans, thus providing many attractive targets that are extensively investigated for drug development. These pathways include the type II fatty acid biosynthesis pathway, which involves 6 distinct enzymes in *Plasmodium* while in human the type I fatty acid biosynthesis pathway involves a multifunctional enzyme, the 1-deoxy D xylulose 5 phosphate (DOXP) isoprenoid biosynthesis pathway that is mevalonate-independent in the malaria parasite contrary to humans, and apicoplast replication, transcription and translation which involve enzymes of bacterial origins (Dahl & Rosenthal, 2008, Goodman & McFadden, 2007, Grawert et al., 2011, Jayabalasingham et al., 2010). Pioneering works led to the emergence of promising antimalarials such as triclosan (believed to target the NADH-dependent enoyl ACP reductase or FabI enzyme), thiolactomycin (targeting FabH and FabB enzymes) and fosmidomycin (targeting the DOXP reductoisomerase) to name the main ones. Also, antibiotics such as tetracyclines and clindamycin, targeting prokaryotic protein synthesis, or quinolone antibiotics and rifampicin, targeting the prokaryotic DNA and RNA machinery, were shown to inhibit *Plasmodium* growth in culture and *in vivo* (Seeber & Soldati-Favre, 2010).

These results stimulated efforts both to genetically validate these putative targets and to improve inhibitor discovery, by solving 3D structures and producing enzymes under recombinant active forms amenable to medium/high throughput screenings (Freundlich et al., 2007, Sato, 2011). In 2008, the genetic inactivation of FabI in *P. falciparum* and in *P. berghei* produced parasite blood stages that were growing normally and were still affected by triclosan (Yu et al., 2008). The FabI gene deletion, on the other hand, blocked the development of the parasite in the liver. Not long later, the genetic inactivation in murine models of other enzymes belonging to the FasII metabolism such as FabB/F confirmed that the FasII pathway was dispensable through the entire parasite development to the exception of the hepatic-blood stage transition phase. These results raised the question of the nature of the parasitic target of triclosan in blood stages. Recently five laboratories reported their failed attempts to inhibit rodent *P. berghei* and *P. chabaudi* proliferation in mice by using similar doses of triclosan (Baschong et al., 2011).

Conversely, recent works focusing on the DOXP non-mevalonate isoprenoid pathway confirmed it appears as a relevant target for antimalarial drug development. Key results include the recent failure to delete the DOXP reductoisomerase gene (Odom & Van Voorhis, 2009). The DOXP metabolic pathway is active in all erythrocytic stages but problems with fosmidomycin, which has long been known to inhibit *Plasmodium* growth *in vitro* and *in* mice (Jomaa et al., 1999), emerged. Due to its short half life that may lead to parasite relapses and/or facilitate selection of resistant parasites, analogues with improved half-lives are actively looked for against this enzyme and the other enzymes of this metabolic pathway (Seeber & Soldati-Favre, 2010). The recent discovery that fosmidomycin is little effective against *Theileria*, *Eimeria* and *Toxoplasma* also raised the question of its bioavailability (Seeber & Soldati-Favre, 2010). This led to the proposal that fosmidomycin and its more active derivative FR900098, both active against *Plasmodium* erythrocytic but not hepatocytic stages, would enter the parasite through new permeation pathways called NPPs (Baumeister et al., 2011). Recently also two triose-phosphate transporters present on the apicoplast membranes have been characterized, PfiTPT/PfAPT1 and PfoTPT/PfATP2, and are being considered as putative targets since they are believed to import from the cytosol into the apicoplast key metabolites to fuel the DOXP pathway (Lim & McFadden, 2010).

2.5.4 Kinases

Malarial kinases but also host cell kinases involved in host-parasite interactions are also currently considered as promising targets (Doerig et al., 2010). The *P. falciparum* theroretical kinome was predicted to comprise 85 to 99 enzymes, depending on the stringency of the computational methods used to identify them, and phylogenetic studies have revealed interesting differences with the human kinome that may be exploited for kinase-targeted drug discovery (Leroy & Doerig, 2008). For example, *P. falciparum* possesses kinases and kinase families such as calcium-dependent protein kinases (CDPK) and the apicomplexan specific FIKK kinase families, that are absent in humans. Important advances in this field have been provided by the fact that many *P. falciparum* kinases have been successfully produced as recombinant active enzymes, allowing medium/high troughput studies, many structures are known or can be deduced by modelling (see http://www.thesgc.com) and several chemical libraries, developed for other pathologies such as cancer may be screened on *P. falciparum* putative targets and parasites. For example, PfCDPK1 that has no ortholog in humans was produced as an active recombinant enzyme and used to screen a library of ~20,000 molecules developed against kinases, from which a purine derivative called purfalcamine active to the low nM range on the enzyme was isolated (Kato et al., 2008). This molecule, able to prevent the *P. falciparum* development in culture had however a low *in vivo* activity on *P. berghei*, possibly due to poor pharmacokinetic parameters. Importantly, not only protein kinases but kinases phosphorylating other substrates such as choline kinase and pantothenate kinases could also be targeted (Leroy & Doerig, 2008). Genetic validation of kinases may be performed by classical gene deletion in *P. falciparum* or rodent *Plasmodium*, but conditional expression systems have also been used as for example using the destabilizing domain and Shield ligand to show the involvement of PfCDPK5 in merozoite egress (Dvorin et al., 2010).

2.5.5 Transporters

Transporters are integral transmembrane proteins that enable the movement of solutes across biological membranes. In *Plasmodium,* they are currently considered as highly promising targets, due to their involvement, as carrier proteins, channels or pumps, in the movement of nutrients, metabolites and ions into and out of the parasite as well as between subcellular compartments within the parasite. They thus regulate essential nutrient uptake into the parasite, homeostasis and disposal of toxic wastes. Host cell transporters modified by the presence of the parasite may also be involved in these biological functions. Of note, malarial transmembrane proteins such as PfCRT, Pgh1, PfNHE1 and possibly PfATP6 are involved in drug-resistance mechanisms.

The recent publication of the theoretical permeome of *P. falciparum* indicated that at least 2.5% of the parasite genome encode transporters, channels and pumps (Martin et al., 2009). Experimental localizations, that have been achieved by using either specific antibodies or epitope-tagged or fluorescent recombinant fusion proteins transfected into parasites, concern few proteins of the parasite surface (PfHT1 or the hexose transporter, PfENT1 or PfNT1, PfMRP, PfAQP), the mitochondrial membrane (ATP/ADP transporter), or the food-vacuole membrane (PfCRT, Pgh1, V-type H+ ATPase and ATP-driven H+ pump). Substrate specificities are also often ill-defined. Even if these could be predicted by orthology for about half of the candidates, experimental validations are still necessary to confirm or discover which they are. Extensive experimental work therefore needs to be done to further exploit such a rich source of potential targets (Staines et al., 2010). Some promising results nonetheless emerged in this field. First, the challenging functional expression of recombinant proteins, which is necessary for the biochemical testing of substrates and inhibitors, has been achieved successfully in *Xenopus laevis* oocytes for several *Plasmodium* transporters. Alternative heterologous systems have also been used such as yeast, *Dictyostelium discoideum* and mammalian cells (Martin et al., 2009). In some cases, cell-free transporter assay systems are used. Recently, recombinant expression of codon-optimized PfHT1 in yeast was performed to permit high-throughput screening of inhibitors (Blume et al., 2010). The P-type ATPases, PfATP4 and PfATP6, and the drug-resistance involved PfCRT and Pgh1 have also been expressed in such heterologous system, opening the road for functional studies (Martin et al., 2009). The number of known 3D-structures remains however extremely low, limited to PfAQP although a model has been proposed for PfHT1 based on the structure of *E. coli* permease (Staines et al., 2010).

Transfection methods have been also critical in this field, in particular to assess the role of PfCRT and Pgh1 in drug resistance, by transfecting *P. falciparum* resistant alleles into sensitive parasites and vice-versa, or by transfecting these alleles in various heterologous expression systems such as yeast (Martin et al., 2009). Gene deletion studies have been also undertaken, but so far for a limited number of candidates. While several genes could be deleted with none or limited impact on parasite asexual growth such as those encoding PfENT1, PfMRP, the *P. berghei* orthologue of the PfAQP, PfKch1 (PfK1) and PfACα, the deletion of genes encoding PfHT1, PfCRT and Pgh1 could not be achieved, suggesting that the two latter ones play essential functions in the parasite biology beside being involved in drug-resistance (Sanchez et al., 2010). Such experiments performed using rodent malaria models further indicated that some candidates, apparently dispensable for the asexual development, turned out important for the development of other parasite stages in insects or liver (Martin et al., 2009, Staines et al., 2004). Among all these candidates, PfHT1 is the only malarial transporter that has been validated both chemically and genetically (Staines et al., 2010). Gene deletion studies and D-glucose derivatives used as inhibitors confirmed the essential role of the hexose transporters for the asexual parasite development and other parasite stages (Blume et al., 2010, Slavic et al., 2011).

3. Renew of phenotypic screening approaches

Advanced antimalarial drug discovery programs revealed four general strategies to discover new drugs (Wu et al., 2011) : 1) To start from specific, validated or not, malaria targets to find new hits (e.g. haem polymerization, enzymes of the pyrimidine synthesis pathway); 2) To synthesize new analogs from known antimalarial pharmacophores (e.g. synthetic endoperoxides (Trioxolanes) or hybrid molecules having two pharmacophores (Trioxaquines)); 3) To start from drugs developed for other diseases whose similar targets are present in malaria parasites (as illustrated by the piggy-back approach undertaken against parasite protein farnesyltransferases using anti-cancer agents targeting protein prenylation developed by pharmaceutical companies); 4) To screen chemicals on whole cell-based assays to identify hits that kill parasite for further optimizations. Most of the current antimalarials were originated from this last phenotypic drug discovery approach. The revolution in molecular biology led to a switch to target-based approaches for drug discovery in pharmaceutical industries. However, this approach failed to deliver the expected results, especially for antimicrobials (Keller et al., 2011, Payne et al., 2007, Sams-Dodd, 2005). In the recent years, the access to large chemical libraries and the improvements of whole cell-based high throughput screening assays led to a renaissance of the phenotypic approach with the forward chemical genetic strategy. Chemical genetics is the study of biological systems using small molecules as tools (O'Connor et al., 2011). Forward chemical genetic uses small molecules to modulate gene-product function leading to a phenotype of interest (parasite killing for example), and the target must be further identified. In contrast, reverse chemical genetic screens specific gene products with libraries of small molecules to identify ligands, which are then tested on cells for phenotypic changes. Over the last few years, reports demonstrated the power of chemical genetic for antimalarial drug discovery. The GlaxoSmithKline (GSK)'s chemical library constituted of nearly 2 million chemical entities was tested upon drug sensitive and multidrug resistant *P. falciparum* strains. More than 8,000 compounds, clustered into 416 molecular frameworks, showed potent antiplasmodial activity. Analysis of historical GSK data suggested that the main target classes affected by these compounds are malaria kinases, proteases and G-protein coupled receptors (Gamo et al., 2010). In a similar study, a library of nearly 310,000 chemicals, designed to cover a large diversity of bioactive compounds, was screened upon drug sensitive and multidrug resistant *P. falciparum* strains (Guiguemde et al., 2010). Amongst hits, 172 were cross-validated by three laboratories using distinct assays. A reverse chemical genetic approach was undertaken with the validated set of compounds using 66 malarial target assays and identified 19 new inhibitors of 4 validated targets. Preliminary pharmacokinetic profiling found most of them suitable for further development. One lead was further evaluated *in vivo* on *P. yoelii*-infected mice and displayed significant antimalarial activity. In another study, the screening of a focused library of about 12,000 natural and synthetic chemicals led to identification of spiroindolone compounds as appropriate candidates for further development (Rottmann et al., 2010). Optimization studies produced NITD609, which is developed by Novartis.

4. *In vivo* antimalarial drug evaluation

Plasmodium species that infect humans are essentially unable to infect non-primate animal models. Historically, *in vivo* evaluation of antimalarial compounds began with the use of avian parasites in birds and simian parasites in monkeys. The discovery by Ignace Vincke and Marcel Lips in 1948 at Keyberg in the then Belgian Congo, of a rodent malaria parasite (*Plasmodium berghei*) which readily infected laboratory mice and rats, greatly facilitated *in vivo* drug screening management. Since then, several other species and subspecies of rodent parasites have been described and employed. With the discovery in the early 90's that the owl monkey (*Aotus trivirgatus*) is susceptible to infection with the human parasites *P. falciparum* and *P. vivax*, the simian models of malaria have regained interest. Infection with *P. falciparum* is now well characterized in both *Aotus* and *Saimiri* monkeys (Collins, 1992), and primate models, because they provide a clear prediction of drug efficacy and pharmacokinetics in humans, are a logical transition to clinical studies. However, there are obvious limitations to their use, and any primary screen dependent upon monkeys appears both wasteful in terms of animal conservation, drug consumption, and ethics. So, the first steps of *in vivo* drug screening typically begins with the use of mouse models of malaria with the rodent parasites *P. berghei, P. yoelii, P. chabaudi* and *P. vinckei*, that have been validated through the evaluation of several antimalarial drugs.

4.1 Rodent models of malaria

Individual parasite species and strains have been well characterized, including duration of cycle, synchronicity, drug sensitivity and course of infection in genetically defined mouse strains. *P. berghei, P. vinckei* and few strains of *P. yoelii* and *P. chabaudi* cause lethal infections in mice, whereas *P. yoelii, P. chabaudi,* and *P. vinckei petterei* are usually cleared after the initial acute parasitaemia or after a subsequent low-grade chronic parasitaemia.

P. berghei - The strains K173, ANKA, NK65 and SP11 are the most frequently used for experimental work. The affinity for immature erythrocytes (reticulocytes) varies according to the strain. ANKA invades preferentially reticulocytes, while NK65 invades indifferently reticulocytes and mature erythrocytes, i.e. normocytes. Both strains are lethal, but ANKA kills the mouse with a low parasitaemia (it rarely exceeds 20%), whereas infection with NK65 induces a continuous increase in parasitaemia until the mouse dies. The erythrocytic cycle is asynchronous and its duration is about 21 h. Schizogony lasts 50 h in hepatocytes. Susceptible mice infected with *P. berghei* ANKA die within two weeks after infection with severe neurological symptoms and cerebral microvascular abnormalities. These are common pathologies to both murine and human infections that make of *P. berghei* ANKA a useful experimental model of cerebral malaria. Resistant mice do not show any neurological symptom but die during the third or fourth week post-infection (p.i.) with high parasitaemia.

P. vinckei - Among four subspecies recognized (*P. vinckei vinckei, P. vinckei petteri, P. vinckei lentum* and *P. vinckei brucechwatti*), *P. v. vinckei* and *P. v. petteri* have been used in some studies for the identification of new antimalarial drugs. Both subspecies preferentially invade normocytes. Schizogony in erythrocytes has a duration time of 24 h and is synchronous. Schizogony in hepatocytes lasts for 60 h or more.

P. yoelii – Three subspecies are recognized: *P. yoelii yoelii, P. yoelii killicki* and *P. yoelii nigeriensis*. *P. yoelii* shows a preference for reticulocytes, but it may also invade normocytes, depending on the virulence of the strain. Duration of the schizogonic cycle is 18 h in erythrocytes. Schizogony is about 45 h long in hepatocytes. The erythrocytic cycle is asynchronous. The parasitaemia of *P. y. yoelii* 17X and 265BY depends mainly on the production of reticulocytes by the host, whereas *P. y. nigeriensis* grows very rapidly by invading all available erythrocytes. Of note, *P. yoelii* is more resistant to chloroquine than are the other species (Beaute-Lafitte et al., 1994). Gametocyte production is constant throughout the infection.

P. chabaudi – Two subspecies of *P. chabaudi* have been identified: *P. chabaudi chabaudi* and *P. chabaudi adami*. This species exhibits many similarities to *P. falciparum*, including analogous blood-stage antigens, invasion of reticulocytes and normocytes, suppression of B- and T-cell responses, and parasite sequestration in liver and spleen which induces parasite withdrawal from the peripheral circulation. The schizogonic cycle of *P. chabaudi* is 24 h long in erythrocytes and is synchronous. It runs 54-58 h in liver. In resistant mice, a rapid parasite multiplication during the first week p.i. is followed by parasite elimination by the fourth week p.i., whereas susceptible mice usually die during the second week p.i.

4.2 Designing an experimental mouse model

Many inbred and outbred strains of mice are available to design a mouse model. Considering that every species and every line or clone of a particular *Plasmodium* species exhibits particular characteristics, the resulting infection may vary greatly within the different laboratory strains of mice. As an example, blood-induced infections of the K173 (N) of *P. berghei* follow a fulminating course in many strains of mouse, but are slow in NMRI mice, and infections with *P. y. yoelii* 17X in Swiss mice are lethal, whereas they resolve in CBA/Ca mice. Scientists should use the most appropriate model for their particular research question and take advantage of their particular knowledge about compounds to be tested, especially in terms of molecular and/or biological targets. A rather rich presentation of experimental malaria infections in different mouse strains, comprising some models for cerebral malaria, can be found in (Sanni et al., 2002).

The difference in the degree of infection, lethality and synchronicity between the rodent plasmodia enlarges the number of possible assays for drug evaluation. For example, parasites that generate high parasitaemia and synchronous infections, like *P. chabaudi* and *P. vinckei*, are more appropriate to study compounds exhibiting stage selectivity. Also, it is important to note that the drug sensitivity of a given rodent *Plasmodium* species may not reflect that of the other rodent species. This can be illustrated by *P. berghei* exhibiting less sensitivity than *P. chabaudi* and *P. vinckei* to iron chelators and lipid biosynthesis inhibitors (Peters & Robinson, 1999, Wengelnik et al., 2002). Drug sensitivity may also not mirror that of *P. falciparum*, as shown in the case of cysteine protease inhibitors, owing to the fact that the enzyme active site is different between rodent plasmodia and *P. falciparum*. This situation has led to question the use of these models in lead optimization (Singh et al., 2002).

Given this, the following criteria must be considered when selecting a mouse model. On the host side, innate factors like peculiarities in pharmacodynamics of the drug; innate immunity; variation between individuals of the same species (strain, age, sex and immune status); environmental factors (temperature and stress, nutrition, intercurrent infections). On the parasite side: variation within a single *Plasmodium* species (variation of sensitivity among different clones, geographic strains, time since isolation of "wild" strain); variation among different *Plasmodium* species; mode and intensity of infection. Also, attention should be paid to drug-dependent factors like the mode of formulation, the route of administration or the drug dosage regimen.

4.3 Current *in vivo* antimalarial tests using rodent models of malaria

4.3.1 Erythrocytic stages of malaria parasites

The most widely used initial test is the "four-day suppressive test", which commonly uses *P. berghei* or *P. chabaudi*. The efficacy of four daily doses of compounds is measured by comparison of mouse survival time and blood parasitaemia on day four p.i. in treated and untreated mice. Compounds identified as being active in those assays can subsequently be progressed through various secondary tests, such as 1) the "dose ranging, full four-day test", in which compounds are tested at a minimum of four different doses to determine effective dose values and get information on oral bioavailability and relative potency of the tested compounds; 2) the "onset/recrudescence" test, in which mice are administered a single dose on day 3 after infection and parasitaemia is monitored daily. Compounds can also be tested for prophylactic activity: the compound is administered prior to infection, and parasitaemia is followed daily.

4.3.2 Other stages of malaria parasites

Several tissue schizontocidal tests (the test of Gregory and Peters (1970) using sporozoites of *P. yoelii nigeriensis*, the test of Rane and Kinnamon with *P. yoelii yoelii*, and the Hill test for causal prophylactic compounds with residual action) have been reported in details (Peters, 1987). Tests that apply to the screening of drugs having gametocidal or sporontocidal action can be found at the same source. A technique such as real time PCR allows quantification of the parasite charge in liver and thus, the inhibitory effect of the molecule tested (Carraz et al., 2006). Recently, the use of a transgenic *P. berghei* parasite expressing the bioluminescent reporter protein luciferase to visualize and quantify parasite development in liver cells in live mice using real-time luminescence imaging was reported (Ploemen et al., 2009). The applicability of real time imaging to assess parasite drug sensitivity in the liver was demonstrated by analysing the effect of primaquine and tafenoquine *in vivo*. The methodology is relatively simple and offers the possibility to analyse liver development in live mice without surgery. It opens up new possibilities for research on *Plasmodium* liver infections and for evaluating the effect of drugs on the liver stage of *Plasmodium*.

4.4 Humanized mice models of malaria

Immunocompromized mice, developed and used in other research contexts, have been used for some years to elaborate new mouse models for human malaria. By grafting them with either human erythrocytes or human hepatocytes, these animals can support, respectively, the asexual blood cycle or the hepatic phase of the human parasite *P. falciparum*. So, drug efficacy and pharmacokinetics can be assessed in an *in vivo* setting against the true parasite target during its blood or hepatic stage development.

4.4.1 The *P. falciparum*-human erythrocyte mouse models

In 2001, the feasibility of evaluating *in vivo* responses to antimalarial drugs in humanised mice models was demonstrated using the *P. falciparum*-human erythrocyte-BXN model, in which Beige Xid Nude (BXN) mice, genetically deficient in T- and B-cell functions and chemically controlled for response of cells involved in innate defences, were grafted with human erythrocytes infected with *P. falciparum* (Moreno et al., 2001). The mice received human erythrocytes infected with drug (chloroquine/quinine/mefloquine) resistant or sensitive strains of *P. falciparum*, and the blood schizonticidal effects of various antimalarial drugs were assessed. Parasite clearance and parasite reduction rate in the mouse model were shown to parallel those reported in humans infected with *P. falciparum*. Since then, improvements of the *P. falciparum* humanized mouse model have been made using NSG mice with improved genetic deficiency of innate immunity. High reproducibility of human erythrocytes grafting and parasite survival could be achieved, along with the possible adjustment of parasitaemia over a range of 1-40% for several weeks (Arnold et al., 2011). In the near future, a model harbouring a hematopoietic stem cell line capable of producing erythroblasts/cytes should replace current models with the advantage of producing reticulocytes to also support *P. vivax*. To date, we are aware of only one work dealing with drug testing in humanised mouse model of malaria, i.e. the one about trioxaquine selection for drug development (Cosledan et al., 2008). The scarcity of reports exemplifies the serious limitations to the use of such malaria models in drug discovery: 1) in most of the models, parasitaemia remains stable only in a minor subset of mice whereas it is rapidly cleared in the majority of the animals, 2) the use of toxic reagents to minimize the mouse innate defence is susceptible to affect the efficacy of antimalarials or effector cells, 3) management of those experimental models is cumbersome and requires specific facilities.

4.4.2 The *P. falciparum*-human hepatocyte mouse models

There have been many attempts to develop laboratory models supporting the survival of human hepatocytes, given that *in vivo* only human cells or those of higher primates are receptive to *P. falciparum*. Invasion by and development of *P. falciparum* in human hepatocyte-transplanted animals was demonstrated in 2006, by combining 1) the use of mice with two genetic deficiencies (uPA-SCID mice) affecting hepatocytes and T and B lymphocytes, and 2) the pharmacological control of their non-adaptive defences, which improved the results of xenotransplantation into mice (Morosan et al., 2006). In these mice, *P. falciparum* sporozoites delivered intravenously infected the transplanted human hepatocytes and developed into liver schizonts up to a size that was comparable to that found in humans and chimpanzees. Alternative approaches to elaborate human hepatocyte-engrafted mouse models have been reported recently. One used the *Fah–/–Rag2–/–Il2rg–/–* mice, the liver of which was very efficiently repopulated (up to approximately 95% of the murine liver) by human hepatocytes under selection pressure by the drug NTBC (2-(2-nitro-4-fluoromethylbenzoyl)-1,3-cyclohexanedione) (Bissig et al., 2010). The suitability of this model for antiviral drug testing after successful infection of the chimeric liver by hepatitis B and C viruses was demonstrated, legitimating to believe in future successful infection by human *Plasmodium* species. Also, very recently, researchers at the MIT developed artificial humanised mouse livers engineered by growing human hepatocytes and human liver endothelial cells with mouse fibroblasts in a three-dimensional polymeric scaffold, and implanted them into mice (Chen et al., 2011). The ectopic livers responded to drugs in a way very similar to the way a human liver does.

4.5 Comments

Obviously those recent experimental models are not yet elaborated enough to meet the requirements for examining the large number of compounds involved in initial drug development. However, they pave the way for more efficient testing of drugs designed for humans. Ultimately, the combination of the immunocompromised mouse model for the liver stage and the model for the blood stage should open access to the complete cycle of the *P. falciparum* development in a small laboratory host, thereby providing an opportunity that should have numerous applications not only in the field of drug testing, pharmacokinetics and toxicology, but also in vaccine development and to investigate some of the biological and physiological aspects of human malaria.

Whatever will be the future of these new models, it seems however that exploration of drug potency using the "classical" rodent models might already be improved by considering some points of interest that we would like to list hereafter. 1) Because rodent malaria species can differ significantly in sensitivity to certain classes of compounds, as illustrated above with iron chelators and lipid biosynthesis inhibitors, it may be recommended to test new compounds on different models. 2) Also, the aspect of synergy between drugs should be considered and examination of therapies in conjunction with antimalarials typically given to treat patients with malaria should be favoured. 3) Notions of chronobiology may help in the selection of an experimental model and in the interpretation of chemotherapy experiments. Indeed, specific characteristics such as the duration of the schizogonic cycle, the time of schizogony or the synchronicity/asynchronicity of the chosen *Plasmodium* species and strain may influence its responsiveness to a drug depending on the time of administration and half-life of the drug (Beaute-Lafitte et al., 1994). This can be easily understood in the case of active compounds that preferentially affect a particular period of the parasite life cycle. Drug administration could be planed such that the peak level of the drug in the blood will be reached at the time the sensitive stage of the parasite is present in the circulation. It is assumed that such timing should increase the efficacy of drug treatment and minimize the dose to be injected. 4) Finally, it is remarkable that most of the drug testing performed in laboratories and promoted as potential therapy is carried out before the onset of malaria symptoms, whereas drug administration to treat human malaria is initiated after the onset of symptoms. Primary screening would gain advantage if new compounds were tested also in this configuration.

5. Conclusions

This last decade, the international mobilization dedicated to antimalarial strategies has regularly increased, allowing many countries to undertake or strengthen effective fight against the parasite, the disease and the vectors, and leading to a slowing-down, even a decline in some place, of malaria all over the world, thanks to the usage of impregnated bed nets and the setting-up of artemisinin combination therapies. However, the resistance of the insect vectors to insecticides and of the parasites to the current antimalarial drugs, especially to artemisinin derivatives, is still increasing and problematic since no new class of antimalarials has been introduced since 1996. The current global antimalarial drug development shows that the pipeline of antimalarials is rather strong in term of initiatives but also rather weak in term of novelty of mechanism of action that is necessary to circumvent resistance. This situation results in an urgent need for new drugs with original mechanisms of action. This last decade has also seen a considerable increase in our understanding of malaria parasite biochemistry that has allowed the identification of many potential targets for new drugs such as apicoplast metabolisms, proteases, kinases, transporters… That has been made possible thanks to the decrypted genomes of several *Plasmodium* species, to our ability to genetically validate potential drug targets and to the access to the transcriptomic and proteomic technologies that offer new opportunities to study the impact of drugs on the entire parasite metabolism.

These advances associated to the setting-up of high-throughput screening platforms on whole-cells or on specific parasite targets, and to the access to large chemical libraries with broad chemical diversity have seen the recent emergence of new potential antimalarial drugs with original molecular frameworks and mechanisms of action, that are auspicious for the future of antimalarial drug development. We are however facing important challenges in the next decade to propose efficient global antimalarial drug development. This will require :

1. Ability to propose efficient heterologous expression and folding systems to produce recombinant active proteins for targets, in order to set up high-throughput screening assays or to obtain 3D-dimensional structure elucidations using X-ray crystallography for drug design.
2. Development of researches on *P. vivax,* which can be considered as a neglected disease when compared to the efforts developed for *P. falciparum* whereas *P. vivax* infection is more widespread and remains an important cause of morbidity.
3. Strengthening researches on drugs acting on the liver parasite stages, including hypnozoites, and the parasite transmission stages, in order to propose an antimalarial drug strategy not only acting on the disease by itself due to the intraerythrocytic parasite development, but also acting on the disease transmission and the disease relapse in the case of *P. vivax.*

Finally, it must be kept in mind that for any promising molecule that will be selected, administration to patients will be the acid test. That is why development of small, easy to manage *in vivo* models as close to humans as possible remains a really challenging part of any therapeutic molecule development. Efforts are currently made to achieve these goals.

6. References

Abiodun, O.O., Gbotosho, G.O., Ajaiyeoba, E.O., Happi, C.T., Hofer, S., Wittlin, S., Sowunmi, A., Brun, R. & Oduola, A.M. (2010). Comparison of SYBR Green I-, PicoGreen-, and [3H]-hypoxanthine-based assays for in vitro antimalarial screening of plants from Nigerian ethnomedicine. *Parasitol Res*, 106, 4, pp. 933-939

Aguero, F., Al-Lazikani, B., Aslett, M., Berriman, M., Buckner, F.S., Campbell, R.K., Carmona, S., Carruthers, I.M., Chan, A.W., Chen, F., Crowther, G.J., Doyle, M.A., Hertz-Fowler, C., Hopkins, A.L., Mcallister, G., Nwaka, S., Overington, J.P., Pain, A., Paolini, G.V., Pieper, U., Ralph, S.A., Riechers, A., Roos, D.S., Sali, A., Shanmugam, D., Suzuki, T., Van Voorhis, W.C. & Verlinde, C.L. (2008). Genomic-scale prioritization of drug targets: the TDR Targets database. *Nat Rev Drug Discov*, 7, 11, pp. 900-907

Alonso, P.L., Brown, G., Arevalo-Herrera, M., Binka, F., Chitnis, C., Collins, F., Doumbo, O.K., Greenwood, B., Hall, B.F., Levine, M.M., Mendis, K., Newman, R.D., Plowe, C.V., Rodriguez, M.H., Sinden, R., Slutsker, L. & Tanner, M. (2011). A research agenda to underpin malaria eradication. *PLoS Med*, 8, 1, pp. e1000406

Aly, A.S. & Matuschewski, K. (2005). A malarial cysteine protease is necessary for *Plasmodium* sporozoite egress from oocysts. *J Exp Med*, 202, 2, pp. 225-230

Arnold, L., Tyagi, R.K., Meija, P., Swetman, C., Gleeson, J., Perignon, J.L. & Druilhe, P. (2011). Further improvements of the *P. falciparum* humanized mouse model. *PLoS One*, 6, 3, pp. e18045

Bacon, D.J., Latour, C., Lucas, C., Colina, O., Ringwald, P. & Picot, S. (2007). Comparison of a SYBR green I-based assay with a histidine-rich protein II enzyme-linked immunosorbent assay for in vitro antimalarial drug efficacy testing and application to clinical isolates. *Antimicrob Agents Chemother*, 51, 4, pp. 1172-1178

Baker, D.A. (2007). Malaria gametocytogenesis. *Mol Biochem Parasitol*, 172, 2, pp. 57-65

Baniecki, M.L., Wirth, D.F. & Clardy, J. (2007). High-throughput *Plasmodium falciparum* growth assay for malaria drug discovery. *Antimicrob Agents Chemother*, 51, 2, pp. 716-723

Baschong, W., Wittlin, S., Inglis, K.A., Fairlamb, A.H., Croft, S.L., Kumar, T.R., Fidock, D.A. & Brun, R. (2011). Triclosan is minimally effective in rodent malaria models. *Nat Med*, 17, 1, pp. 33-34

Basco, L.K. (2003). Molecular epidemiology of malaria in Cameroon. XV. Experimental studies on serum substitutes and supplements and alternative culture media for in vitro drug sensitivity assays using fresh isolates of *Plasmodium falciparum*. *Am J Trop Med Hyg*, 69, 2, pp. 168-173

Basco, L.K. (2004). Molecular epidemiology of malaria in cameroon. XX. Experimental studies on various factors of in vitro drug sensitivity assays using fresh isolates of *Plasmodium falciparum*. *Am J Trop Med Hyg*, 70, 5, pp. 474-480

Bauer, H., Fritz-Wolf, K., Winzer, A., Kuhner, S., Little, S., Yardley, V., Vezin, H., Palfey, B., Schirmer, R.H. & Davioud-Charvet, E. (2006). A fluoro analogue of the menadione derivative 6-[2'-(3'-methyl)-1',4'-naphthoquinolyl]hexanoic acid is a suicide substrate of glutathione reductase. Crystal structure of the alkylated human enzyme. *J Am Chem Soc*, 128, 33, pp. 10784-10794

Baumeister, S., Wiesner, J., Reichenberg, A., Hintz, M., Bietz, S., Harb, O.S., Roos, D.S., Kordes, M., Friesen, J., Matuschewski, K., Lingelbach, K., Jomaa, H. & Seeber, F. (2011). Fosmidomycin uptake into *Plasmodium* and *Babesia*-infected erythrocytes is facilitated by parasite-induced new permeability pathways. *PLoS One*, 6, 5, pp. e19334

Beaute-Lafitte, A., Altemayer-Caillard, V., Chabaud, A.G. & Landau, I. (1994). *Plasmodium yoelii nigeriensis*: biological mechanisms of resistance to chloroquine. *Parasite*, 1, 3, pp. 227-233

Bennett, T.N., Paguio, M., Gligorijevic, B., Seudieu, C., Kosar, A.D., Davidson, E. & Roepe, P.D. (2004). Novel, rapid, and inexpensive cell-based quantification of antimalarial drug efficacy. *Antimicrob Agents Chemother*, 48, 5, pp. 1807-1810

Bergmann-Leitner, E.S., Duncan, E.H., Burge, J.R., Spring, M. & Angov, E. (2008). Miniaturization of a high-throughput pLDH-based *Plasmodium falciparum* growth inhibition assay for small volume samples from preclinical and clinical vaccine trials. *Am J Trop Med Hyg*, 78, 3, pp. 468-471

Beutler, E. & Duparc, S. (2007). Glucose-6-phosphate dehydrogenase deficiency and antimalarial drug development. *Am J Trop Med Hyg*, 77, 4, pp. 779-789

Bhaumik, P., Horimoto, Y., Xiao, H., Miura, T., Hidaka, K., Kiso, Y., Wlodawer, A., Yada, R.Y. & Gustchina, A. (2011). Crystal structures of the free and inhibited forms of plasmepsin I (PMI) from *Plasmodium falciparum*. *J Struct Biol*, 175, 1, pp. 73-84

Biagini, G.A., O'neill, P.M., Nzila, A., Ward, S.A. & Bray, P.G. (2003). Antimalarial chemotherapy: young guns or back to the future? *Trends Parasitol*, 19, 11, pp. 479-487

Bissig, K.D., Wieland, S.F., Tran, P., Isogawa, M., Le, T.T., Chisari, F.V. & Verma, I.M. (2010). Human liver chimeric mice provide a model for hepatitis B and C virus infection and treatment. *J Clin Invest*, 120, 3, pp. 924-930

Blackman, M.J. (2008). Malarial proteases and host cell egress: an 'emerging' cascade. *Cell Microbiol*, 10, 10, pp. 1925-1934

Blume, M., Hliscs, M., Rodriguez-Contreras, D., Sanchez, M., Landfear, S., Lucius, R., Matuschewski, K. & Gupta, N. (2010). A constitutive pan-hexose permease for the *Plasmodium* life cycle and transgenic models for screening of antimalarial sugar analogs. *FASEB J*, 25, 4, pp. 1218-1229

Boddey, J.A., Hodder, A.N., Gunther, S., Gilson, P.R., Patsiouras, H., Kapp, E.A., Pearce, J.A., De Koning-Ward, T.F., Simpson, R.J., Crabb, B.S. & Cowman, A.F. (2010). An aspartyl protease directs malaria effector proteins to the host cell. *Nature*, 463, 7281, pp. 627-631

Briolant, S., Parola, P., Fusai, T., Madamet-Torrentino, M., Baret, E., Mosnier, J., Delmont, J.P., Parzy, D., Minodier, P., Rogier, C. & Pradines, B. (2007). Influence of oxygen on asexual blood cycle and susceptibility of *Plasmodium falciparum* to chloroquine: requirement of a standardized in vitro assay. *Malar J*, 6, pp. 44

Buchholz, K., Burke, T.A., Williamson, K.C., Wiegand, R.C., Wirth, D.F. & Marti, M. (2011). A high-throughput screen targeting malaria transmission stages opens new avenues for drug development. *J Infect Dis*, 203, 10, pp. 1445-1453

Carraz, M., Jossang, A., Franetich, J.F., Siau, A., Ciceron, L., Hannoun, L., Sauerwein, R., Frappier, F., Rasoanaivo, P., Snounou, G. & Mazier, D. (2006). A plant-derived morphinan as a novel lead compound active against malaria liver stages. *PLoS Med*, 3, 12, pp. e513

Chattopadhyay, R., Velmurugan, S., Chakiath, C., Andrews Donkor, L., Milhous, W., Barnwell, J.W., Collins, W.E. & Hoffman, S.L. (2010). Establishment of an in vitro assay for assessing the effects of drugs on the liver stages of *Plasmodium vivax* malaria. *PLoS One*, 5, 12, pp. e14275

Chen, A.A., Thomas, D.K., Ong, L.L., Schwartz, R.E., Golub, T.R. & Bhatia, S.N. (2011). Humanized mice with ectopic artificial liver tissues. *Proc Natl Acad Sci U S A*, 108, 29, pp. 11842-11847

Chevalley, S., Coste, A., Lopez, A., Pipy, B. & Valentin, A. (2010). Flow cytometry for the evaluation of anti-plasmodial activity of drugs on *Plasmodium falciparum* gametocytes. *Malar J*, 9, pp. 49

Collier, R. (2009). WHO reports progress in malaria control. *CMAJ*, 182, 2, pp. E105-106

Collins, W.E. (1992). South American monkeys in the development and testing of malarial vaccines-a review. *Mem Inst Oswaldo Cruz*, 87 Suppl 3, pp. 401-406

Cosledan, F., Fraisse, L., Pellet, A., Guillou, F., Mordmuller, B., Kremsner, P.G., Moreno, A., Mazier, D., Maffrand, J.P. & Meunier, B. (2008). Selection of a trioxaquine as an antimalarial drug candidate. *Proc Natl Acad Sci U S A*, 105, 45, pp. 17579-17584

Crabb, B.S., De Koning-Ward, T.F. & Gilson, P.R. (2011). Toward forward genetic screens in malaria-causing parasites using the piggyBac transposon. *BMC Biol*, 9, pp. 21

Dahl, E.L. & Rosenthal, P.J. (2008). Apicoplast translation, transcription and genome replication: targets for antimalarial antibiotics. *Trends Parasitol*, 24, 6, pp. 279-284

Deharo, E., Garcia, R.N., Oporto, P., Gimenez, A., Sauvain, M., Jullian, V. & Ginsburg, H. (2002). A non-radiolabelled ferriprotoporphyrin IX biomineralisation inhibition test for the high throughput screening of antimalarial compounds. *Exp Parasitol*, 100, 4, pp. 252-256

Delhaes, L., Lazaro, J.E., Gay, F., Thellier, M. & Danis, M. (1999). The microculture tetrazolium assay (MTA): another colorimetric method of testing *Plasmodium falciparum* chemosensitivity. *Ann Trop Med Parasitol*, 93, 1, pp. 31-40

Desjardins, R.E., Canfield, C.J., Haynes, J.D. & Chulay, J.D. (1979). Quantitative assessment of antimalarial activity in vitro by a semiautomated microdilution technique. *Antimicrob Agents Chemother*, 16, 6, pp. 710-718

Doerig, C. & Meijer, L. (2007). Antimalarial drug discovery: targeting protein kinases. *Expert Opin Ther Targets*, 11, 3, pp. 279-290

Doerig, C., Abdi, A., Bland, N., Eschenlauer, S., Dorin-Semblat, D., Fennell, C., Halbert, J., Holland, Z., Nivez, M.P., Semblat, J.P., Sicard, A. & Reininger, L. (2010). Malaria: targeting parasite and host cell kinomes. *Biochim Biophys Acta*, 1804, 3, pp. 604-612

Druilhe, P., Moreno, A., Blanc, C., Brasseur, P.H. & Jacquier, P. (2001). A colorimetric in vitro drug sensitivity assay for *Plasmodium falciparum* based on a highly sensitive double-site lactate dehydrogenase antigen-capture enzyme-linked immunosorbent assay. *Am J Trop Med Hyg*, 64, 5-6, pp. 233-241

Dvorin, J.D., Martyn, D.C., Patel, S.D., Grimley, J.S., Collins, C.R., Hopp, C.S., Bright, A.T., Westenberger, S., Winzeler, E., Blackman, M.J., Baker, D.A., Wandless, T.J. & Duraisingh, M.T. (2010). A plant-like kinase in *Plasmodium falciparum* regulates parasite egress from erythrocytes. *Science*, 328, 5980, pp. 910-912

Eggleson, K.K., Duffin, K.L. & Goldberg, D.E. (1999). Identification and characterization of falcilysin, a metallopeptidase involved in hemoglobin catabolism within the malaria parasite *Plasmodium falciparum*. *J Biol Chem*, 274, 45, pp. 32411-32417.

Eksi, S., Czesny, B., Greenbaum, D.C., Bogyo, M. & Williamson, K.C. (2004). Targeted disruption of *Plasmodium falciparum* cysteine protease, falcipain 1, reduces oocyst production, not erythrocytic stage growth. *Mol Microbiol*, 53, 1, pp. 243-250

Enserink, M. (2010). Redrawing Africa's malaria map. *Science*, 328, 5980, pp. 842

Florent, I., Marechal, E., Gascuel, O. & Brehelin, L. (2010). Bioinformatic strategies to provide functional clues to the unknown genes in *Plasmodium falciparum* genome. *Parasite*, 17, 4, pp. 273-283

Freundlich, J.S., Wang, F., Tsai, H.C., Kuo, M., Shieh, H.M., Anderson, J.W., Nkrumah, L.J., Valderramos, J.C., Yu, M., Kumar, T.R., Valderramos, S.G., Jacobs, W.R., Jr., Schiehser, G.A., Jacobus, D.P., Fidock, D.A. & Sacchettini, J.C. (2007). X-ray structural analysis of *Plasmodium falciparum* enoyl acyl carrier protein reductase as a pathway toward the optimization of triclosan antimalarial efficacy. *J Biol Chem*, 282, 35, pp. 25436-25444

Gamo, F.J., Sanz, L.M., Vidal, J., De Cozar, C., Alvarez, E., Lavandera, J.L., Vanderwall, D.E., Green, D.V., Kumar, V., Hasan, S., Brown, J.R., Peishoff, C.E., Cardon, L.R. & Garcia-Bustos, J.F. (2010). Thousands of chemical starting points for antimalarial lead identification. *Nature*, 465, 7296, pp. 305-310

Gego, A., Silvie, O., Franetich, J.F., Farhati, K., Hannoun, L., Luty, A.J., Sauerwein, R.W., Boucheix, C., Rubinstein, E. & Mazier, D. (2006). New approach for high-throughput screening of drug activity on *Plasmodium* liver stages. *Antimicrob Agents Chemother*, 50, 4, pp. 1586-1589

Goodman, C.D. & Mcfadden, G.I. (2007). Fatty acid biosynthesis as a drug target in apicomplexan parasites. *Curr Drug Targets*, 8, 1, pp. 15-30

Grawert, T., Groll, M., Rohdich, F., Bacher, A. & Eisenreich, W. (2011). Biochemistry of the non-mevalonate isoprenoid pathway. *Cell Mol Life Sci*, DOI: 10.1007/s00018-011-0753-z

Grellier, P., Depoix, D., Schrevel, J. & Florent, I. (2008). Discovery of new targets for antimalarial chemotherapy. *Parasite*, 15, 3, pp. 219-225

Grimberg, B.T. (2011). Methodology and application of flow cytometry for investigation of human malaria parasites. *J Immunol Methods*, 367, 1-2, pp. 1-16

Guiguemde, W.A., Shelat, A.A., Bouck, D., Duffy, S., Crowther, G.J., Davis, P.H., Smithson, D.C., Connelly, M., Clark, J., Zhu, F., Jimenez-Diaz, M.B., Martinez, M.S., Wilson, E.B., Tripathi, A.K., Gut, J., Sharlow, E.R., Bathurst, I., El Mazouni, F., Fowble, J.W., Forquer, I., Mcginley, P.L., Castro, S., Angulo-Barturen, I., Ferrer, S., Rosenthal, P.J., Derisi, J.L., Sullivan, D.J., Lazo, J.S., Roos, D.S., Riscoe, M.K., Phillips, M.A., Rathod, P.K., Van Voorhis, W.C., Avery, V.M. & Guy, R.K. (2010). Chemical genetics of *Plasmodium falciparum*. *Nature*, 465, 7296, pp. 311-315

Hegge, S., Kudryashev, M., Barniol, L. & Frischknecht, F. (2010). Key factors regulating *Plasmodium berghei* sporozoite survival and transformation revealed by an automated visual assay. *FASEB J*, 24, 12, pp. 5003-5012

Humberstone, A.J., Cowman, A.F., Horton, J. & Charman, W.N. (1998). Effect of altered serum lipid concentrations on the IC50 of halofantrine against *Plasmodium falciparum*. *J Pharm Sci*, 87, 2, pp. 256-258

Huy, N.T., Uyen, D.T., Maeda, A., Trang, D.T., Oida, T., Harada, S. & Kamei, K. (2007). Simple colorimetric inhibition assay of heme crystallization for high-throughput screening of antimalarial compounds. *Antimicrob Agents Chemother*, 51, 1, pp. 350-353

Hyde, J.E. (2007). Targeting purine and pyrimidine metabolism in human apicomplexan parasites. *Curr Drug Targets*, 8, 1, pp. 31-47

Jayabalasingham, B., Menard, R. & Fidock, D.A. (2010). Recent insights into fatty acid acquisition and metabolism in malarial parasites. *F1000 Biol Rep*, 2, pp. 24

Jomaa, H., Wiesner, J., Sanderbrand, S., Altincicek, B., Weidemeyer, C., Hintz, M., Turbachova, I., Eberl, M., Zeidler, J., Lichtenthaler, H.K., Soldati, D. & Beck, E. (1999). Inhibitors of the nonmevalonate pathway of isoprenoid biosynthesis as antimalarial drugs. *Science*, 285, 5433, pp. 1573-1576.

Kato, N., Sakata, T., Breton, G., Le Roch, K.G., Nagle, A., Andersen, C., Bursulaya, B., Henson, K., Johnson, J., Kumar, K.A., Marr, F., Mason, D., Mcnamara, C., Plouffe, D., Ramachandran, V., Spooner, M., Tuntland, T., Zhou, Y., Peters, E.C., Chatterjee, A., Schultz, P.G., Ward, G.E., Gray, N., Harper, J. & Winzeler, E.A. (2008). Gene expression signatures and small-molecule compounds link a protein kinase to *Plasmodium falciparum* motility. *Nat Chem Biol*, 4, 6, pp. 347-356

Keller, T.H., Shi, P.Y. & Wang, Q.Y. (2011). Anti-infectives: can cellular screening deliver? *Curr Opin Chem Biol*, 15, 4, pp. 529-533

Klemba, M., Gluzman, I. & Goldberg, D.E. (2004). A *Plasmodium falciparum* dipeptidyl aminopeptidase I participates in vacuolar hemoglobin degradation. *J Biol Chem*, 279, 41, pp. 43000-43007

Kocken, C.H., Ozwara, H., Van Der Wel, A., Beetsma, A.L., Mwenda, J.M. & Thomas, A.W. (2002). *Plasmodium knowlesi* provides a rapid in vitro and in vivo transfection system that enables double-crossover gene knockout studies. *Infect Immun*, 70, 2, pp. 655-660

Kosaisavee, V., Suwanarusk, R., Nosten, F., Kyle, D.E., Barrends, M., Jones, J., Price, R., Russell, B. & Lek-Uthai, U. (2006). *Plasmodium vivax*: isotopic, PicoGreen, and microscopic assays for measuring chloroquine sensitivity in fresh and cryopreserved isolates. *Exp Parasitol*, 114, 1, pp. 34-39

Ku, M.J., Dossin, F.M., Choi, Y., Moraes, C.B., Ryu, J., Song, R. & Freitas-Junior, L.H. (2011). Quantum dots: a new tool for anti-malarial drug assays. *Malar J*, 10, pp. 118

Lacroix, C., Giovannini, D., Combe, A., Bargieri, D.Y., Spath, S., Panchal, D., Tawk, L., Thiberge, S., Carvalho, T.G., Barale, J.C., Bhanot, P. & Menard, R. (2011). FLP/FRT-mediated conditional mutagenesis in pre-erythrocytic stages of *Plasmodium berghei*. *Nat Protoc*, 6, 9, pp. 1412-1428

Leroy, D. & Doerig, C. (2008). Drugging the *Plasmodium* kinome: the benefits of academia-industry synergy. *Trends Pharmacol Sci*, 29, 5, pp. 241-249

Lim, L. & Mcfadden, G.I. (2010). The evolution, metabolism and functions of the apicoplast. *Philos Trans R Soc Lond B Biol Sci*, 365, 1541, pp. 749-763

Limenitakis, J. & Soldati-Favre, D. (2011). Functional genetics in Apicomplexa: potentials and limits. *FEBS Lett*, 585, 11, pp. 1579-1588

Liu, J., Istvan, E.S., Gluzman, I.Y., Gross, J. & Goldberg, D.E. (2006). *Plasmodium falciparum* ensures its amino acid supply with multiple acquisition pathways and redundant proteolytic enzyme systems. *Proc Natl Acad Sci U S A*, 103, 23, pp. 8840-8845

Mahmoudi, N., Ciceron, L., Franetich, J.F., Farhati, K., Silvie, O., Eling, W., Sauerwein, R., Danis, M., Mazier, D. & Derouin, F. (2003). In vitro activities of 25 quinolones and fluoroquinolones against liver and blood stage *Plasmodium* spp. *Antimicrob Agents Chemother*, 47, 8, pp. 2636-2639

Mahmoudi, N., Garcia-Domenech, R., Galvez, J., Farhati, K., Franetich, J.F., Sauerwein, R., Hannoun, L., Derouin, F., Danis, M. & Mazier, D. (2008). New active drugs against liver stages of *Plasmodium* predicted by molecular topology. *Antimicrob Agents Chemother*, 52, 4, pp. 1215-1220

Makler, M.T., Ries, J.M., Williams, J.A., Bancroft, J.E., Piper, R.C., Gibbins, B.L. & Hinrichs, D.J. (1993). Parasite lactate dehydrogenase as an assay for *Plasmodium falciparum* drug sensitivity. *Am J Trop Med Hyg*, 48, 6, pp. 739-741

Makler, M.T., Piper, R.C. & Milhous, W.K. (1998). Lactate dehydrogenase and the diagnosis of malaria. *Parasitol Today*, 14, 9, pp. 376-377

Mambu, L. & Grellier, P. (2008). Antimalarial compounds of traditionally used medicinal plants, In: *Bioactive natural products, detection, isolation, and structural determination*, 2nd edition, Molyneux, R.J. & Colgate, S.M., pp. 491, CRC Press

Martin, R.E., Ginsburg, H. & Kirk, K. (2009). Membrane transport proteins of the malaria parasite. *Mol Microbiol*, 74, 3, pp. 519-528

Mather, M.W., Henry, K.W. & Vaidya, A.B. (2007). Mitochondrial drug targets in apicomplexan parasites. *Curr Drug Targets*, 8, 1, pp. 49-60

Mazier, D., Beaudoin, R.L., Mellouk, S., Druilhe, P., Texier, B., Trosper, J., Miltgen, F., Landau, I., Paul, C., Brandicourt, O. & Et Al. (1985). Complete development of hepatic stages of *Plasmodium falciparum* in vitro. *Science*, 227, 4685, pp. 440-442

Mazier, D., Franetich, J.F., Carraz, M., Silvie, O. & Pino, P. (2004). Models for studying effects of herbal antimalarials at different stages of the *Plasmodium* life cycle, In: *Traditional medicinal plants and malaria, Willcox, M., Bodeker, G. & Rasoanaivo, P.*, pp. 271, CRC Press, Boca raton

Mcgowan, S., Porter, C.J., Lowther, J., Stack, C.M., Golding, S.J., Skinner-Adams, T.S., Trenholme, K.R., Teuscher, F., Donnelly, S.M., Grembecka, J., Mucha, A., Kafarski, P., Degori, R., Buckle, A.M., Gardiner, D.L., Whisstock, J.C. & Dalton, J.P. (2009). Structural basis for the inhibition of the essential *Plasmodium falciparum* M1 neutral aminopeptidase. *Proc Natl Acad Sci U S A*, 106, 8, pp. 2537-2542

Mckerrow, J.H., Rosenthal, P.J., Swenerton, R. & Doyle, P. (2008). Development of protease inhibitors for protozoan infections. *Curr Opin Infect Dis*, 21, 6, pp. 668-672

Mcrobert, L., Jiang, S., Stead, A. & Mcconkey, G.A. (2005). *Plasmodium falciparum*: interaction of shikimate analogues with antimalarial drugs. *Exp Parasitol*, 111, 3, pp. 178-181

Moreno, A., Badell, E., Van Rooijen, N. & Druilhe, P. (2001). Human malaria in immunocompromised mice: new in vivo model for chemotherapy studies. *Antimicrob Agents Chemother*, 45, 6, pp. 1847-1853

Morosan, S., Hez-Deroubaix, S., Lunel, F., Renia, L., Giannini, C., Van Rooijen, N., Battaglia, S., Blanc, C., Eling, W., Sauerwein, R., Hannoun, L., Belghiti, J., Brechot, C., Kremsdorf, D. & Druilhe, P. (2006). Liver-stage development of *Plasmodium falciparum*, in a humanized mouse model. *J Infect Dis*, 193, 7, pp. 996-1004

Mwakingwe, A., Ting, L.M., Hochman, S., Chen, J., Sinnis, P. & Kim, K. (2009). Noninvasive real-time monitoring of liver-stage development of bioluminescent *Plasmodium* parasites. *J Infect Dis*, 200, 9, pp. 1470-1478

Ncokazi, K.K. & Egan, T.J. (2005). A colorimetric high-throughput beta-hematin inhibition screening assay for use in the search for antimalarial compounds. *Anal Biochem*, 338, pp. 306-319

Noedl, H., Wernsdorfer, W.H., Miller, R.S. & Wongsrichanalai, C. (2002). Histidine-rich protein II: a novel approach to malaria drug sensitivity testing. *Antimicrob Agents Chemother*, 46, 6, pp. 1658-1664

Noedl, H., Se, Y., Schaecher, K., Smith, B.L., Socheat, D. & Fukuda, M.M. (2008). Evidence of artemisinin-resistant malaria in western Cambodia. *N Engl J Med*, 359, 24, pp. 2619-2620

O'connor, C.J., Laraia, L. & Spring, D.R. (2011). Chemical genetics. *Chem Soc Rev*, 40, 8, pp. 4332-4345

O'neill, P.M., Ward, S.A., Berry, N.G., Jeyadevan, J.P., Biagini, G.A., Asadollaly, E., Park, B.K. & Bray, P.G. (2006). A medicinal chemistry perspective on 4-aminoquinoline antimalarial drugs. *Curr Top Med Chem*, 6, 5, pp. 479-507

Odom, A.R. & Van Voorhis, W.C. (2009). Functional genetic analysis of the *Plasmodium falciparum* deoxyxylulose 5-phosphate reductoisomerase gene. *Mol Biochem Parasitol*, 170, 2, pp. 108-111

Olliaro, P. & Wells, T.N. (2009). The global portfolio of new antimalarial medicines under development. *Clin Pharmacol Ther*, 85, 6, pp. 584-595

Palmer, C.J., Lindo, J.F., Klaskala, W.I., Quesada, J.A., Kaminsky, R., Baum, M.K. & Ager, A.L. (1998). Evaluation of the OptiMAL test for rapid diagnosis of *Plasmodium vivax* and *Plasmodium falciparum* malaria. *J Clin Microbiol*, 36, 1, pp. 203-206

Parvanova, I., Epiphanio, S., Fauq, A., Golde, T.E., Prudencio, M. & Mota, M.M. (2009). A small molecule inhibitor of signal peptide peptidase inhibits *Plasmodium* development in the liver and decreases malaria severity. *PLoS One*, 4, 4, pp. e5078

Payne, D.J., Gwynn, M.N., Holmes, D.J. & Pompliano, D.L. (2007). Drugs for bad bugs: confronting the challenges of antibacterial discovery. *Nat Rev Drug Discov*, 6, 1, pp. 29-40

Peatey, C.L., Skinner-Adams, T.S., Dixon, M.W., Mccarthy, J.S., Gardiner, D.L. & Trenholme, K.R. (2009). Effect of antimalarial drugs on *Plasmodium falciparum* gametocytes. *J Infect Dis*, 200, 10, pp. 1518-1521

Peters, W. (1987). Techniques of drug evaluation I: primary screening, In : *Chemotherapy and drug resistance in Malaria*, Vol. 1, Jovanovich , H.B., pp 97, Academic Press, Oval road, London

Peters, W. & Robinson, B.L. (1999). The chemotherapy of rodent malaria. LVI. Studies on the development of resistance to natural and synthetic endoperoxides. *Ann Trop Med Parasitol*, 93, 4, pp. 325-329

Ploemen, I.H., Prudencio, M., Douradinha, B.G., Ramesar, J., Fonager, J., Van Gemert, G.J., Luty, A.J., Hermsen, C.C., Sauerwein, R.W., Baptista, F.G., Mota, M.M., Waters, A.P., Que, I., Lowik, C.W., Khan, S.M., Janse, C.J. & Franke-Fayard, B.M. (2009). Visualisation and quantitative analysis of the rodent malaria liver stage by real time imaging. *PLoS One*, 4, 11, pp. e7881

Ponpuak, M., Klemba, M., Park, M., Gluzman, I.Y., Lamppa, G.K. & Goldberg, D.E. (2007). A role for falcilysin in transit peptide degradation in the *Plasmodium falciparum* apicoplast. *Mol Microbiol*, 63, 2, pp. 314-334

Prabhu, P. & Patravale, V. (2011). Novel Targets for Malaria Therapy. *Curr Drug Targets*, pp.

Ringwald, P., Meche, F.S., Bickii, J. & Basco, L.K. (1999). In vitro culture and drug sensitivity assay of *Plasmodium falciparum* with nonserum substitute and acute-phase sera. *J Clin Microbiol*, 37, 3, pp. 700-705

Rosenthal, P.J. (2010). Falcipains and other cysteine proteases of malaria parasites, In: *Falcipains and other cysteine proteases of malaria parasites, Advances in Experimental Medicine and Biology, vol.712,* Robinson, W. and Dalton, JP., pp. 30, Landes Biosciences and Springer Science+Business Media, LCC, 233 Spring Street, New York, New York, USA.

Rottmann, M., Mcnamara, C., Yeung, B.K., Lee, M.C., Zou, B., Russell, B., Seitz, P., Plouffe, D.M., Dharia, N.V., Tan, J., Cohen, S.B., Spencer, K.R., Gonzalez-Paez, G.E., Lakshminarayana, S.B., Goh, A., Suwanarusk, R., Jegla, T., Schmitt, E.K., Beck, H.P., Brun, R., Nosten, F., Renia, L., Dartois, V., Keller, T.H., Fidock, D.A., Winzeler, E.A. & Diagana, T.T. (2010). Spiroindolones, a potent compound class for the treatment of malaria. *Science*, 329, 5996, pp. 1175-1180

Rush, M.A., Baniecki, M.L., Mazitschek, R., Cortese, J.F., Wiegand, R., Clardy, J. & Wirth, D.F. (2009). Colorimetric high-throughput screen for detection of heme crystallization inhibitors. *Antimicrob Agents Chemother*, 53, 6, pp. 2564-2568

Russo, I., Babbitt, S., Muralidharan, V., Butler, T., Oksman, A. & Goldberg, D.E. (2010). Plasmepsin V licenses *Plasmodium* proteins for export into the host erythrocyte. *Nature*, 463, 7281, pp. 632-636

Sahu, N.K., Sahu, S. & Kohli, D.V. (2008). Novel molecular targets for antimalarial drug development. *Chem Biol Drug Des*, 71, 4, pp. 287-297

Sams-Dodd, F. (2005). Target-based drug discovery: is something wrong? *Drug Discov Today*, 10, 2, pp. 139-147

Sanni, L.A., Fonseca, L.F. & Langhome, J. (2002). Mouse models for erythrocytic-stage malaria, In: *Methods in molecular medicine, Vol. 72: Malaria methods and protocols*, Doolan, D.L., pp 57, Humana Press, Inc., Totowa, NJ

Sanchez, C.P., Dave, A., Stein, W.D. & Lanzer, M. (2010). Transporters as mediators of drug resistance in *Plasmodium falciparum*. *Int J Parasitol*, 40, 10, pp. 1109-1118

Sato, S. & Wilson, R.J. (2005). The plastid of *Plasmodium* spp.: a target for inhibitors. *Curr Top Microbiol Immunol*, 295, pp. 251-273

Sato, S. (2011). The apicomplexan plastid and its evolution. *Cell Mol Life Sci*, 68, 8, pp. 1285-1296

Seeber, F. & Soldati-Favre, D. (2010). Metabolic pathways in the apicoplast of apicomplexa. *Int Rev Cell Mol Biol*, 281, pp. 161-228

Semenov, A., Olson, J.E. & Rosenthal, P.J. (1998). Antimalarial synergy of cysteine and aspartic protease inhibitors. *Antimicrob Agents Chemother*, 42, 9, pp. 2254-2258

Sijwali, P.S., Koo, J., Singh, N. & Rosenthal, P.J. (2006). Gene disruptions demonstrate independent roles for the four falcipain cysteine proteases of *Plasmodium falciparum*. *Mol Biochem Parasitol*, 150, 1, pp. 96-106

Sims, P.F. & Hyde, J.E. (2006). Proteomics of the human malaria parasite *Plasmodium falciparum*. *Expert Rev Proteomics*, 3, 1, pp. 87-95

Singh, A., Shenai, B.R., Choe, Y., Gut, J., Sijwali, P.S., Craik, C.S. & Rosenthal, P.J. (2002). Critical role of amino acid 23 in mediating activity and specificity of vinckepain-2, a papain-family cysteine protease of rodent malaria parasites. *Biochem J*, 368, 1, pp. 273-281

Singh, A.P., Zhang, Y., No, J.H., Docampo, R., Nussenzweig, V. & Oldfield, E. (2010). Lipophilic bisphosphonates are potent inhibitors of *Plasmodium* liver-stage growth. *Antimicrob Agents Chemother*, 54, 7, pp. 2987-2993

Singh, K., Agarwal, A., Khan, S.I., Walker, L.A. & Tekwani, B.L. (2007). Growth, drug susceptibility, and gene expression profiling of *Plasmodium falciparum* cultured in medium supplemented with human serum or lipid-rich bovine serum albumin [corrected]. *J Biomol Screen*, 12, 8, pp. 1109-1114

Skinner-Adams, T.S., Stack, C.M., Trenholme, K.R., Brown, C.L., Grembecka, J., Lowther, J., Mucha, A., Drag, M., Kafarski, P., Mcgowan, S., Whisstock, J.C., Gardiner, D.L. & Dalton, J.P. (2009). *Plasmodium falciparum* neutral aminopeptidases: new targets for anti-malarials. *Trends Biochem Sci*, 35, 1, pp. 53-61

Slavic, K., Straschil, U., Reininger, L., Doerig, C., Morin, C., Tewari, R. & Krishna, S. (2010). Life cycle studies of the hexose transporter of *Plasmodium* species and genetic validation of their essentiality. *Mol Microbiol*, 75, 6, pp. 1402-1413

Slavic, K., Krishna, S., Derbyshire, E.T. & Staines, H.M. (2011). Plasmodial sugar transporters as anti-malarial drug targets and comparisons with other protozoa. *Malar J*, 10, pp. 165

Sologub, L., Kuehn, A., Kern, S., Przyborski, J., Schillig, R. & Pradel, G. (2011). Malaria proteases mediate inside-out egress of gametocytes from red blood cells following parasite transmission to the mosquito. *Cell Microbiol*, 13, 6, pp. 897-912

Staines, H.M., Powell, T., Thomas, S.L. & Ellory, J.C. (2004). *Plasmodium falciparum*-induced channels. *Int J Parasitol*, 34, 6, pp. 665-673

Staines, H.M., Derbyshire, E.T., Slavic, K., Tattersall, A., Vial, H. & Krishna, S. (2010). Exploiting the therapeutic potential of *Plasmodium falciparum* solute transporters. *Trends Parasitol*, 26, 6, pp. 284-296

Tasdemir, D., Sanabria, D., Lauinger, I.L., Tarun, A., Herman, R., Perozzo, R., Zloh, M., Kappe, S.H., Brun, R. & Carballeira, N.M. (2010). 2-Hexadecynoic acid inhibits plasmodial FAS-II enzymes and arrests erythrocytic and liver stage *Plasmodium* infections. *Bioorg Med Chem*, 18, 21, pp. 7475-7485

Trager, W. & Jensen, J.B. (1976). Human malaria parasites in continuous culture. *Science*, 193, 4254, pp. 673-675

Trenholme, K.R., Brown, C.L., Skinner-Adams, T.S., Stack, C., Lowther, J., To, J., Robinson, M.W., Donnelly, S.M., Dalton, J.P. & Gardiner, D.L. (2010). Aminopeptidases of malaria parasites: new targets for chemotherapy. *Infect Disord Drug Targets*, 10, 3, pp. 217-225

Udomsangpetch, R., Kaneko, O., Chotivanich, K. & Sattabongkot, J. (2008). Cultivation of *Plasmodium vivax*. *Trends Parasitol*, 24, 2, pp. 85-88

Van Voorhis, W.C., Rivas, K.L., Bendale, P., Nallan, L., Horney, C., Barrett, L.K., Bauer, K.D., Smart, B.P., Ankala, S., Hucke, O., Verlinde, C.L., Chakrabarti, D., Strickland, C., Yokoyama, K., Buckner, F.S., Hamilton, A.D., Williams, D.K., Lombardo, L.J., Floyd, D. & Gelb, M.H. (2007). Efficacy, Pharmacokinetics, and Metabolism of Tetrahydroquinoline Inhibitors of *Plasmodium falciparum* Protein Farnesyltransferase. *Antimicrob Agents Chemother*, 51, 10, pp. 3659-3671

Wegscheid-Gerlach, C., Gerber, H.D. & Diederich, W.E. (2010). Proteases of *Plasmodium falciparum* as potential drug targets and inhibitors thereof. *Curr Top Med Chem*, 10, 3, pp. 346-367

Weissbuch, I. & Leiserowitz, L. (2008). Interplay between malaria, crystalline hemozoin formation, and antimalarial drug action and design. *Chem Rev*, 108, 11, pp. 4899-4914

Wengelnik, K., Vidal, V., Ancelin, M.L., Cathiard, A.M., Morgat, J.L., Kocken, C.H., Calas, M., Herrera, S., Thomas, A.W. & Vial, H.J. (2002). A class of potent antimalarials and their specific accumulation in infected erythrocytes. *Science*, 295, 5558, pp. 1311-1314

Wiesner, J. & Jomaa, H. (2007). Isoprenoid biosynthesis of the apicoplast as drug target. *Curr Drug Targets*, 8, 1, pp. 3-13

Wu, T., Nagle, A.S. & Chatterjee, A.K. (2011). Road towards new antimalarials - overview of the strategies and their chemical progress. *Curr Med Chem*, 18, 6, pp. 853-871

Wu, Y., Wang, X., Liu, X. & Wang, Y. (2003). Data-mining approaches reveal hidden families of proteases in the genome of malaria parasite. *Genome Res*, 13, 4, pp. 601-616.

Yu, M., Kumar, T.R., Nkrumah, L.J., Coppi, A., Retzlaff, S., Li, C.D., Kelly, B.J., Moura, P.A., Lakshmanan, V., Freundlich, J.S., Valderramos, J.C., Vilcheze, C., Siedner, M., Tsai, J.H., Falkard, B., Sidhu, A.B., Purcell, L.A., Gratraud, P., Kremer, L., Waters, A.P., Schiehser, G., Jacobus, D.P., Janse, C.J., Ager, A., Jacobs, W.R., Jr., Sacchettini, J.C., Heussler, V., Sinnis, P. & Fidock, D.A. (2008). The fatty acid biosynthesis enzyme FabI plays a key role in the development of liver-stage malarial parasites. *Cell Host Microbe*, 4, 6, pp. 567-578

Permissions

The contributors of this book come from diverse backgrounds, making this book a truly international effort. This book will bring forth new frontiers with its revolutionizing research information and detailed analysis of the nascent developments around the world.

We would like to thank Dr Omolade O. Okwa, for lending her expertise to make the book truly unique. She has played a crucial role in the development of this book. Without her invaluable contribution this book wouldn't have been possible. She has made vital efforts to compile up to date information on the varied aspects of this subject to make this book a valuable addition to the collection of many professionals and students.

This book was conceptualized with the vision of imparting up-to-date information and advanced data in this field. To ensure the same, a matchless editorial board was set up. Every individual on the board went through rigorous rounds of assessment to prove their worth. After which they invested a large part of their time researching and compiling the most relevant data for our readers. Conferences and sessions were held from time to time between the editorial board and the contributing authors to present the data in the most comprehensible form. The editorial team has worked tirelessly to provide valuable and valid information to help people across the globe.

Every chapter published in this book has been scrutinized by our experts. Their significance has been extensively debated. The topics covered herein carry significant findings which will fuel the growth of the discipline. They may even be implemented as practical applications or may be referred to as a beginning point for another development. Chapters in this book were first published by InTech; hereby published with permission under the Creative Commons Attribution License or equivalent.

The editorial board has been involved in producing this book since its inception. They have spent rigorous hours researching and exploring the diverse topics which have resulted in the successful publishing of this book. They have passed on their knowledge of decades through this book. To expedite this challenging task, the publisher supported the team at every step. A small team of assistant editors was also appointed to further simplify the editing procedure and attain best results for the readers.

Our editorial team has been hand-picked from every corner of the world. Their multi-ethnicity adds dynamic inputs to the discussions which result in innovative outcomes. These outcomes are then further discussed with the researchers and contributors who give their valuable feedback and opinion regarding the same. The feedback is then collaborated with the researches and they are edited in a comprehensive manner to aid the understanding of the subject.

Apart from the editorial board, the designing team has also invested a significant amount of their time in understanding the subject and creating the most relevant covers. They scrutinized every image to scout for the most suitable representation of the subject and create an appropriate cover for the book.

The publishing team has been involved in this book since its early stages. They were actively engaged in every process, be it collecting the data, connecting with the contributors or procuring relevant information. The team has been an ardent support to the editorial, designing and production team. Their endless efforts to recruit the best for this project, has resulted in the accomplishment of this book. They are a veteran in the field of academics and their pool of knowledge is as vast as their experience in printing. Their expertise and guidance has proved useful at every step. Their uncompromising quality standards have made this book an exceptional effort. Their encouragement from time to time has been an inspiration for everyone.

The publisher and the editorial board hope that this book will prove to be a valuable piece of knowledge for researchers, students, practitioners and scholars across the globe.

List of Contributors

John C. Igweh
Delta State University, Abraka Nigeria, Nigeria

Omolade O. Okwa
Department of Zoology, Parasitology Unit, Lagos State University (LASU), Lagos, Nigeria

Guido Favia Irene Ricci, Patrizia Scuppa, Claudia Damiani, Paolo Rossi, Aida Capone, Chenoa De Freece, Matteo Valzano, Alessia Cappelli, Michela Mosca and Ulisse Ulissi
School of Bioscience & Biotechnology, University of Camerino, Camerino (MC), Italy

V. Choumet
Institut Pasteur, France

Alfonso Marzal
University of Extremadura, Spain

Hiroko Asahi
Department of Parasitology, National Institute of Infectious Diseases, Japan

R.K. Tyagi
Department of Global Health, College of Public Health, University of South Florida, Tampa, Florida, USA. Malaria Vaccine Development Laboratory, Institute Pasteur Paris, France

N.K. Garg
Shantha Biotechnics Ltd., (A Part of Sanofi Aventis Group), Hyderabad, AP, India

T. Sahu
National Institute of Allergy and Infectious Diseases, National Institutes of Health, Rockville, MD, USA

P. Prabha
Gene Regulation Laboratory, School Of Biotechnology, Jawaharlal Nehru University, New Delhi, India

Alassane Mbengue and Catherine Braun-Breton
University Montpellier II, CNRS UMR5235, University Montpellier I, Dynamique des Interactions Membranaires Normales et Pathologiques, France

Xue Yan Yam
University Montpellier II, CNRS UMR5235, University Montpellier I, Dynamique des

Interactions Membranaires Normales et Pathologiques, France School of Biological Sciences, Nanyang Technological University, Singapore

Adeola Orogade
Ahmadu Bello University Teaching Hospital, Shika Zaria, Nigeria

Sam M. Kinyanjui
KEMRI-Wellcome Trust Research Programme, Kilifi, Kenya

Alyssa E. Barry
Walter and Eliza Hall Institute for Medical Research, Australia Department of Medical Biology, University of Melbourne, Australia

John C. Reeder
Burnet Institute, Australia Monash University, Australia

James Beeson, Freya J.I. Fowkes and Alicia Arnott
Burnet Institute, Australia

Elke S. Bergmann-Leitner, Elizabeth H. Duncan and Evelina Angov
Department of Molecular Parasitology, Division of Malaria Vaccine Development, Walter Reed Army Institute of Research, USA

Pieter B. Burger and Fourie Joubert
University of Pretoria, South Africa

Alison Machado, Cheikh Loucoubar, Laura Grange, Jean-François Bureau, Anavaj Sakuntabhai and Richard Paul
Unité de Génétique Fonctionnelle des Maladies Infectieuses, Institut Pasteur, France

Grellier Philippe, Deregnaucourt Christiane and Florent Isabelle
National Museum of Natural History, UMR 7245 CNRS, Team APE, Paris, France